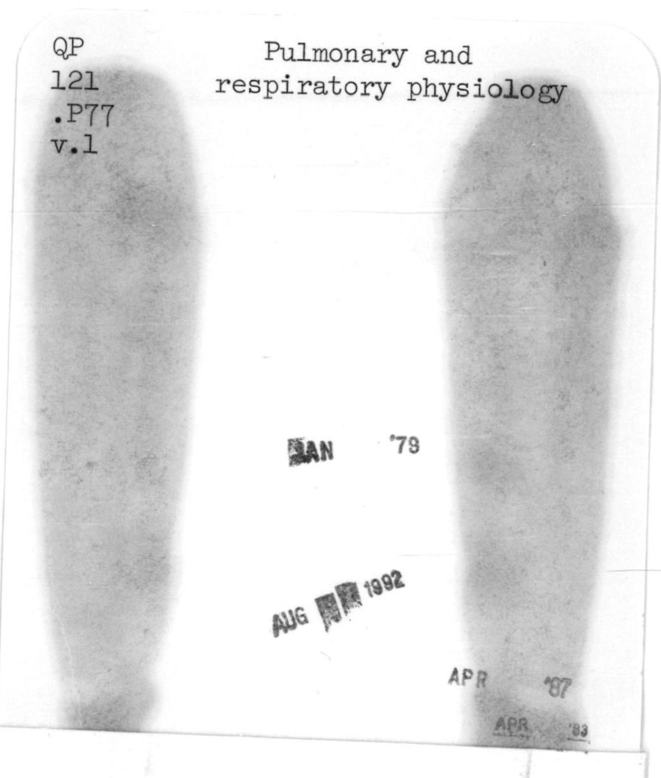
QP
121
.P77
v.1
Pulmonary and
respiratory physiology
'79
AUG 1992
APR '87

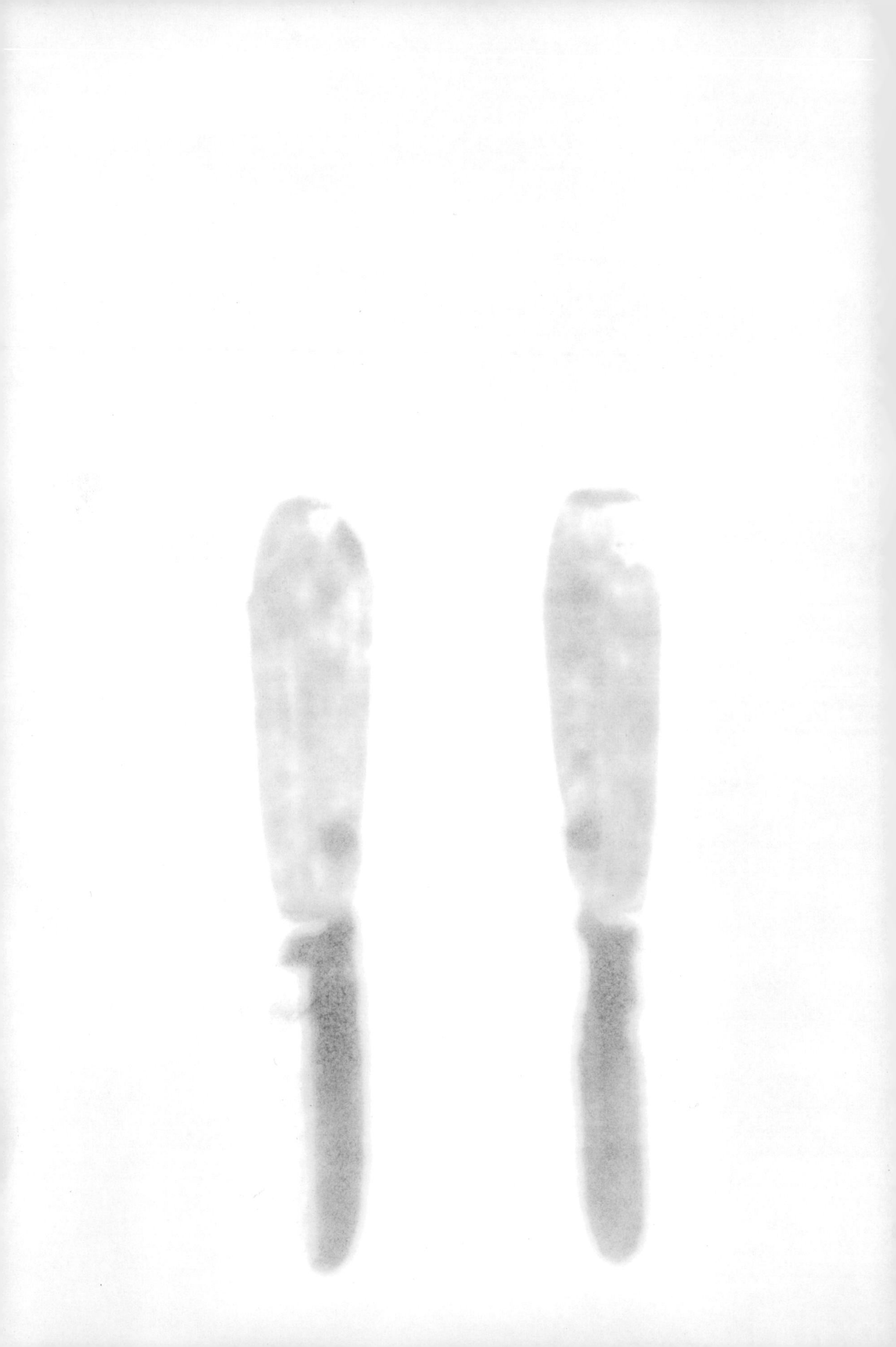

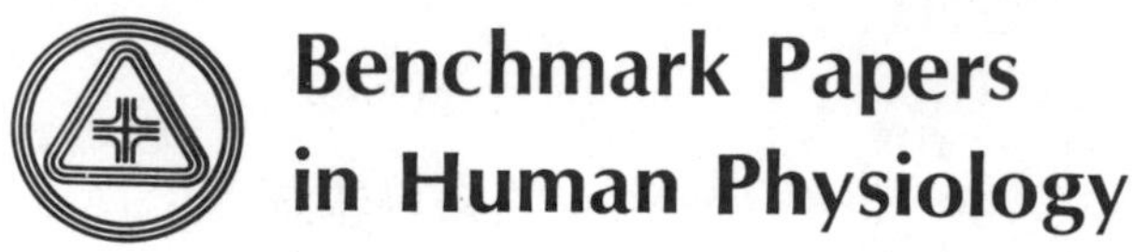

Benchmark Papers in Human Physiology

Series Editor: L. L. Langley
School of Medicine
University of Missouri–Kansas City

PUBLISHED VOLUMES

HOMEOSTASIS: Origins of the Concept
L. L. Langley
CONTRACEPTION
L. L. Langley
MICROCIRCULATION
Mary P. Wiedeman
CARDIOVASCULAR PHYSIOLOGY
James V. Warren
PULMONARY AND RESPIRATORY PHYSIOLOGY, PART I
Julius H. Comroe, Jr.
PULMONARY AND RESPIRATORY PHYSIOLOGY, PART II
Julius H. Comroe, Jr.

RELATED TITLES IN OTHER BENCHMARK SERIES

HORMONES AND SEXUAL BEHAVIOR (Benchmark Papers in Animal Behavior, Vol. 1)
Carol Sue Carter

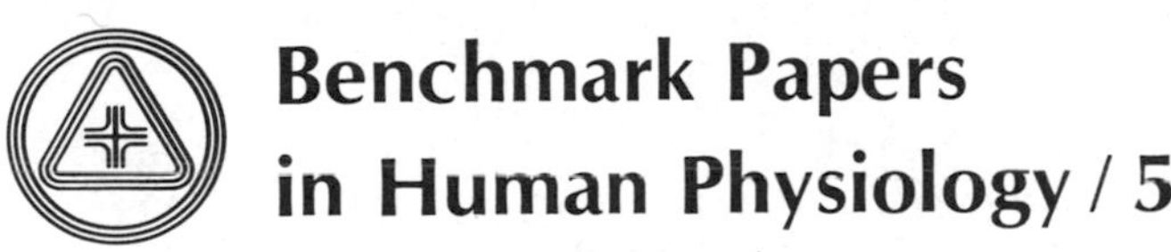

A BENCHMARK® Books Series

PULMONARY AND RESPIRATORY PHYSIOLOGY Part I

Edited by

Julius H. Comroe, Jr.
University of California
San Francisco

With the assistance of Karen Kreller

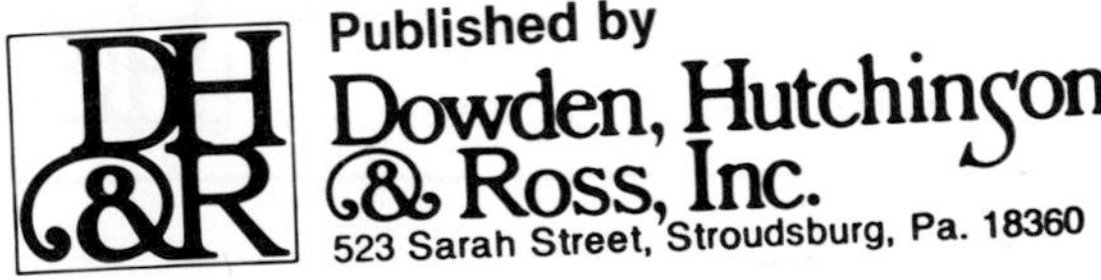

Distributed by ACADEMIC PRESS

Benchmark Papers in Human Physiology, Volume 5
Library of Congress Catalog Card Number: 75–33085
ISBN: 0–87933–189–5

78 77 76 1 2 3 4 5
Manufactured in the United States of America.

LIBRARY OF CONGRESS CATALOGING IN PUBLICATION DATA

Main entry under title:
Pulmonary and respiratory physiology; pt. 1
(Benchmark papers in human physiology/5)
Includes indexes.
1. Lungs—Addresses, essays, lectures. 2. Pulmonary circulation—Addresses, essays, lectures.
3. Respiration —Addresses, essays, lectures.
I. Comroe, Julius Hiram, 1911– II. Series.
QP121.P77 pt. 1 612'.2'08s [612'.22] 75–33085
ISBN 0–87933–189–5

Distributed by
ACADEMIC PRESS
A Subsidiary of Harcourt Brace Jovanovich, Publishers

ACKNOWLEDGMENTS AND PERMISSIONS

ACKNOWLEDGMENTS

AMERICAN PHILOSOPHICAL SOCIETY—*Michael Servetus, A Translation of his Geographical, Medical and Astrological Writings with Introductions and Notes*
Christianismi Restitutio

LONG'S COLLEGE BOOK COMPANY—*Barometric Pressure: Researches in Experimental Physiology*
Excerpt

PERMISSIONS

The following papers have been reprinted or translated with the permission of the authors and copyright holders.

ACTA PHYSIOLOGICA SCANDINAVICA, KAROLINSKA INSTITUTET
Acta Physiologica Scandinavica
Observations on the Pulmonary Arterial Blood Pressure in the Cat
Skandinavisches Archiv fuer Physiologie
Measurements of the Blood Flow Through the Lungs of Man

AMERICAN MEDICAL ASSOCIATION—*American Medical Association Journal of Diseases of Children*
Surface Properties in Relation to Atelectasis and Hyaline Membrane Disease

AMERICAN PHYSIOLOGICAL SOCIETY
The American Journal of Physiology
The Pressure-Volume Diagram of the Thorax and Lung
Journal of Applied Physiology
Mechanical Factors in Distribution of Pulmonary Ventilation
Mechanics of Breathing in Man
Physical Properties of Human Lungs Measured During Spontaneous Respiration
Pulmonary "Capillary" Pressure in Man
Relationship Between Maximum Expiratory Flow and Degree of Lung Inflation

AMERICAN SOCIETY FOR CLINICAL INVESTIGATION—*The Journal of Clinical Investigation*
The Elastic Properties of the Emphysematous Lung and Their Clinical Significance
Mechanics of Airflow in Health and in Emphysema
A New Method for Measuring Airway Resistance in Man Using a Body Plethysmograph: Values in Normal Subjects and in Patients with Respiratory Disease
Pulmonary Capillary Blood Flow in Man
Regional Pulmonary Function Studied with $Xenon^{133}$

Acknowledgments and Permissions

BLACKWELL SCIENTIFIC PUBLICATIONS LTD.—*Movement of the Heart and Blood in Animals*
Excerpts

FRANK CASS & CO. LTD.—*Essays: Physical and Chemical*
On the Burning of Phosphorus, and the Formation of Its Acid

COLUMBIA UNIVERSITY PRESS—*The Physical Treatises of Pascal: The Equilibrium of Liquids and the Weight of the Mass of the Air*
Torricelli's Letters on the Pressure of the Atmosphere

THE JOHNS HOPKINS UNIVERSITY PRESS—*Bulletin of the Johns Hopkins Hospital*
Mechanisms of Airway Obstruction

J. B. LIPPINCOTT COMPANY—*Annals of Surgery*
Commentary on the Anatomy of the Canon of Avicenna

E & S LIVINGSTONE LTD.—*Quarterly Journal of Experimental Physiology*
5-Hydroxytryptamine. Pharmacological Action and Destruction in Perfused Lungs

MACMILLAN JOURNALS LTD.—*Nature*
Properties, Function, and Origin of the Alveolar Lining Layer

THE ROYAL SOCIETY, LONDON—*Proceedings of the Royal Society*
Properties, Function, and Origin of the Alveolar Lining Layer

THE ROYAL SOCIETY OF EDINBURGH
Medico-Physical Works
Excerpts
The Discovery of Oxygen, Part 2, Experiments by Carl Wilhelm Scheele (1777)
Chemical Treatise on Air and Fire

THE ROYAL SOCIETY OF MEDICINE—*Proceedings of the Royal Society of Medicine*
Epistle II: About the Lungs

SOCIETY FOR EXPERIMENTAL BIOLOGY AND MEDICINE—*Proceedings of the Society for Experimental Biology and Medicine*
Catheterization of the Right Auricle in Man
Surface Tension of Lung Extracts

SPRINGER-VERLAG, BERLIN, HEIDELBERG, NEW YORK
Archiv fuer Pathologische Anatomie und Physiologie und fuer Klinische Medizin
The Intrapleural Pressure in Living Healthy Man
Klinische Wochenschrift
The Catheterization of the Right Side of the Heart
Pfluegers Archiv fuer die Gesamte Physiologie
The Behavior of Pleural Pressure with Breathing and the Causes of Its Variability
The Resistance to Flow in the Human Air Passages and the Influence of the Irregular Branching of the Bronchial System on the Course of Respiration in Different Regions in the Lungs
The Pneumotachograph: An Apparatus for Determining the Velocity of Respired Air
Zeitschrift fuer die Gesamte Experimentelle Medizin
New Notions on a Fundamental Principal of Respiratory Mechanics: The Retractibility of the Lung, Dependent on the Surface Tension in the Alveoli
Zeitschrift fuer Klinische Medizin
A Method for Measuring Pulmonary Elasticity in Living Man, Especially in Emphysema

SERIES EDITOR'S PREFACE

I have known Julius Comroe long enough to have a full reservoir of trepidation splashing about whenever I approach him with a request. To undertake a Benchmark volume requires a major time commitment. J. C. is noted for the careful, precise manner in which he protects the utilization of his hours. For these reasons I hesitated, thought of others who might do a volume on respiration, but the more I considered the matter, the more certain I became that Julius Comroe had to be approached first. If I became inundated and drowned in my trepidation, so be it. To my utter astonishment and exuberant delight, he did not tell me I was crazy, or that his back ached too much, or that he had endless commitments, or that I should contact so and so, or that the project was hardly worth the time and effort. With his usual alacrity, he immediately recognized that a collection of the key papers which over time have given rise to our current concepts of the physiology of respiration would be a needed and major contribution. He agreed to undertake it.

Julius Comroe is a marvelous mixture of brillance and erudition, humor and seriousness, warmth and formidableness. He has not only drawn freely and copiously from his field; he has made major contributions to it. He thinks with startling clarity. His lectures, his research, his writing provide irrefragable proof. As the senior statesman in this field, he is the "one" to edit this volume.

At the onset we agreed that the usual format of about 25 papers and a total of some 400 pages would suffice. It did not. In fact, 800 pages proved to be too few, but the basic laws of economics had to intervene. Beyond cavil, articles of true Benchmark significance are not included. As Comroe points out in his Preface, selection is not simple and there is rarely unanimity of thought concerning which papers to include or exclude. Yet, unless a reader has a particular axe to grind, he must agree that the classic papers are here and that they are presented in a highly logical sequence. What better place to begin a study of respiration than with the discovery of the respiratory gases, or to conclude with a consideration of the transport of these gases in the blood?

If I have given the impression that from the conception of this volume through its completion all has been sweetness and sunshine, complete accord, and mutual admiration among the series editor, the volume editor, and the publisher, I have given the wrong impression. The volume grew too large and the publisher grew unhappy, Julius insisted on including "nonrespiratory functions of the lungs" and I disagreed; letters weren't answered quickly enough and the volume editor fired off a few of his classic missiles. The letters got answered, nonrespiratory functions stayed in, and the volume grew. I wonder why I thought it would be otherwise?

L. L. LANGLEY

PREFACE

The idea of selecting 50 or 60 papers that have had an important influence on the advance of respiratory physiology is a superb one. But the selection itself is difficult. Respiration means many things—ventilation, dead space, alveolar ventilation, mechanics of breathing, regulation of respiration, diffusion, pulmonary blood flow, matching of blood and gas, transport of oxygen and carbon dioxide, nonrespiratory functions of the lungs—to name some of the most important. And each has had its own historical development. So the limitations of space mean that only a small fraction of significant papers can be included.

What is a significant paper? I thought at first that I might solve this problem (or at least shift responsibility away from a single editor) by preparing a fairly complete list of 30 candidate articles in one subdivision of respiratory physiology and asking eight recognized authorities in this field to vote "Definitely yes," or "Maybe," or "Definitely no" on the question "Include each article or not?" They expanded my list of 30 to 40 but only one of the new total got a unanimous "Yes"; three more got seven "Yes" votes, and the rest got one, two, three, or four "Yes" votes. Since I finally selected 27 articles in this field, obviously the final responsibility was mine.

I hesitated for a long time over including recent studies to stand alongside Harvey, Boyle, and Lavoisier, but when one of my postdoctoral fellows, in the introduction to a research seminar in 1974, referred to "some *very old* studies published in 1952," I decided that they, too, were ready to be included.

My final selections do not always fit the classic Benchmark formula of reproducing all or most of an article exactly as originally published. The two volumes do include facsimile reproductions of 44 complete articles, but they also include selected portions of 72 additional articles. The device of including short or long selections from many articles has permitted me to provide a thread of continuity to the fabric of respiratory physiology over several hundred years; it has also prevented the sin of excluding articles simply because they were too long to reproduce in full (the longest was 984 pages!). I have also included references to a few articles that were fit to print but didn't "fit to print."

Preface

I want to express my appreciation to the University of California San Francisco Library and librarians for their invaluable help in locating hard-to-find volumes, to William Bunker for his skillful photography of many yellowing pages, and to Aida Cordano and Daniel Benton for library and secretarial assistance.

JULIUS H. COMROE, JR.

CONTENTS

Acknowledgments and Permissions v
Series Editor's Preface vii
Preface ix
Contents by Author xvii

Introduction 1

I: AIR, OXYGEN, AND CARBON DIOXIDE

Editor's Comments on Papers 1 Through 11 6

DISCOVERY OF CARBON DIOXIDE AND OXYGEN

1 VAN HELMONT, J. B.: *Oriatricke, or Physick Refined* 13
J. C., Sometime of M. H. Oxon, London, trans., Lodowick Loyd, 1662, p. 106

2 BLACK, J.: *Experiments upon Magnesia Alba, Quick-Lime and Other Alcaline Substances* 14
William Creech, Edinburgh, 1796, pp. 28–32, 72–73

3 MAYOW, J.: *Medico-Physical Works* 17
E. and S. Livingstone Ltd. for the Alembic Club, 1957, pp. 75–76, 84–85

4 PRIESTLEY, J.: Of Dephlogisticated Air, and of the Constitution of the Atmosphere 20
Experiments and Observations on Different Kinds of Air, Vol. 2, J. Johnson, London, 1775, pp. 29–31, 43–44, 46, 99–102

5 SCHEELE, C. W.: Chemical Treatise on Air and Fire 26
The Discovery of Oxygen, Part 2, Experiments by Carl Wilhelm Scheele (1777), E. and S. Livingstone Ltd. for the Alembic Club, 1952, pp. 5–8

6 LAVOISIER, A.: On the Burning of Phosphorus, and the Formation of Its Acid 31
Essays: Physical and Chemical, T. Henry, trans., Vol. 1, 2nd ed., Frank Cass & Co. Ltd., 1970, pp. 377–379, 416–417

TOTAL AND PARTIAL PRESSURE OF GASES

7 **TORRICELLI, E.:** Torricelli's Letters on the Pressure of the Atmosphere 34
The Physical Treatises of Pascal: The Equilibrium of Liquids and the Weight of the Mass of the Air, I. H. B. and A. G. H. Spiers, trans., Columbia University Press, 1937, pp. 163–166

8 **BOYLE, R.:** A Defence of the Doctrine Touching the Spring and Weight of the Air 38
The Works of the Honourable Robert Boyle, Vol. 1, London, 1772, pp. 156, 157–159, 160

9 **HENRY, W.:** Experiments on the Quantity of Gases Absorbed by Water, at Different Temperatures, and Under Different Pressures 42
Abstracts Philos. Trans. R. Soc. Lond., **1,** 103–104 (1800–1814)

10A **DALTON, J.:** Experimental Enquiry into the Proportion of the Several Gases or Elastic Fluids, Constituting the Atmosphere 44
Manch. Philos. Soc. Mem., **1,** 244–245 (1805)

10B **DALTON, J.:** On the Tendency of Elastic Fluids to Diffusion Through Each Other 45
Manch. Philos. Soc. Mem., **1,** 259–262 (1805)

10C **DALTON, J.:** On the Absorption of Gases by Water and Other Liquids 49
Manch. Philos. Soc. Mem., **1,** 282–284 (1805)

11 **BERT, P.:** *Barometric Pressure: Researches in Experimental Physiology* 51
M. A. Hitchcock and F. A. Hitchcock, trans., College Book Company, 1943, pp. 980–984

II: MECHANICAL PROPERTIES OF THE LUNGS AND THORAX

Editor's Comments on Papers 12 Through 37 56

ELASTIC PROPERTIES OF LUNGS

12 **HOOKE, R.:** Lectures De Potentia Restitutiva, or of Spring 68
Early Science in Oxford, Vol. 8, R. T. Gunther, Oxford, 1931, pp. 333–335

13 **ARON, E.:** The Intrapleural Pressure in Living Healthy Man 73
Translated from *Arch. Pathol. Anat. Physiol. Klin. Med.,* **160,** 228, 230, 231 (1900)

14 **WIRZ, K.:** The Behavior of Pleural Pressure with Breathing and the Causes of Its Variability 75
Translated from *Pfluegers Arch.,* **199,** 47, 52 (1923)

15 **NEERGAARD, K. VON, and K. WIRZ:** A Method for Measuring Pulmonary Elasticity in Living Man, Especially in Emphysema 77
Translated from *Z. Klin. Med.,* **105,** 43 (1927)

16 **CHRISTIE, R. V.:** The Elastic Properties of the Emphysematous Lung and Their Clinical Significance 79
J. Clin. Invest., **13**(2), 295–299, 318–320 (1934)

17 **BUYTENDIJK, H. J.:** Esophagael Pressure and Lung Elasticity 86
Translated from *Oesophagusdruk en Longelasticiteit,* Drukkerij I. Oppenheim N. V., 1949, pp. 13–14, 24–25, 34–37, 48, 55, 126

18 **DORNHORST, A. C., and G. L. LEATHART:** A Method of Assessing the Mechanical Properties of Lungs and Air-Passages 92
Lancet, **2,** 109–111 (1952)

19 **RAHN, H., A. B. OTIS, L. E. CHADWICK, and W. O. FENN:** The Pressure-Volume Diagram of the Thorax and Lung 94
Am. J. Physiol., **146**(6), 161–178 (1946)

20 **OTIS, A. B., W. O. FENN, and H. RAHN:** Mechanics of Breathing in Man 112
J. Appl. Physiol., **2**(11), 592–607 (1950)

21 **MEAD, J., and J. L. WHITTENBERGER:** Physical Properties of Human Lungs Measured During Spontaneous Respiration 128
J. Appl. Physiol., **5**(12), 784–786, 793–796 (1952–1953)

22 **OTIS, A. B., C. B. McKERROW, R. A. BARTLETT, J. MEAD, M. B. McILROY, N. J. SELVERSTONE, and E. P. RADFORD, Jr.:** Mechanical Factors in Distribution of Pulmonary Ventilation 134
J. Appl. Physiol., **8**(4), 427–443 (1956)

AIRWAY RESISTANCE

23 **POISEUILLE, J. L. M.:** Experimental Studies on the Movement of Fluids Through Tubes of Very Small Diameter 151
Translated from *C.R. Acad Sci.*, **11**, 961–967, and 1041–1048 (1840)

24 **ROHRER, F.:** The Resistance to Flow in the Human Air Passages and the Influence of the Irregular Branching of the Bronchial System on the Course of Respiration in Different Regions of the Lungs 161
Translated from *Pfluegers Arch.*, **162,** 225–227, 252–256, 292–299 (1915)

25 **FLEISCH, A.:** The Pneumotachograph; An Apparatus for Determining the Velocity of Respired Air 173
Translated from *Pfluegers Arch.*, **209,** 715–716 (1925)

26 **DuBOIS, A. B., S. Y. BOTELHO, and J. H. COMROE, Jr.:** A New Method for Measuring Airway Resistance in Man Using a Body Plethysmograph: Values in Normal Subjects and in Patients with Respiratory Disease 175
J. Clin. Invest., **35**(3), 327–335 (1956)

27 **DAYMAN, H.:** Mechanics of Airflow in Health and in Emphysema 184
J. Clin. Invest., **30**(11), 1175, 1182–1184, 1187–1190 (1951)

28 **CAMPBELL, E. J. M., H. B. MARTIN, and R. L. RILEY:** Mechanisms of Airway Obstruction 191
Bull. Johns Hopkins Hosp., **101**(6), 329–343 (1957)

29 **HYATT, R. E., D. P. SCHILDER, and D. L. FRY:** Relationship Between Maximum Expiratory Flow and Degree of Lung Inflation 206
J. Appl. Physiol., **13**(3), 331–336 (1958)

SURFACE TENSION: PULMONARY SURFACTANT

30 LAPLACE, P. S.: Theory of Capillary Action 212
Traité de Mécanique Céleste, Vol. 4, N. Bowditch, trans., Hilliard, Gray, Little & Wilkins, Boston, 1829–1839, pp. 688–689, 1009, 1017

31 NEERGAARD, K. VON: New Notions on a Fundamental Principle of Respiratory Mechanics: The Retractile Force of the Lung, Dependent on the Surface Tension in the Alveoli 214
Translated from *Z. Gesamte Exp. Med.,* **66,** 373–394 (1929)

32 MACKLIN, C. C.: The Pulmonary Alveolar Mucoid Film and the Pneumonocytes 235
Lancet, **266,** 1099, 1101 (May 1954)

33 PATTLE, R. E.: Properties, Function, and Origin of the Alveolar Lining Layer 237
Nature, (Lond.) **175,** 1125–1126 (June 1955)

34 CLEMENTS, J. A.: Surface Tension of Lung Extracts 239
Proc. Soc. Exp. Biol. Med., **95,** 170–172 (1957)

35 PATTLE, R. E.: Properties, Function, and Origin of the Alveolar Lining Layer 242
Proc. R. Soc. Lond., **B148,** 217–218, 220–221, 222–224, 226, 229–231, 232, 233–234, 236, 238–240 (1958)

36 AVERY, M. E., and J. MEAD: Surface Properties in Relation to Atelectasis and Hyaline Membrane Disease 256
A.M.A. J. Dis. Child., **97,** 517–523 (May 1959)

37 CLEMENTS, J. A.: Surface Phenomena in Relation to Pulmonary Function 263
Physiologist, **5**(1), 12–28 (1962)

III: THE PULMONARY CIRCULATION

Editor's Comments on Papers 38 Through 52 282

DISCOVERY AND EARLY OBSERVATIONS

38 IBN NAFĪS: Commentary on the Anatomy of the Canon of Avicenna 287
"A Forgotten Chapter in the History of the Circulation of the Blood," *Ann. Surg.,* **104**(1), 3, 5, 7 (1936)

39 SERVETUS, M.: Christianismi Restitutio 290
Michael Servetus, A Translation of his Geographical, Medical and Astrological Writings with Introductions and Notes, C. D. O'Malley, trans., American Philosophical Society, 1953, pp. 204–205

40 HARVEY, W.: *Movement of the Heart and Blood in Animals* 293
K. Franklin, trans., Blackwell Scientific Publications Ltd., 1957, pp. 51–56, 87

41 MALPIGHI, M.: Epistle II: About the Lungs 301
Proc. R. Soc. Med., J. Young, ed., **23,** 7–11 (1929–1930)

42 **HOOKE, R.:** An Account of an Experiment Made by M. Hook, of Preserving Animals Alive by Blowing Through Their Lungs with Bellows 306
Philos. Trans., **2,** 539–540 (1667)

43 **LOWER, R.:** *Tractatus de Corde: Item De Motu & Colore Sanguinis et Chyli in cum Transitu* 309
Elzevir edition, 1669, p. 176. English excerpt: On the Color of the Blood. K. J. Franklin, trans., *Early Science in Oxford,* Vol. 9, Clarendon Press, 1932

PRESSURE AND FLOW

44 **KROGH, A., and J. LINDHARD:** Measurements of the Blood Flow Through the Lungs of Man 310
Skand. Arch. Physiol., **27,** 100–105, 106–109, 118–121, 124–125 (1912)

45 **LEE, G. DE J., and A. B. DuBOIS:** Pulmonary Capillary Blood Flow in Man 324
J. Clin. Invest., **34**(9), 1380–1390 (1955)

46 **FORSSMANN, W.:** The Catheterization of the Right Side of the Heart 335
Translated from *Klin. Wochenschr.,* **8**(45), 2085–2087 (1929)

47 **COURNAND, A., and H. A. RANGES:** Catheterization of the Right Auricle in Man 341
Proc. Soc. Exp. Biol. Med., **46**(3), 462–466 (1941)

48 **HELLEMS, H. K., F. W. HAYNES, and L. DEXTER:** Pulmonary "Capillary" Pressure in Man 346
J. Appl. Physiol., **2**(1), 24–29(1949–1950)

49 **VON EULER, U. S., and G. LILJESTRAND:** Observations on the Pulmonary Arterial Blood Pressure in the Cat 352
Acta Physiol. Scand., **12,** 301–306, 309–312, 316–320 (1946)

50 **BALL, W. C., Jr., P. B. STEWART, L. G. S. NEWSHAM, and D. V. BATES:** Regional Pulmonary Function Studied with Xenon^{133} 366
J. Clin. Invest., **41**(3), 519–525, 527–529, 530–531 (1962)

NONRESPIRATORY FUNCTIONS

51 **COLIN, G.-C.:** On the Absorption in Airways 375
Translated from *Traité de Physiologie Comparée des Animaux,* 2nd ed., J.-B. Baillière et Fils, Vol. 2, 1873, pp. 108–111

52 **GADDUM, J. H., C. O. HEBB, A. SILVER, and A. A. B. SWAN:** 5-Hydroxytryptamine. Pharamacological Action and Destruction in Perfused Lungs 379
Q.J. Exp. Physiol., **38,** 255–262 (1953)

Author Citation Index 389
Subject Index 395
About the Editor 398

CONTENTS BY AUTHOR

Aron, E., 73
Avery, M. E., 256
Ball, W. C., Jr., 366
Bartlett, R. A., 134
Bates, D. V., 366
Bert, P., 51
Black, J., 14
Boyle, R., 38
Botelho, S. Y., 175
Buytendijk, H. J., 86
Campbell, E. J. M., 191
Chadwick, L. E., 94
Christie, R. V., 79
Clements, J. A., 239, 263
Colin, G.-C., 375
Comroe, J. H., Jr., 175
Cournand, A., 341
Dalton, J., 44, 45, 49
Dayman, H., 184
Dexter, L., 346
Dornhorst, A. C., 92
DuBois, A. B., 175, 324
Fenn, W. O., 94, 112
Fleisch, A., 173
Forssmann, W., 335
Fry, D. L., 206
Gaddum, J. H., 379
Harvey, W., 293
Haynes, F. W., 346
Hebb, C. O., 379
Hellems, H. K., 346
Henry, W., 42
Hooke, R., 68, 306
Hyatt, R. E., 206
Ibn Nafīs, 287
Krogh, A., 310
Laplace, P. S., 212
Lavoisier, A., 31
Leathart, G. L., 92
Lee, G. de J., 324
Liljestrand, G., 352
Lindhard, J., 310
Lower, R., 309
Macklin, C. C., 235
Malpighi, M., 301
Martin, H. B., 191
Mayow, J., 17
McIlroy, M. B., 134
McKerrow, C. B., 134
Mead, J., 128, 134, 256
Neergaard, K. von, 77, 214
Newsham, L. G. S., 366
Otis, A. B., 94, 112, 134
Pattle, R. E., 237, 242
Poiseuille, J. L. M., 151
Priestley, J., 20
Radford, E. P., Jr., 134
Rahn, H., 94, 112
Ranges, H. A., 341
Riley, R. L., 191
Rohrer, F., 161
Scheele, C. W., 26
Schilder, D. P., 206
Selverstone, N. J., 134
Servetus, M., 290
Silver, A., 379

Stewart, P. B., 366
Swan, A. A. B., 379
Torricelli, E., 34
Van Helmont, J. B., 13
Von Euler, U. S., 352
Whittenberger, J. L., 128
Wirz, K., 75, 77

INTRODUCTION

The lungs have many functions. Their main function, of course, is to serve as a meeting place for fresh air and mixed venous blood where the proper amount of oxygen can leave the air to enter the blood and the proper amount of carbon dioxide can move from blood to air. The meeting place, the alveolar capillary membranes, is an extremely thin tissue (less than 0.1 μm thick) with a vast area (70 m^2) that permits ready exchange of gases. The "proper amount" exchanged, however, requires control mechanisms that can sense a need for more or less air and send messages to the brain to increase or decrease ventilation to match the need.

The ultimate function of pulmonary gas exchange is to provide proper gas exchange between every cell in the body and its capillary blood. Thus gas exchange must involve transport of oxygen in arterial blood to tissues, its release to cells on demand, and the transport of carbon dioxide by venous blood back to the pulmonary circulation.

The pulmonary circulation is an integral part of the lungs, and the amount and distribution of pulmonary capillary blood flow is as important to gas exchange as is the amount and distribution of fresh air to the alveoli. To function properly, the lungs need two systems: one supplies air; the other supplies blood. The respiratory system uses an *air* pump, which draws fresh air through hundreds of millions of small air sacs (alveoli). The circulatory system uses a *blood* pump, which drives the entire cardiac output through hundreds of millions of fine, thin-walled blood tubes (capillaries) that surround the alveoli. That these two pumps can distribute blood and air in the same ratio to all parts of both lungs simultaneously is an amazing feat of engineering. The two systems have much in common: each is a low-resistance system and each can greatly increase flow when needed. The blood pump can increase its output from 4 liters/min (in man at rest) to as much as 30–40 liters/min (in man during maximal exercise). The air pump can increase its output from 5 or 6 liters/min to as much as 120–140 liters/min. The same laws for pressure, flow, and resistance hold for both systems; Poiseuille's law, formulated from data obtained on the flow of water through fine tubes, also holds for air flow.

There are differences between the two systems. The blood pump, the right ventricle, is a positive pressure pump that pushes blood in only one direction; valves in the system prevent backflow when the pump is filling for its next stroke. The air pump is a negative (subatmospheric) rather than a positive pump. A positive pressure air pump would, by muscular effort, compress the thorax and lungs to push air out of the lungs (expiration) and then allow fresh air to enter when, during muscle relaxation, the thorax and lungs returned to their initial position. The real air pump, however, actively enlarges the thorax during inspiration, which lowers the pressure to less than atmospheric in the pleural cavity and alveoli so that air, at atmospheric pressure, must flow in; the thorax and lungs then recoil passively to their resting position to push air out. The air pump, on demand, can be both a positive and negative pressure pump to produce active expiratory effort as well as active inspiration.

The air pump also differs from the blood pump in that it has no valves; instead of flowing *through* the lungs as does the blood, air flows back and forth through the same tubes. Thus some inspired air never reaches alveoli and is "wasted" ventilation; it remains in tubes (dead space) where no gas exchange occurs. Dead space in the system increases the total ventilation and muscular effort required to provide a needed alveolar gas flow; however, the use of one set of tubes instead of two (one for air entering and another for air leaving) allows more space in the thorax for alveoli and their gas-exchange membranes.

Section I of this volume deals first with the discovery of oxygen and carbon dioxide and then with the formulation of the gas laws. The seventeenth-century studies of Torricelli and Boyle on air pressure marked the beginning of the revolution in physics;

the discovery of oxygen by Lavoisier in the eighteenth century set the chemical revolution into motion; and John Dalton's work on partial pressure of gases in the early nineteenth century marked the beginning of atomic theory.

Sections II and III of this volume present important papers on the air and blood pumps and their mechanical properties, and on the characteristics of the air and blood tubes. One section deals with the recent discovery that recoil of the lungs occurs only in part because of recoil of elastic fibers that are stretched during inspiration; these studies show that an important component in recoil is a unique surfactant synthesized in type II alveolar cells.

Several of the papers on pulmonary circulation emphasize that the lung does more than exchange gases. Fluids and small molecules can cross alveolar–capillary membranes and enter blood. And the endothelial cells of the pulmonary vessels are much more than a lining: they can take up materials from blood and either store, inactivate, or activate these, and they can synthesize new substances and release these or other materials into pulmonary capillary blood. Recent studies on type II alveolar cells and pulmonary endothelium show that the lung is a metabolically active organ and does not consist simply of conduits for the flow of blood and gas pumped with energy supplied by contractions of the right ventricle and the thoracic muscles.

I

AIR, OXYGEN, AND CARBON DIOXIDE

Papers 1 Through 11

DISCOVERY OF CARBON DIOXIDE AND OXYGEN

1 **VAN HELMONT**
Excerpt from *Oriatricke, or Physick Refined*

2 **BLACK**
Excerpts from *Experiments upon Magnesia Alba, Quick-Lime, and Other Alcaline Substances*

3 **MAYOW**
Excerpts from *Medico-Physical Works*

4 **PRIESTLEY**
Excerpts from *Of Dephlogisticated Air, and of the Constitution of the Atmosphere*

5 **SCHEELE**
Excerpt from *Chemical Treatise on Air and Fire*

6 **LAVOISIER**
Excerpts from *On the Burning of Phosphorus, and the Formation of Its Acid*

TOTAL AND PARTIAL PRESSURE OF GASES

7 **TORRICELLI**
Torricelli's Letters on the Pressure of the Atmosphere

8 **BOYLE**
Excerpts from *A Defense of the Doctrine Touching the Spring and Weight of the Air*

9 **HENRY**
Experiments on the Quantity of Gases Absorbed by Water, at Different Temperatures, and Under Different Pressures

10A **DALTON**
Excerpt from *Experimental Enquiry into the Proportion of the Several Gases or Elastic Fluids, Constituting the Atmosphere*

10B **DALTON**
Excerpt from *On the Tendency of Elastic Fluids to Diffusion Through Each Other*

10c DALTON
Excerpt from *On the Absorption of Gases by Water and Other Liquids*

11 BERT
Excerpt from *Barometric Pressure: Researches in Experimental Physiology*

EDITOR'S COMMENTS

In the 1970s, it is hard to transport ourselves backward to the time when oxygen and carbon dioxide were unknown and the gas laws had not yet been formulated. The rediscovery of carbon dioxide (1755) and the discovery of oxygen (1775) marked the beginning of quantitative chemistry (the chemical revolution); measurement of the pressure of air (1644) and of its "spring" (1669) marked the beginning of a revolution in physics.

DISCOVERY OF CARBON DIOXIDE AND OXYGEN

Paper 1 presents the initial discovery of carbon dioxide by Jean Van Helmont. According to Michael Foster, Van Helmont was two men: one, a man who observed, measured, weighed, used instruments of exact research, and reached conclusions by accurate quantitative means; the other, a mystic and a speculative dreamer who wove a fantastic scheme of powers and forces ruling the universe and called on invisible, supernatural agencies to explain natural phenomenon. Little wonder that the two paragraphs reproduced here, found among many hundreds of pages of fanciful, mystical writing, had no impact on chemistry. But Van Helmont did introduce the word "gas," did discover carbon dioxide, formed by the combustion of charcoal ($C + O_2 \rightarrow CO_2$), and did note its similarity to gas formed in the fermentation of grapes. He called carbon dioxide "gas sylvestre" or "wild gas."

Carbon dioxide had to be rediscovered in 1755 (Paper 2)—this time by Joseph Black, who put chemistry on a scientific basis and set the stage for the discovery of oxygen. Black weighed chemical substances before and after reactions, noted gain or loss in weight, and accounted for the change. Working with limestone (calcium carbonate) and magnesia alba (magnesium carbonate), he noted that each lost weight on heating. Limestone changes to quicklime (CaO) and "the air which quicklime attracts is . . . different from common elastic air . . . . To this I have given the name *fixed air.*" Fixed air extinguished both flame and life.

John Mayow (Paper 3) came very close to discovering oxygen in 1674. He demonstrated that only *part* of air was necessary for life and that part was removed both by respiration and by fire (combustion). He called this part "nitro-aerial spirits." He enclosed an animal and a lighted lamp in a vessel (fortunately, over water that absorbed CO_2), so arranged that air could not enter. The lamp died first (because, as Mayow pointed out, it exhausted the particles immediately around the flame); the mouse died a little later (later because its breathing brought in particles from a distance). He stated that gills of fish function as lungs and that fish survive in water only because water contains nitro-aerial spirits (he observed that fish cannot live in boiled water since boiling removes the vital substance). However, Mayow did not realize that the vital substance was a gas that could be isolated.

The discovery of oxygen came 100 years after Mayow's observations. On August 1, 1774, Joseph Priestley, using a 12-in. "burning glass" facing the summer sun, heated mercuric oxide and so released a gas:

$$2Hg + O_2\ (\text{air}) \xrightarrow{\text{heat}} 2HgO$$

$$2HgO \xrightarrow{\text{intense heat}} 2Hg + O_2$$

This he reported to the Royal Society in March 1775 (Paper 4). On March 8, 1775, he exposed a mouse to gas he had released from mercuric oxide and found the gas "was much better than common air." Priestley was the first man to breathe pure oxygen, the first to note the beauty and vivacity of a flame in oxygen, and the first to suggest the use of oxygen and flame to melt platinum and to explode gunpowder. But he never renounced the phlogiston theory and till his death he thought of oxygen as "dephlogisticated air." And yet it was Priestley who wrote: "We may take a maxim so strongly for granted, that the plainest evidence of sense will not intirely change and often hardly modify our persuasions; and the more ingenious a man is, the more effectively he is entangled in his errors." (It is beyond the scope of these comments to explain Stahl's "phlogiston" theory, a completely erroneous but persuasive and dominant hypothesis, which entangled

Priestley and prevented him from discovering the true nature of the substance that he had prepared.)

Carl Wilhelm Scheele also prepared oxygen; he called it "fire-air." His experiments were probably completed by 1773 but his treatise, "Fire and Air," was not published till 1777 (Paper 5). Fascinated by fire, Scheele realized that "to fathom this beautiful phenomenon" he had to learn about air, and this led him to experiments that produced oxygen. In 1774 Scheele suggested in a letter to Lavoisier that he heat dry silver carbonate with a burning glass and collect the gas; "you will see how much air is produced in which a candle will burn and an animal will live." Scheele also demonstrated the effect of light on silver granules and so provided a basis for the later development of photography. But he too was enmeshed in the phlogiston reasoning.

Antoine Lavoisier was not. With a mind uncommitted to any existing doctrine, he identified "highly respirable air" (Paper 6), then recognized it as "vital air," and finally named it "oxygen." This put an end to the phlogiston doctrine and permitted Lavoisier and others to develop a whole new system of modern quantitative chemistry.

Lavoisier's experiments on oxygen were performed over a 6 to 7 year period. He had indirect help from Black's experiments with fixed air, from Scheele's observations, and from Priestley. In 1774, Priestley visited Lavoisier in Paris and described his new air (prepared by heating mercuric oxide), in which a candle burned more brightly. Later Lavoisier performed a critical experiment in which he heated mercury for 12 days and found that one fifth of the air in a connecting chamber had been used up; the residual air extinguished lighted candles and asphyxiated animals.

It is difficult to select one paper to reproduce from a long sequence. Lavoisier's 1775 memoir has been frequently cited. Paper 6, read before the Royal Academy on April 26 (sometimes called the Easter Memoir of 1775), was immediately published in *Journal de Physique* in May 1775 (p. 429). It was read again before the Academy on August 8, 1778, with a few very important changes, and then published in the *Mémoires de l'Académie des Sciences* in 1778. Conant (1957, pp. 77–84) has called attention to these few changes in his brilliant analysis of the crucial experiments performed between 1775 and 1778. To point six in the 1775 version (see p. 33), Lavoisier added in 1778: "Charcoal burned in it with a radiance almost like that of phosphorus and all combustible bodies in general were consumed with astonishing speed."

And in point six, he changed "All these circumstances convinced me fully that this air was not only *common air* . . ." to "All these circumstances convinced me fully that this air, *far from being fixed air,* was in a *state more respirable and more combustible* . . . ." In 1775, Lavoisier had said in fact that the gas he obtained from mercuric oxide was *both* "common air" and "purer than common air"; in 1778, he decided, without equivocation, that it was neither "common air" nor "fixed air" but "highly respirable air"; later he called it "oxygen."

TOTAL AND PARTIAL PRESSURE OF GASES

The torr, a unit of measure now widely used to signify mm Hg of total or partial pressure, was named after Evangelista Torricelli. In 1644, Torricelli, in a letter to M. Ricci, told of his discovery of the mercury barometer and of what later was called a Torricellian vacuum between the top of the mercury column and the top of the closed tube (Paper 7). Although it was known that air had weight, Torricelli, a pupil of Galileo, seems to have been the first to propose that "we live submerged at the bottom of an ocean of the element air."

Galileo had an interest in the practical problem of pumping water but he never connected it with the weight of air. In "Dialogues Concerning Two New Sciences" (1638), Galileo has a character say

> I once saw a cistern which had been provided with a pump . . . this pump worked perfectly so long as the water in the cistern stood above a certain level; but below this level, the pump failed to work . . . . The workman whom I called in to repair it told me the defect was not in the pump but in the water, which had fallen too low; he added it was not possible by a pump . . . to lift water a hair's breadth above 18 cubits [about 33 feet].

Torricelli provided the explanation by his classic and simple experiment of substituting mercury for water, thus creating a manageable experimental setting. Later, Pascal (1648) measured barometric pressure at the foot and top of a mountain and solidified the concept of a "sea of air."

Robert Boyle (Paper 8) is best known to respiratory physiologists for Boyle's law, which states that at a given temperature the pressure and volume of gases are inversely related: $P \times V$ = constant or $P_1/P_2 = V_2/V_1$. But he had varied interests, many to be sure associated with his development of pumps. He extracted gas from blood by a vacuum pump; he experimented with artificial ventilation and determined that sound was transmitted poorly or not at all in a vacuum. Of considerable interest is that he used his own funds to publish Newton's *Principia*. He was one of the original "invisible college" at Oxford, which also included Newton, Hooke, Lower, and Mayow, that later (1660) became the Royal College and developed the first formal system of communicating the experiments of one scientist to another. The early volumes of *Philosophical Transactions of the Royal College* (beginning in 1666) are amazing in the range of interests of the members: circulation of the blood, Copernican hypotheses, comets, valves in veins, telescopes, fall of heavy bodies, extracorporeal arterialization of the blood, transfusions, earthquakes, elephants, preservation of embryos, whale fishing.

Boyle was the leading exponent in England of the new *experimental* philosophy; note (pp. 40 and 41) that his theoretical concepts are supported by detailed tables of data relating pressure and volume. Note also from these tables that Boyle required measurements of absolute pressure of air (from Torricelli's earlier work) to establish Boyle's law. Conant has pointed out that, in contrast, it is hard to tell whether some of Pascal's so-called experiments on pneumatics were ever performed.

William Henry was an English chemist best known for his law which states that the amount of gas that dissolves in a liquid is proportional to the partial pressure of the gas above the liquid. Henry published his treatise in 1803 (only the abstract is reproduced as Paper 9). It is difficult to know whether John Dalton's first experiments on solubility of gases in liquids preceded Henry's (since Dalton's experiments of 1802 and 1803 were not published until 1805), but Dalton states in his 1803 communication that

> I had the result of Mr. William Henry's experience (1803) on the subject before me; . . . by the reciprocal communications since, we have been enabled to bring the results of our experiments to a near agreement . . . . There are two very important facts contained in the second article. The first is, that the quantity of gas absorbed is as the density or pressure—this was discovered by Mr. William Henry, before either he or I had formed any theory on the subject.

Dalton (Papers 10A–10C) scarcely needed credit for his studies on the solubility of gases in liquids or even for Dalton's law of partial pressures (the partial pressure of a gas in a mixture of gases is the pressure it would exert if all the other gases in the mixture were absent). Dalton's fame is secure for his atomic theory presented in the first volume of *A New System of Chemical Philosophy* (2 volumes, 1808–1827) in which he emphasized relative atomic weights and presented a symbolic system for approaching chemical reactions. He used experiments on gases as a convenient and accessible approach to atomic theory and the quantitative aspects of physical and chemical interactions between molecules. His 1803 treatise, *On the Absorption of Gases,* contains in an appendix (p. 287) a "Table of the relative weights of the ultimate particles of gaseous and other bodies"; this was his first publication dealing with atomic theory. Throughout the early history of science, we come across giants who had little formal education; Dalton was one of these, although he taught in a village school at the age of 12!

Paul Bert (Paper 11) was best known during his lifetime for his pioneer studies on skin grafting. His obituary in the *Lancet* (November 20, 1886) does not mention *La Pression barométrique* or even that he was a great physiologist, although he had worked under Claude Bernard and later succeeded him as professor of physiology at the Faculté des Sciences, Paris. Bert's great work on the study of man at high and low pressures (1178 pages and 89 figures) applied for the first time Dalton's law of partial pressure to human respiration and circulation. Bert proved beyond doubt, in studies in low-pressure chambers, that high-altitude sickness was due to low partial pressure of oxygen and not to a decrease in total barometric pressure. Bert also studied the effect of high pressures and caisson disease and was the first to relate partial pressure of oxygen to the oxygen content of blood (the first oxygen dissociation curve, which is reproduced as Paper 52 in *Pulmonary and Respiratory Physiology, Part II: Regulation of Breathing—Clinical Pulmonary Physiology,* Dowden, Hutchinson & Ross, Inc., Stroudsburg, Pa. (in press).

REFERENCES

Conant, James B. (ed.). *Harvard Case Histories in Experimental Science,* Vol. 1. Cambridge, Mass.: Harvard University Press, 1957. Case 1, Robert Boyle's Experiments in Pneumatics, pp. 3–62; Case 2, The Overthrow of the Phlogiston Theory, pp. 67–115; Case 4, The Atomic-Molecular Theory, pp. 217–321.

1

Reprinted from *Oriatricke, or Physick Refined,* by J. B. Van Helmont. J. C., Sometime of M. H. Oxon, London, trans., Lodowick Loyd, 1662, p. 106

ORIATRICKE, OR PHYSICK REFINED

Jean Baptiste Van Helmont

[*Editor's Note:* In the original, material precedes this excerpt.]

13 Moreover, every coal which is made of the co-melting of Sulphur and *Salt* (working a-
mong themſelves in time of burning) although it be roaſted even to its laſt day in a bright
burning Furnace, the Veſſel being ſhut, it is fired indeed; but there is true fire in the Veſſel, no otherwiſe than in the coal not being ſhut up; yet nothing of it is waſted, it not being
able to be conſumed, through the hindering of its eflux. Therefore the live coal, and generally whatſoever bodies do not immediately depart into water, nor yet are fixed, do neceſſa-
rily belch forth a wild ſpirit or breath. Suppoſe thou, that of *62* pounds of Oaken coal, one
pound of aſhes is compoſed: Therefore the *61* remaining pounds, are the wild ſpirit, which
alſo being fired, cannot depart, the Veſſel being ſhut.
I call this Spirit, unknown hitherto, by the new name of Gas, which can neither be con-
14 ſtrained by Veſſels, nor reduced into a viſible body, unleſs the ſeed being firſt extinguiſhed.
But Bodies do contain this Spirit, and do ſometimes wholly depart into ſuch a Spirit, not indeed, becauſe it is actually in thoſe very bodies (for truly it could not be detained, yea the
whole compoſed body ſhould flie away at once) but it is a Spirit grown together, coagula-
ted after the manner of a body, and is ſtirred up by an attained ferment, as in Wine, the juyce
15 of unripe Grapes, bread, hydromel or water and Honey, *&c.* Or by a ſtrange addition, as I
ſhall ſometime ſhew concerning *Sal Armoniack*: or at length, by ſome alterative diſpoſi-
tion, ſuch as is roaſting in reſpect of an Apple: For the Grape is kept and dried, being un-
hurt; but its skin being once burſt, and wounded, it ſtraightway conceiveth a ferment of
boyling up, and from hence the beginning of a tranſmutation. Therefore the Wines of
Grapes, Apples, berries, Honey, and likewiſe flowers and leaves being pounced, a ferment
being ſnatched to them, they begin to boyl and be hot, whence ariſeth a Gas; but from Ray-
ſins bruiſed, and uſed, for want of a ferment, a Gas is not preſently granted.

[*Editor's Note:* Material has been omitted at this point.]

2

EXPERIMENTS

UPON

MAGNESIA ALBA, QUICK-LIME,

AND OTHER

ALCALINE SUBSTANCES;

By JOSEPH BLACK, M. D
Professor of Chemistry in the University of Edinburgh.

To which is annexed,

An Essay on the Cold produced by Evaporating Fluids,

AND

Of some other means of producing Cold;

By WILLIAM CULLEN, M. D.
Late Professor of the Practice of Physic in the University of Edinburgh.

Extracted from Essays and Observations, Physical and Literary, Read before a Society in Edinburgh, Anno 1755.

EDINBURGH:
PRINTED FOR WILLIAM CREECH.

1796.

Reprinted from *Experiments upon Magnesia Alba, Quick-Lime, and Other Alcaline Substances* by Joseph Black. William Creech, Edinburgh, 1796, pp. 28–32, 72–73

By the following experiments, I propofed to know whether this fubftance could be reduced to a quick-lime.

An ounce of *magnefia* was expofed in a crucible, for about an hour, to fuch a heat as is fufficient to melt copper. When taken out, it weighed three drams and one fcruple, or had loft $\frac{7}{12}$ of its former weight.

I repeated, with the *magnefia* prepared in this manner, moft of thofe experiments I had already made upon it before calcination, and the refult was as follows——

It diffolves in all the acids, and with thefe compofes falts exactly fimilar to thofe defcribed in the firft fet of experiments: But, what is particularly to be remarked, it is diffolved without any the leaft degree of effervefcence.

It flowly precipitates the corrofive fublimate of mercury, in the form of a black powder.

It feparates the volatile alkali in falt-ammoniac from the acid, when it is mixed with a warm folution of that falt. But it does not feparate an acid from a calcareous earth, nor does it introduce the leaft change upon lime-water.

Lastly, when a dram of it is digefted with an ounce of water in a bottle for fome hours, it does not make any the leaft change in the water. The *magnefia*, when dried, is found to have gained ten grains; but it neither effervefces with acids, nor does it fenfibly affect lime-water.

Observing *magnefia* to lofe fuch a remarkable proportion of its weight in the fire, my next attempts were directed to the inveftigation of this volatile part; and, among other experiments, the following feemed to throw fome light upon it——

Three ounces of *magnefia* were diftilled in a glafs retort and receiver, the fire being gradually increafed until the *magnefia* was obfcurely red hot. When all was cool, I found only five drams of a whitifh water in the receiver, which had a faint fmell of the fpirit of hartshorn, gave a green colour to the juice of violets, and rendered the folutions of corrofive fublimate, and of filver, very flightly turbid. But it did not fenfibly effervefce with acids.

The *magnefia*, when taken out of the retort, weighed an ounce, three drams, and thirty grains, or had loft more than the half of its weight. It ftill effervefced pretty brifkly with acids, though not fo ftrongly as before this operation.

The fire fhould have been raifed here to the degree requifite for the perfect calcination of *magnefia*. But, even from this imperfect experiment, it is evident, that, of the volatile parts contained in that powder, a ſmall proportion only is water; the reſt cannot, it ſeems, be retained in veſſels, under a viſible form. Chemiſts have often obſerved, in their diſtillations, that part of a body has vaniſhed from their ſenſes, notwithſtanding the utmoſt care to retain it; and they have always found, upon further inquiry, that ſubtile part to be air, which having been impriſoned in the body, under a ſolid form, was ſet free, and rendered fluid and elaſtic by the fire. We may therefore ſafely conclude, that the volatile matter, loſt in the calcination of *magneſia*, is moſtly air; and hence the calcined *magneſia* does not emit air, or make an effervеſcence when mixed with acids.

[*Editor's Note:* Material has been omitted at this point.]

it is evident, that the air which quick-lime attracts, is of a different kind from that which is mixed with water. And that it is alſo different from common elaſtic air, is ſufficiently proved by daily experience; for lime-water, which ſoon attracts air, and forms a cruſt when expoſed in open and ſhallow veſſels, may be preſerved, for any time, in bottles which are but ſlightly corked, or cloſed in ſuch a manner as would allow free acceſs to elaſtic air, were a vacuum formed in the bottle. Quick-lime, therefore, does not attract air when in its moſt ordinary form, but is capable of being joined to one particular ſpecies only, which is diſperſed through the atmoſphere, either in the ſhape of an exceedingly ſubtle powder, or more probably in that of an elaſtic fluid. To this I have given the name of *fixed air*, and perhaps very improperly; but I thought it better to uſe a word already familiar in philoſophy, than to invent a new name, before we be more fully acquainted with the nature and properties of this ſubſtance, which will probably be the ſubject of my further inquiry.

[*Editor's Note:* Material has been omitted at this point.]

3

Reprinted from *Medico-Physical Works (Being a Translation of Tractatus Quinque Medico-Physici)* by John Mayow, 1674. E. and S. Livingstone Ltd., for the Alembic Club, Edinburgh, 1957, pp. 75–76, 84–85

MEDICO-PHYSICAL WORKS

John Mayow

[*Editor's Note:* In the original, material precedes this excerpt.]

Hence it is manifest that air is deprived of its elastic force by the breathing of animals very much in the same way as by the burning of flame. And indeed we must believe that animals and fire draw particles of the same kind from the air, as is further confirmed by the following experiment.

For let any animal be enclosed in a glass vessel along with a lamp so that the entrance of air from without is prevented, which is easily done if the orifice of the inverted glass be immersed in water in the manner already described. When this is done we shall soon see the lamp go out and the animal will not long survive the fatal torch. For I have ascertained by experiment that an animal enclosed in a glass vessel along with a lamp will not breathe much longer than half the time it would otherwise have lived.

Nor is there any reason for supposing that the animal is suffocated by the smoke of the lamp, for scarcely any smoke will emanate from it if spirit of wine is used, and indeed the animal will live in the glass for some time after the extinction of the lamp—that is, after the fumes have entirely disappeared—so that it is by no means to be supposed that it has been suffocated by the fumes of the lamp. But since the air enclosed in the glass is in part deprived of its nitro-aërial particles by the burning of the lamp, as has already been pointed out, it cannot support long the breathing of the animal, hence not only the lamp but also the animal soon expires for want of nitro-aërial particles.

But the reason why an animal can live for some time after the extinction of the lamp seems to be this. It is only by a continuous and moreover an abundant and rapid stream of nitro-aërial particles that a lamp is sustained. Consequently if the succession of nitro-aërial particles be but for a moment interrupted, or if they are not supplied in due abundance, the flame will immediately sink down and expire. Hence as soon as the nitro-aërial particles begin to come but sparsely and slowly to the flame it presently goes out. But a smaller ration of aërial nourishment and that introduced at intervals will suffice for animals ; so that an animal can be sustained by the aërial particles remaining after the extinction of the flame. It supports this view that the movement of the subsiding lungs conduces not a little to draw in the aërial particles if any remain in the said glass and to carry them into the blood of the breathing animal. Hence it results that the animal does not die until the aërial particles have been entirely exhausted. And hence it is that the air in which an animal is suffocated is contracted in volume by more than twice as much as that in which a lamp goes out, as was formerly pointed out.

[*Editor's Note:* Material has been omitted at this point.]

Further, in what has been already said the reason is to be sought why lamp and animal when placed in the aforesaid glass vessels expire even when air in sufficient abundance seems to be contained in them. It must not be supposed here that of the air enclosed in those vessels a part has been entirely consumed while the rest remains unchanged, because if that were so there would be nothing to hinder the animal from still breathing in it. But it must rather be thought that nearly all the particles of the air have undergone some change, and that they have been deprived to such an extent of nitro-aërial particles that the air has become quite unfit to sustain life and flame.

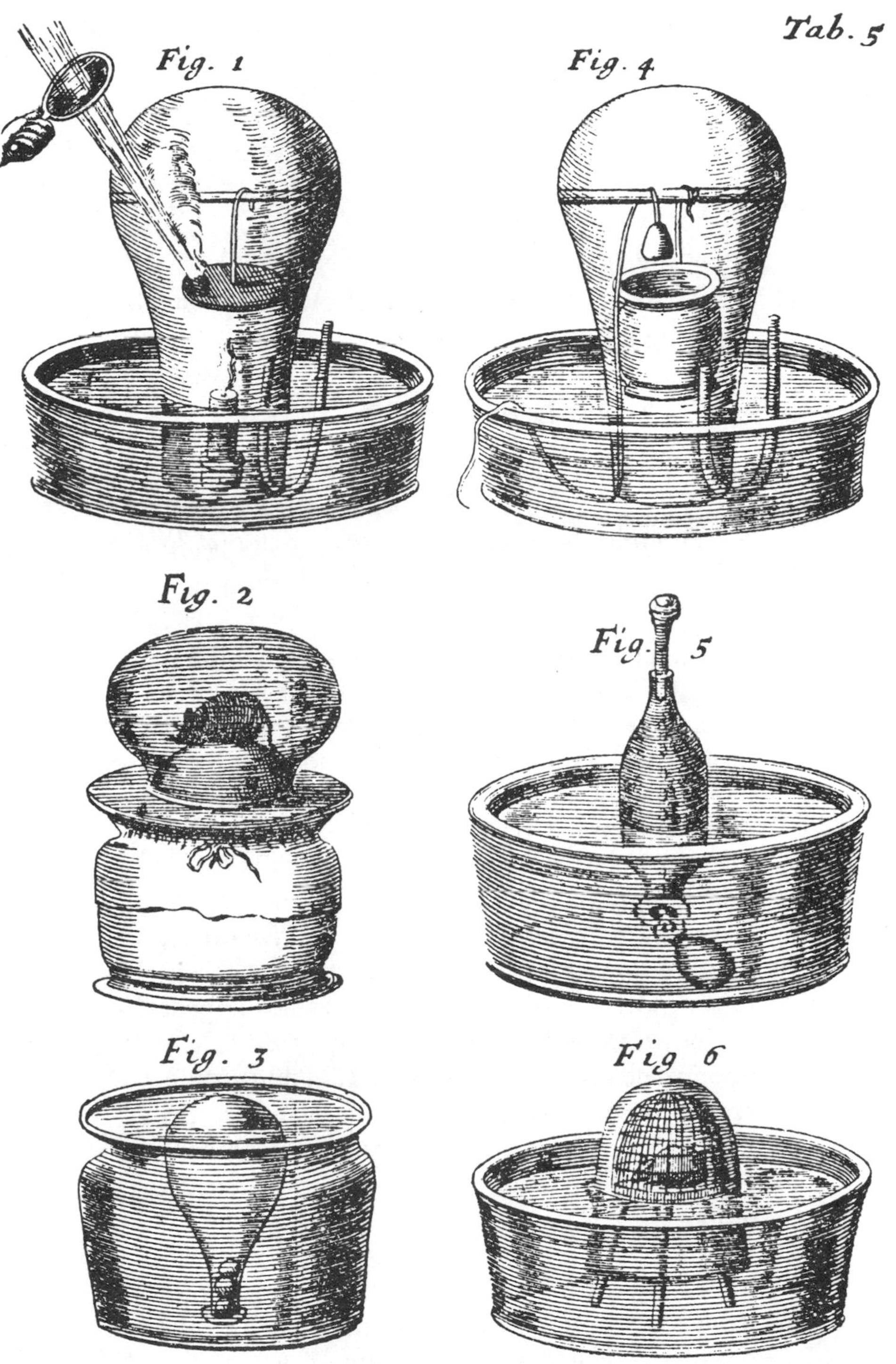

Figures showing lighting a candle in an air-filled inverted glass (Fig. 1), and a mouse in a similar air-filled container (Figs. 2 and 6).

4

Reprinted from *Experiments and Observations on Different Kinds of Air* by Joseph Priestley, Vol. 2. J. Johnson, London, 1775, pp. 29–31, 43–44, 46, 99–102

EXPERIMENTS AND OBSERVATIONS ON DIFFERENT KINDS OF AIR

Joseph Priestley

SECTION III.

Of DEPHLOGISTICATED *Air, and of the conſtitution of the Atmoſphere,*

The contents of this ſection will furniſh a very ſtriking illuſtration of the truth of a remark, which I have more than once made in my philoſophical writings, and which can hardly be too often repeated, as it tends greatly to encourage philoſophical inveſtigations; viz. that more is owing to what we call *chance*, that is, philoſophically ſpeaking, to the obſervation of *events ariſing from unknown cauſes*, than to any proper *deſign*, or pre-conceived *theory* in this buſineſs. This does not appear in the works of thoſe who write *ſynthetically* upon theſe ſubjects; but would, I doubt not, appear very ſtrikingly in thoſe who are the moſt celebrated for their philoſophical acumen, did they write *analytically* and ingenuouſly.

For my own part, I will frankly acknowledge, that, at the commencement of the experiments recited in this ſection, I was ſo far from having formed any hypotheſis that led to the diſcoveries I made in purſuing them, that they would have appeared very improbable to me had I been told of them; and when the decifive facts did at length obtrude themfelves upon my notice, it was very flowly, and with great hefitation, that I yielded to the evidence of my fenfes. And yet, when I re-confider the matter, and compare my laft difcoveries relating to the conftitution of the atmofphere with the firft, I fee the clofeft and the eafieft connexion in the world between them, fo as to wonder that I fhould not have been led immediately from the one to the other. That this was not the cafe, I attribute to the force of prejudice, which, unknown to ourfelves, biaffes not only our *judgments*, properly fo called, but even the perceptions of our fenfes: for we may take a maxim fo ftrongly for granted, that the plaineft evidence of fenfe will not intirely change, and often hardly modify our perfuafions; and the more ingenious a man is, the more effectually he is entangled in his errors; his ingenuity only helping him to deceive himfelf, by evading the force of truth.

There are, I believe, very few maxims in philofophy that have laid firmer hold upon the mind, than that air, meaning atmofpherical air (free from various foreign matters, which were always fuppofed to be diffolved, and intermixed with it) is *a fimple elementary fubftance*, indeftructible, and unalterable, at leaft as much fo as water is fuppofed to be. In the courfe of my inquiries, I was, however, foon fatisfied that atmofpherical air is not an unalterable thing; for that the phlogifton with which it becomes loaded from bodies burning in it, and animals breathing it, and various other chemical proceffes, fo far alters and depraves it, as to render it altogether unfit for inflammation, refpiration, and other purpofes to which it is fubfervient; and I had difcovered that agitation in water, the proceſs of vegetation, and probably other natural proceſſes, by taking out the ſuperfluous phlogiſton, reſtore it to its original purity. But I own I had no idea of the poſſibility of going any farther in this way, and thereby procuring air purer than the beſt common air. I might, indeed, have naturally imagined that ſuch would be air that ſhould contain leſs phlogiſton than the air of the atmoſphere; but I had no idea that ſuch a compoſition was poſſible.

[*Editor's Note:* Material omitted at this point.]

I cannot, at this diſtance of time, recollect what it was that I had in view in making this experiment; but I know I had no expectation of the real iſſue of it. Having acquired a conſiderable degree of readineſs in making experiments of this kind, a very ſlight and evaneſcent motive would be ſufficient to induce me to do it. If, however, I had not happened, for ſome other purpoſe, to have had a lighted candle before me, I ſhould probably never have made the trial; and the whole train of my future experiments relating to this kind of air might have been prevented.

[*Editor's Note:* Material omitted at this point.]

On the 8th of this month I procured a mouſe, and put it into a glaſs veſſel, containing two ounce-meaſures of the air from mercurius calcinatus. Had it been common air, a full-grown mouſe, as this was, would have lived in it about a quarter of an hour. In this air, however, my mouſe lived a full half hour; and though it was taken out ſeemingly dead, it appeared to have been only exceedly chilled; for, upon being held to the fire, it preſently revived, and appeared not to have received any harm from the experiment.

By this I was confirmed in my conclufion, that the air extracted from mercurius calcinatus, &c. was, *at leaft*, *as good* as common air; but I did not certainly conclude that it was any *better*; becaufe, though one moufe would live only a quarter of an hour in a given quantity of air, I knew it was not impoffible but that another moufe might have lived in it half an hour; fo little accuracy is there in this method of afcertaining the goodnefs of air.

[*Editor's Note:* Material omitted at this point.]

Being now fully fatisfied that this air, even after the moufe had breathed it half an hour, was much better than common air; and having a quantity of it ftill left, fufficient for the experiment, viz. an ounce-meafure and a half, I put the moufe into it; when I obferved that it feemed to feel no fhock upon being put into it, evident figns of which would have been vifible, if the air had not been very wholefome; but that it remained perfectly at its eafe another full half hour, when I took it out quite lively and vigorous. Meafuring the air the next day, I found it to be reduced from $1\frac{1}{2}$ to $\frac{2}{3}$ of an ounce-meafure. And after this, if I remember well (for in my *regifter* of the day I only find it noted, that it was *confiderably diminifhed* by nitrous air) it was nearly as good as common air. It was evident, indeed, from the moufe having been taken out quite vigorous, that the air could not have been rendered very noxious.

[*Editor's Note:* Material omitted at this point.]

The dipping of a lighted candle into a jar filled with dephlogifticated air is alone a very beautiful experiment. The ftrength and vivacity of the flame is ftriking, and the heat produced by the flame, in thefe circumftances is is alſo remarkably great. But this experiment is more pleaſing, when the air is only little more than twice as good as common air; for when it is highly dephlogiſticated, the candle burns with a crackling noiſe, as if it was full of ſome combuſtible matter.

It may be inferred, from the very great exploſions made in dephlogiſticated air, that, were it poſſible to fire gunpowder in it, leſs than a tenth part of the charge, in all caſes, would ſuffice; the force of an exploſion in this kind of air, far exceeding what might have been expected from the purity of it, as ſhewn in other kinds of trial. But I do not ſee how it is poſſible to make this application of it. I ſhould not, however, think it difficult to confine gunpowder in bladders, with the interſtices of the grains filled with this, inſtead of common air; and ſuch bladders of gunpowder might, perhaps, be uſed in mines, or for blowing up rocks, in digging for metals, &c.

Nothing, however, would be eaſier than to augment the force of fire to a prodigious degree, by blowing it with dephlogiſticated air inſtead of common air. This I have tried, in the preſence of my friend Mr. Magellan, by filling a bladder with it, and puffing it, through a ſmall glaſs-tube, upon a piece of lighted wood: but it would be very eaſy to ſupply a pair of bellows with it from a large reſervoir.

Poſſibly much greater things might be effected by chymiſts, in a variety of reſpects, with the prodigious heat which this air may be the means of affording them. I had no ſooner mentioned the diſcovery of this kind of air to my friend Mr. Michell, than this uſe of it occurred to him. He obſerved that poſſibly *platina* might be melted by means of it.

From the greater ſtrength and vivacity of the flame of a candle, in this pure air, it may be conjectured, that it might be peculiarly ſalutary to the lungs in certain morbid caſes, when the common air would not be ſufficient to carry off the phlogiſtic putrid effluvium faſt enough. But, perhaps, we may alſo infer from theſe experiments, that though pure dephlogiſticated air might be very uſeful as a *medicine*, it might not be ſo proper for us in the uſual healthy ſtate of the body: for, as a candle burns out much faſter in dephlogiſticated than in common air, ſo we might, as may be ſaid, *live out too faſt*, and the animal powers be too ſoon exhauſted in this pure kind of air. A moraliſt, at leaſt, may ſay, that the air which nature has provided for us is as good as we deſerve.

My reader will not wonder, that, after having aſcertained the ſuperior goodneſs of dephlogiſticated air by mice living in it, and the other teſts above mentioned, I ſhould have the curioſity to taſte it myſelf. I have gratified that curioſity, by breathing it, drawing it through a glaſs-ſyphon, and, by this means, I reduced a large jar full of it to the ſtandard of common air. The feeling of it to my lungs was not ſenſibly different from that of common air; but I fancied that my breaſt felt peculiarly light and eaſy for ſome time afterwards. Who can tell but that, in time, this pure air may become a faſhionable article in luxury. Hitherto only two mice and myſelf have had the privilege of breathing it.

[*Editor's Note:* Material omitted at this point.]

5

Carl Wilhelm Scheele's

d. Königl. Schwed. Acad. d. Wissenschaft. Mitgliedes,

Chemische Abhandlung

von der

Luft und dem Feuer.

Nebst einem Vorbericht

von

Torbern Bergman,

Chem. und Pharm. Prof. und Ritter; verschied. Societ. Mitglied.

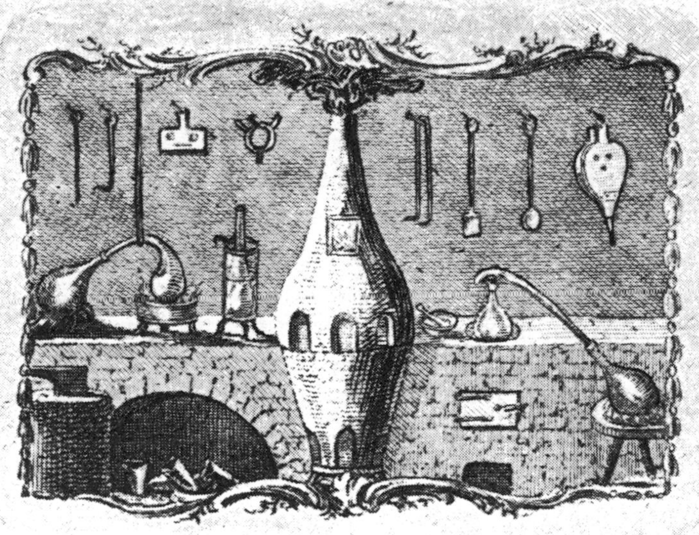

Upsala und Leipzig,

Verlegt von Magn. Swederus, Buchhändler; zu finden bey S. L. Crusius.

1777.

Reprinted from *The Discovery of Oxygen, Part 2, Experiments by Carl Wilhelm Scheele* (1777). E. and S. Livingstone Ltd., for the Alembic Club, Edinburgh, 1952, pp. 5–8

CHEMICAL TREATISE ON AIR AND FIRE.*

1. IT is the object and chief business of chemistry to skilfully separate substances into their constituents, to discover their properties, and to compound them in different ways.

How difficult it is, however, to carry out such operations with the greatest accuracy, can only be unknown to one who either has never undertaken this occupation, or at least has not done so with sufficient attention.

2. Hitherto chemical investigators are not agreed as to how many elements or fundamental materials compose all substances. In fact this is one of the most difficult problems; some indeed hold that there remains no further hope of searching out the elements of substances. Poor comfort for those who feel their greatest pleasure in the investigation of natural things! Far is he mistaken, who endeavours to confine chemistry, this noble science, within such narrow bounds! Others believe that earth and phlogiston are the things from which all material nature has derived its origin. The majority seem completely attached to the peripatetic elements.

3. I must admit that I have bestowed no little trouble upon this matter in order to obtain a clear conception of it. One may reasonably be amazed at the numerous ideas and conjectures which authors have recorded on the subject, especially when they give a decision respecting the fiery phenomenon; and this very matter was

---

* **Carl Wilhelm Scheele's Chemische Abhandlung von der Luft und dem Feuer. Upsala und Leipzig, 1777.**

[*Editor's Note:* The title page is reproduced from *The Collected Papers of Carl Wilhelm Scheele,* L. Dobbin, trans., G. Bell & Sons Ltd., London, 1931.]

of the greatest importance to me. I perceived the necessity of a knowledge of fire, because without this it is not possible to make any experiment; and without fire and heat it is not possible to make use of the action of any solvent. I began accordingly to put aside all explanations of fire; I undertook a multitude of experiments in order to fathom this beautiful phenomenon as fully as possible. I soon found, however, that one could not form any true judgment regarding the phenomena which fire presents, without a knowledge of the air. I saw, after carrying out a series of experiments, that air really enters into the mixture of fire, and with it forms a constituent of flame and of sparks. I learned accordingly that a treatise like this, on fire, could not be drawn up with proper completeness without taking the air also into consideration.

4. Air is that fluid invisible substance which we continually breathe, which surrounds the whole surface of the earth, is very elastic, and possesses weight. It is always filled with an astonishing quantity of all kinds of exhalations, which are so finely subdivided in it that they are scarcely visible even in the sun's rays. Water vapours always have the preponderance amongst these foreign particles. The air, however, is also mixed with another elastic substance resembling air, which differs from it in numerous properties, and is, with good reason, called aerial acid by Professor Bergman. It owes its presence to organised bodies, destroyed by putrefaction or combustion.

5. Nothing has given philosophers more trouble for some years than just this delicate acid or so-called fixed air. Indeed it is not surprising that the conclusions which one draws from the properties of this elastic acid are not favourable to all who are prejudiced by previously conceived opinions. These defenders of the Paracelsian

doctrine believe that the air is in itself unalterable; and, with Hales, that it really unites with substances thereby losing its elasticity; but that it regains its original nature as soon as it is driven out of these by fire or fermentation. But since they see that the air so produced is endowed with properties quite different from common air, they conclude, without experimental proofs, that this air has united with foreign materials, and that it must be purified from these admixed foreign particles by agitation and filtration with various liquids. I believe that there would be no hesitation in accepting this opinion, if one could only demonstrate clearly by experiments that a given quantity of air is capable of being completely converted into fixed or other kind of air by the admixture of foreign materials; but since this has not been done, I hope I do not err if I assume as many kinds of air as experiment reveals to me. For when I have collected an elastic fluid, and observe concerning it that its expansive power is increased by heat and diminished by cold, while it still uniformly retains its elastic fluidity, but also discover in it properties and behaviour different from those of common air, then I consider myself justified in believing that this is a peculiar kind of air. I say that air thus collected must retain its elasticity even in the greatest cold, because otherwise an innumerable multitude of varieties of air would have to be assumed, since it is very probable that all substances can be converted by excessive heat into a vapour resembling air.

6. Substances which are subjected to putrefaction or to destruction by means of fire diminish, and at the same time consume, a part of the air; sometimes it happens that they perceptibly increase the bulk of the air, and sometimes finally that they neither increase nor diminish a given quantity of air—phenomena which are certainly remarkable. Conjectures can here determine nothing

with certainty, at least they can only bring small satisfaction to a chemical philosopher, who must have his proofs in his hands. Who does not see the necessity of making experiments in this case, in order to obtain light concerning this secret of nature?

7. General properties of ordinary air.

(1.) Fire must burn for a certain time in a given quantity of air. (2.) If, so far as can be seen, this fire does not produce during combustion any fluid resembling air, then, after the fire has gone out of itself, the quantity of air must be diminished between a third and a fourth part. (3.) It must not unite with common water. (4.) All kinds of animals must live for a certain time in a confined quantity of air. (5.) Seeds, as for example peas, in a given quantity of similarly confined air, must strike roots and attain a certain height with the aid of some water and of a moderate heat.

Consequently, when I have a fluid resembling air in its external appearance, and find that it has not the properties mentioned, even when only one of them is wanting, I feel convinced that it is not ordinary air.

[*Editor's Note:* Material has been omitted at this point.]

6

Reprinted from *Essays: Physical and Chemical* by Antoine Lavoisier, T. Henry, trans., 1776, Vol. 1, 2nd ed. Frank Cass & Co. Ltd., 1970; pp. 377–379, 416–417

ESSAYS: PHYSICAL AND CHEMICAL

Antoine Lavoisier

CHAPTER IX.

ON THE BURNING OF PHOSPHORUS, AND THE FORMATION OF ITS ACID.

EXPERIMENT I.

THE BURNING OF PHOSPHORUS UNDER A RECEIVER INVERTED IN WATER.

EIGHT grains of Kunkel's phoſphorus were placed on a little agate cup which was put under a glaſs receiver inverted in water, and a thin covering of oil was introduced to the ſurface of the water by means of a crooked funnel: this apparatus is the ſame as that repreſented fig. 8. I then threw upon the phoſphorus the focus of a glaſs lens of eight inches diameter.

THE phoſphorus was ſoon fuſed, and then

kindled, yielding a beautiful flame; at the ſame time a great quantity of white vapours aroſe, which ſettled on the internal ſurface of the receiver and tarniſhed it. Theſe vapours afterwards ran in ***deliquium***, and formed drops of clear limpid liquor. At firſt, the water in the receiver rather fell, from the rarefaction occaſioned by the heat; but it preſently began to reaſcend ſenſibly, even during the burning, and when the veſſels were grown cold it ſettled at one inch five lines above its firſt level.

THE internal diameter of this receiver was $4\frac{2}{10}$ inches; and conſequently the abſorption of air had been $19\frac{2}{3}$ inches. Having taken the cup from under the receiver, a yellow matter was found at the bottom which was nothing but the phoſphorus half decompoſed; I waſhed and dried it, after which it weighed between one and two grains, and therefore there had been only, in reality, between ſix and ſeven grains of phoſphorus burnt, and the abſorption of air had been about three inches for every grain of phoſphorus.

THE part of the receiver above the water contained about 109 cubic inches. The abſorption, then, of air was $\frac{2}{11}$, or, what is the ſame thing, between a fifth and ſixth of the whole quantity of air contained under the receiver.

[*Editor's Note:* Material has been omitted at this point.]

Number I—A Memoir: On the Nature of the Principle Which Is Combined with Metals During Their Calcination, and Occasions an Increase in Their Weight

Read before the Royal Academy, April 26th, 1775, by Antoine Lavoisier

[*Editor's Note:* Material has been omitted at this point.]

HAVING thus fixed the firſt reſults, nothing now remained, but to ſubmit the ſeventy-eight cubic inches of air which I had obtained to all the trials proper for determining its nature, and I diſcovered with much ſurprize, 1ſt. that it was not capable of combination with water by agitation; 2dly. that it did not precipitate lime-water; 3dly. that it did not unite with fixed or volatile alkalis; 4thly. that it did not, at all, diminiſh their cauſtic quality; 5thly. that it would ſerve again for the calcination of metals; 6thly. that it was diminiſhed like common air, by addition of one-third of nitrous air; laſtly, that it had none of the properties of fixed air: far from being fatal, like it, to animals, it ſeemed, on the contrary, more proper for the purpoſes of reſpiration; candles and burning bodies were not only *not* extinguiſhed by it, but burned with an enlarged flame in a very remarkable manner; the light they gave was much greater and clearer than in common air. All theſe circumſtances fully convinced me that this air was not only common air, but that it was even more reſpirable, more combuſtible, and conſequently more pure even than the air in which we live.

7

Reprinted from *The Physical Treatises of Pascal; The Equilibrium of Liquids and the Weight of the Mass of the Air* (1663), I. H. B. Spiers and A. G. H. Spiers, trans. Columbia University Press, New York, 1937, pp. 163–166

TORRICELLI'S LETTERS ON THE PRESSURE OF THE ATMOSPHERE

Translated from the text of Loria and Vassura[1] by Vincenzo Cioffari.

---

1. Letter of Torricelli to Michelangelo Ricci

Florence, June 11, 1644.

MY MOST illustrious Sir and most cherished Master: Several weeks ago I sent some demonstrations of mine on the area of the cycloid to Signor Antonio Nardi, entreating him to send them directly to you or to Signor Magiotti after he had seen them. I have already intimated to you that a certain physical experiment was being performed on the vacuum; not simply to produce a vacuum, but to make an instrument which would show the changes in the air, which is at times heavier and thicker and at times lighter and more rarefied. Many have said that a vacuum cannot be produced,

[1] Gino Loria e Giuseppe Vassura: *Opere di Evangelista Torricelli* (Faenza, 1919), III, 186 *seq.*

others that it can be produced, but with repugnance on the part of Nature and with difficulty; so far, I know of no one who has said that it can be produced without effort and without resistance on the part of Nature. I reasoned in this way: if I were to find a plainly apparent cause for the resistance which is felt when one needs to produce a vacuum, it seems to me that it would be vain to try to attribute that action, which patently derives from some other cause, to the vacuum; indeed, I find that by making certain very easy calculations, the cause I have proposed (which is the weight of the air) should in itself have a greater effect than it does in the attempt to produce a vacuum. I say this because some Philosopher, seeing that he could not avoid the admission that the weight of the air causes the resistance which is felt in producing a vacuum, did not say that he admitted the effect of the weight of the air, but persisted in asserting that Nature also contributes at least to the abhorrence of a vacuum. We live submerged at the bottom of an ocean of the element air, which by unquestioned experiments is known to have weight,[2] and so much, indeed, that near the surface of the earth where it is most dense, it weighs [volume for volume] about the four-hundredth part of the weight of water. Those who have written about twilight, moreover, have observed that the vaporous and visible air rises above us about fifty or fifty-four miles; I do not, however, believe its height is as great as this, since if it were, I could show that the vacuum would have to offer much greater resistance than it does—even though there is in their favor the argument that the weight referred to by Galileo applies to the air in very low places where men and animals live, whereas that on the tops of high mountains begins to be distinctly rare and of much less weight than the four-hundredth part of the weight of water.

We have made many glass vessels like the following marked A and B with necks two cubits.[3] We filled these with quicksilver,

[2] See note, p. 73, n. 5.

[3] *Braccia;* each closely 23 inches. The "vessels" A and B, according to Torricelli, are the parts *above* the "necks" BC, AD, in the figure (p. 165).

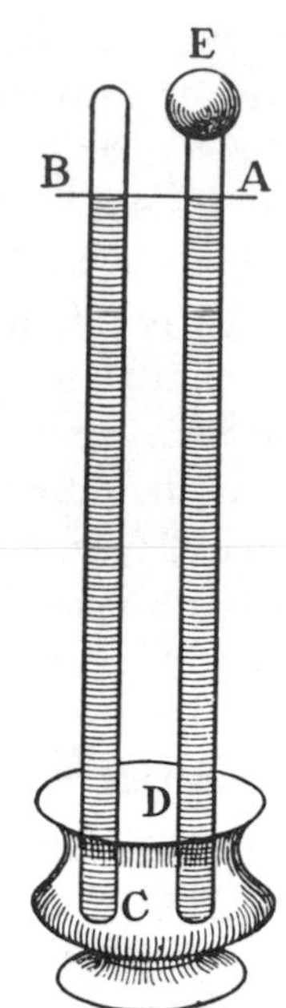

and then, the mouths being stopped with a finger and being inverted in a basin where there was quicksilver C, they seemed to become empty and nothing happened in the vessel that was emptied; the neck AD, therefore, remained always filled to the height of a cubit and a quarter and an inch besides. To show that the vessel was perfectly empty, the underlying basin was filled with water up to D, and as the vessel was slowly raised, when its mouth reached the water, one could see the quicksilver fall from the neck, whereupon with a violent impetus the vessel was filled with water completely to the mark E. This experiment was performed when the vessel AE was empty and the quicksilver, although very heavy, was held up in the neck AD. The force which holds up that quicksilver against its nature to fall down again, has been believed hitherto to be inside of the vessel AE, and to be due either to vacuum or to that material [mercury] highly rarefied; but I maintain that it is external and that the force comes from without. On the surface of the liquid which is in the basin, there gravitates a mass of air fifty miles high; is it therefore to be wondered at if in the glass CE, where the mercury is not attracted nor indeed repelled, since there is nothing there, it enters and rises to such an extent as to come to equilibrium with the weight of this outside air which presses upon it? Water also, in a similar but much longer vessel, will rise up to almost eighteen cubits, that is, as much further than the quicksilver rises as quicksilver is heavier than water, in order to come to equilibrium with the same force, which presses alike the one and the other.

The above conclusion was confirmed by an experiment made at the same time with a vessel A and a tube B, in which the quicksilver always came to rest at the same level, AB. This is an almost certain indication that the force was not within;

because if that were so, the vessel AE would have had greater force, since within it there was more rarefied material to attract the quicksilver, and a material much more powerful than that in the very small space B, on account of its greater rarefaction. I have since tried to consider from this point of view all the kinds of repulsions which are felt in the various effects attributed to vacuum, and thus far I have not encountered anything which does not go [to confirm my opinion]. I know that you will think up many objections, but I also hope that, as you think about them, you will overcome them. I must add that my principal intention—which was to determine with the instrument EC when the air was thicker and heavier and when it was more rarefied and light—has not been fulfilled; for the level AB changes from another cause (which I never would have believed), namely, on account of heat and cold; and changes very appreciably, exactly as if the vase AE were full of air.[4]

37

8

THE

WORKS

OF THE HONOURABLE

ROBERT BOYLE.

In SIX VOLUMES.

To which is prefixed

The LIFE of the AUTHOR.

VOLUME THE FIRST.

A NEW EDITION.

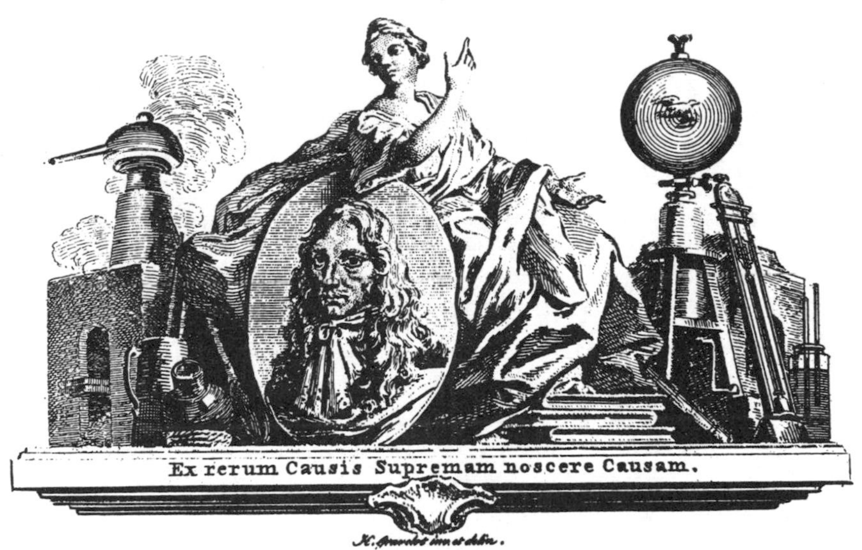

LONDON.

Printed for J. and F. Rivington, L. Davis, W. Johnston, S. Crowder, T. Payne, G. Kearsley, J. Robson, B. White, T. Becket and P. A. De Hondt, T. Davies, T. Cadell, Robinson and Roberts, Richardson and Richardson, J. Knox, W. Woodfall, J. Johnson, and T. Evans. MDCCLXXII.

Reprinted from *The Works of the Honourable Robert Boyle* (1669), Vol. 1. London, 1772, pp. 156, 157–159, 160

A Defence of the Doctrine touching the SPRING *and* WEIGHT *of the* AIR.

CHAP. V.

Two new Experiments touching the meaſure of the force of the ſpring of air compreſſed and dilated.

THE other thing, that I would have conſidered touching our adverſary's hypotheſis is, that it is needleſs. For whereas he denies not, that the air has ſome weight and ſpring, but affirms, that it is very inſufficient to perform ſuch great matters as the counterpoiſing of a mercurial cylinder of 29 inches, as we teach that it may; we ſhall now endeavour to manifeſt by experiments purpoſely made, that the ſpring of the air is capable of doing far more than it is neceſſary for us to aſcribe to it, to ſolve the phænomena of the Torricellian experiment.

WE took then a long glaſs-tube, which, by a dexterous hand and the help of a lamp, was in ſuch a manner crooked at the bottom, that the part turned up was almoſt parallel to the reſt of the tube, and the orifice of this ſhorter leg of the ſiphon (if I may ſo call the whole inſtrument) being hermetically ſealed, the length of it was divided into inches (each of which was ſubdivided into eight parts) by a ſtreight liſt of paper, which containing thoſe diviſions, was carefully paſted all along it. Then putting in as much quickſilver as ſerved to fill the arch or bended part of the ſiphon, that the mercury ſtanding in a level might reach in the one leg to the bottom of the divided paper, and juſt to the ſame height or horizontal line in the other; we took care, by frequently inclining the tube, ſo that the air might freely paſs from one leg into the other by the ſides of the mercury (we took, I ſay, care) that the air at laſt included in the ſhorter cylinder ſhould be of the ſame laxity with the reſt of the air about it. This done, we began to pour quickſilver into the longer leg of the ſiphon, which by its weight preſſing up that in the ſhorter leg, did by degrees ſtreighten the included air: and continuing this pouring in of quickſilver till the air in the ſhorter leg was by condenſation reduced to take up but half the ſpace it poſſeſſed (I ſay, poſſeſſed, not filled) before; we caſt our eyes upon the longer leg of the glaſs, on which was likewiſe paſted a liſt of paper carefully divided into inches and parts, and we obſerved, not without delight and ſatisfaction, that the quickſilver in that longer part of the tube was 29 inches higher than the other. Now that this obſervation does both very well agree with and confirm our hypotheſis, will be eaſily diſcerned by him, that takes notice what we teach; and Monſieur *Paſchal* and our Engliſh friend's experiments prove, that the greater the weight is that leans upon the air, the more forcible is its endeavour of dilatation, and conſequently its power of reſiſtance (as other ſprings are ſtronger when bent by greater weights). For this being conſidered, it will appear to agree rarely-well with the hypotheſis, that as according to it the air in that degree of denſity and correſpondent meaſure of reſiſtance, to which the weight of the incumbent atmoſphere had brought it, was able to counterbalance and refift the preffure of a mercurial cylinder of about 29 inches, as we are taught by the Torricellian experiment; fo here the fame air being brought to a degree of denfity about twice as great as that it had before, obtains a fpring twice as ftrong as formerly. As may appear by its being able to fuftain or refift a cylinder of 29 inches in the longer tube, together with the weight of the atmofpherical cylinder, that leaned upon thofe 29 inches of mercury; and, as we juft now inferred from the Torricellian experiment, was equivalent to them.

[*Editor's Note:* Material has been omitted at this point.]

A table of the condenfation of the air.

A	*A*	*B*	*C*	*D*	*E*
48	12	00	Added to $22\frac{1}{8}$ makes	$29\frac{2}{16}$	$29\frac{2}{16}$
46	$11\frac{1}{2}$	$01\frac{7}{16}$		$30\frac{9}{16}$	$33\frac{6}{16}$
44	11	$02\frac{13}{16}$		$31\frac{15}{16}$	$31\frac{12}{16}$
42	$10\frac{1}{2}$	$04\frac{6}{16}$		$33\frac{8}{16}$	$33\frac{1}{7}$
40	10	$06\frac{3}{16}$		$35\frac{5}{16}$	35- -
38	$9\frac{1}{2}$	$07\frac{14}{16}$		37	$36\frac{15}{19}$
36	9	$10\frac{2}{16}$		$39\frac{5}{16}$	$38\frac{7}{8}$
34	$8\frac{1}{2}$	$12\frac{8}{16}$		$41\frac{10}{16}$	$41\frac{2}{17}$
32	8	$15\frac{1}{16}$		$44\frac{3}{16}$	$43\frac{11}{16}$
30	$7\frac{1}{2}$	$17\frac{15}{16}$		$47\frac{1}{16}$	$46\frac{3}{5}$
28	7	$21\frac{3}{16}$		$50\frac{5}{16}$	50- -
26	$6\frac{1}{2}$	$25\frac{3}{16}$		$54\frac{5}{16}$	$53\frac{10}{13}$
24	6	$29\frac{11}{16}$		$58\frac{13}{16}$	$58\frac{2}{8}$
23	$5\frac{3}{4}$	$32\frac{3}{16}$		$61\frac{5}{16}$	$60\frac{18}{23}$
22	$5\frac{1}{2}$	$34\frac{15}{16}$		$64\frac{1}{16}$	$63\frac{6}{11}$
21	$5\frac{1}{4}$	$37\frac{15}{16}$		$67\frac{1}{16}$	$66\frac{4}{7}$
20	5	$41\frac{9}{16}$		$70\frac{11}{16}$	70- -
19	$4\frac{3}{4}$	45- -		$74\frac{2}{16}$	$73\frac{11}{19}$
18	$4\frac{1}{2}$	$48\frac{12}{16}$		$77\frac{14}{16}$	$77\frac{2}{3}$
17	$4\frac{1}{4}$	$53\frac{11}{16}$		$82\frac{12}{16}$	$82\frac{4}{17}$
16	4	$58\frac{2}{16}$		$87\frac{14}{16}$	$87\frac{3}{8}$
15	$3\frac{3}{4}$	$63\frac{15}{16}$		$93\frac{1}{16}$	$93\frac{1}{5}$
14	$3\frac{1}{2}$	$71\frac{5}{16}$		$100\frac{7}{16}$	$99\frac{6}{7}$
13	$3\frac{1}{4}$	$78\frac{11}{16}$		$107\frac{13}{16}$	$107\frac{7}{13}$
12	3	$88\frac{7}{16}$		$117\frac{9}{16}$	$116\frac{4}{8}$

AA. The number of equal fpaces in the fhorter leg, that contained the fame parcel of air diverfly extended.

B. The height of the mercurial cylinder in the longer leg, that compreffed the air into thofe dimenfions.

C. The height of the mercurial cylinder, that counterbalanced the preffure of the atmofphere.

D. The aggregate of the two laft columns *B* and *C*, exhibiting the preffure fuftained by the included air.

E. What that preffure fhould be according to the hypothefis, that fuppofes the preffures and expanfions to be in reciprocal proportion.

For the better underftanding of this experiment, it may not be amifs to take notice of the following particulars:

1. That the tube being fo tall, that we could not conveniently make ufe of it in a chamber, we were fain to ufe it on a pair of ftairs, which yet were very lightfome, the tube being for prefervation's fake by ftrings fo fufpended, that it did fcarce touch the box prefently to be mentioned.

2. The lower and crooked part of the pipe was placed in a fquare wooden box, of a good largenefs and depth, to prevent the lofs of the quickfilver, that might fall afide in the transfufion from the veffel into the pipe, and to receive the whole quickfilver in cafe the tube fhould break.

3. That we were two to make the obfervation together, the one to take notice at the bottom, how the quickfilver rofe in the fhorter cylinder, and the other to pour in at the top of the longer; it being very hard and troublefome for one man alone to do both accurately.

4. That the quickfilver was poured in but by little and little, according to the direction of him that obferved below; it being far eafier to pour in more, than to take out any, in cafe too much at once had been poured in.

5. THAT at the beginning of the operation, that we might the more truly difcern where the quickfilver refted from time to time, we made ufe of a fmall looking-glafs, held in a convenient pofture to reflect to the eye what we defired to difcern.

6. THAT when the air was fo compreffed, as to be crouded into lefs than a quarter of the fpace it poffeffed before, we tried whether the cold of a linen cloth dipped in water would then condenfe it. And it fometimes feemed a little to fhrink, but not fo manifeftly as that we dare build any thing upon it. We then tried likewife, whether heat would, notwithftanding fo forcible a compreffure, dilate it; and approaching the flame of a candle to that part where the air was pent up, the heat had a more fenfible operation than the cold had before; fo that we fcarce doubted, but that the expanfion of the air would, notwithftanding the weight that oppreft it, have been made confpicuous, if the fear of unfeafonably breaking the glafs had not kept us from increafing the heat.

[*Editor's Note:* Material has been omitted at this point.]

And to let you fee, that we did not (as a little above) inconfiderately mention the weight of the incumbent atmofpherical cylinder as a part of the weight refifted by the imprifoned air, we will here annex, that we took care, when the mercurial cylinder in the longer leg of the pipe was about an hundred inches high, to caufe one to fuck at the open orifice; whereupon (as we expected) the mercury in the tube did notably afcend.

And therefore we fhall render this reafon of it, that the preffure of the incumbent air being in part taken off by its expanding itfelf into the fucker's dilated cheft; the imprifoned air was thereby enabled to dilate itfelf manifeftly, and repel the mercury, that compreft it, till there was an equality of force betwixt the ftrong fpring of that compreft air on the one part, and the tall mercurial cylinder, together with the contiguous dilated air, on the other part.

Now, if to what we have thus delivered concerning the compreffion of the air, we add fome obfervations concerning its fpontaneous expanfion, it will the better appear, how much the phænomena of thefe mercurial experiments depend upon the differing meafures of ftrength to be met with in the air's fpring, according to its various degrees of compreffion and laxity.

[*Editor's Note:* Material has been omitted at this point.]

A table of the rarefaction of the air.

A. The number of equal fpaces at the top of the tube, that contained the fame parcel of air.

B. The height of the mercurial cylinder, that together with the fpring of the included, air counterbalanced the preffure of the atmofphere.

C. The preffure of the atmofphere.

D. The complement of *B* to *C*, exhibiting the preffure fuftained by the included air.

E. What that preffure fhould be, according to the hypothefis.

A	*B*	*C*	*D*	*E*
1	$00\frac{0}{0}$	Subftracted from $29\frac{3}{4}$ leaves	$29\frac{3}{4}$	$29\frac{3}{4}$
$1\frac{1}{2}$	$10\frac{5}{8}$		$19\frac{1}{8}$	$19\frac{5}{6}$
2	$15\frac{3}{8}$		$14\frac{3}{8}$	$14\frac{7}{8}$
3	$20\frac{2}{8}$		$9\frac{4}{8}$	$9\frac{15}{12}$
4	$22\frac{5}{8}$		$7\frac{1}{8}$	$7\frac{7}{16}$
5	$24\frac{1}{8}$		$5\frac{5}{8}$	$5\frac{19}{20}$
6	$24\frac{7}{8}$		$4\frac{7}{8}$	$4\frac{27}{26}$
7	$25\frac{4}{8}$		$4\frac{2}{8}$	$4\frac{1}{4}$
8	$26\frac{0}{0}$		$3\frac{6}{8}$	$3\frac{23}{32}$
9	$26\frac{3}{8}$		$3\frac{3}{8}$	$3\frac{11}{86}$
10	$26\frac{6}{8}$		$3\frac{0}{0}$	$2\frac{39}{40}$
12	$27\frac{1}{8}$		$2\frac{5}{8}$	$2\frac{23}{48}$
14	$27\frac{4}{8}$		$2\frac{2}{8}$	$2\frac{1}{8}$
16	$27\frac{6}{8}$		$2\frac{0}{0}$	$1\frac{55}{64}$
18	$27\frac{7}{8}$		$1\frac{7}{8}$	$1\frac{47}{72}$
20	$28\frac{0}{0}$		$1\frac{6}{8}$	$1\frac{9}{80}$
24	$28\frac{2}{8}$		$1\frac{4}{8}$	$1\frac{23}{96}$
28	$28\frac{3}{8}$		$1\frac{3}{8}$	$1\frac{1}{16}$
32	$28\frac{4}{8}$		$1\frac{2}{8}$	$0\frac{119}{128}$

[*Editor's Note:* Material has been omitted at this point.]

9

Reprinted from *Abstracts Philos. Trans. R. Soc. Lond.*, **1**, 103–104 (1800–1814)

EXPERIMENTS ON THE QUANTITY OF GASES ABSORBED BY WATER, AT DIFFERENT TEMPERATURES, AND UNDER DIFFERENT PRESSURES

(Read December 23, 1802)

William Henry

After a short recapitulation of what has of late been done by Mr. Cavendish, Dr. Priestley, Dr. Nooth, and others, respecting the impregnation of water with different gases, our author observes, that the circumstance of the different degrees of temperature and pressure had not been as yet sufficiently attended to. Dr. Priestley, indeed, had long since remarked, that, in an exhausted receiver, Pyrmont water will actually boil at a common temperature, by the copious discharge of its air; and that hence it is very probable, that by means of a condensing engine, water might be much more highly impregnated with the virtues of the Pyrmont spring: but this conjecture remained as yet to be proved by experiments; and this is the task our author has undertaken in the present paper.

This paper consists of two sections; the first treating of the quantities of gases absorbed by water under the usual pressure of the atmosphere; and the second, of the influence of pressure in promoting the absorption of gases. The apparatus contrived for these experiments may be described as a siphon, of which one side, or leg, is a glass vessel of comparatively a considerable diameter, and the other a long glass tube of about a quarter of an inch bore; the junction of these two parts at the bottom being a short pipe of India rubber, well secured by proper integuments of leather, thus forming a joint, which admits of the vessel being briskly agitated. This vessel has a stop-cock both at top and bottom, in order to insert and emit fluids and gases; and both the vessel and tube are accurately graduated. It may now be understood, that a known quantity of water and of a certain gas being put in the vessel, and the tube being filled to a certain extent with mercury, the absorption of the gas will be accurately measured by the column of mercury in the tube. Those who are particularly interested in this inquiry will find in the paper various precautions and additional contrivances, all tending to insure the success and accuracy of the investigation.

The first experiments were made on the absorption of carbonic acid gas by water: and here a singular disagreement was observed in the first trials made under exactly the same circumstances. It soon occurred that this might be owing to the variable amount of the residua of the gas, after the absorption; and this was actually confirmed by the observation, that, of a greater quantity of gas, more would be absorbed than of a smaller, though both quantities were sufficient for saturation of equal quantities of water. This was found to be owing to the quantity of common air, which will ever be extricated from the water, though it be ever so pure, and which will form a greater proportion of the smaller than of the greater dose of the residuary gas.

A table of nine experiments is next given, in which are entered the temperature, the quantities of water and gas, the quantities of gas absorbed, the residua, and the quantities absorbed by 100 inches of water. The two extreme results are, that, at the temperature of 55°, 13 measures of water, exposed to 32 measures of gas, absorbed 14 measures, leaving a residuum of 18 measures; so that the absorption of 100 measures of water would be 108 measures of gas. In the temperature of 110°, 20 measures of water, exposed to 20 measures of gas, absorbed 9 and left 11; so that 45 in 100 was the total of the absorption.

A series of experiments on other less absorbable gases have afforded for one temperature, viz. 60°, and in 100 cubic inches of water, the following results:—nitrous gas 5 inches, oxygenous gas 2·63, phosphorated hydrogen gas 2·14, azotic gas 1·20, and hydrogen gas 1·08. Some experiments are next described on the quantity of atmospherical air that may be extricated from water; the general result of which is, that 100 cubic inches of common spring water will yield 4·76 of gas; which, being analysed, was found to consist of 3·38 carbonic acid, and 1·38 atmospherical air.

The object of the second section being to ascertain the ratio between the addition of pressure and the increased absorption of gases by water, Mr. Henry made some alteration in his apparatus, which consisted chiefly in lengthening the tube, so that, by the addition of mercury, any required addition of pressure might be obtained on the water and gases.

The results of a series of at least fifty experiments on a variety of gases were, that under equal circumstances of temperature, water takes up, in all cases, the same volume of condensed gas as of gas under ordinary pressure; but that as the spaces occupied by every gas are inversely as the compressing force, it follows that water takes up of gas, condensed by one, two, or three additional atmospheres, a quantity which, ordinarily compressed, would be equal to twice, thrice, &c. the volume absorbed under the common pressure of the atmosphere.

10A

Reprinted from *Manch. Philos. Soc. Mem.*, **1**, 244–245 (1805)

EXPERIMENTAL ENQUIRY *into the* PROPORTION *of the several* GASES *or* ELASTIC FLUIDS, *constituting the* ATMOSPHERE.

By JOHN DALTON.

Read Nov 12, 1802.

IN a former paper which I submitted to this society, " on the constitution of mixed gases," I adopted such proportions of the simple elastic fluids to constitute the atmosphere as were then current, not intending to warrant the accuracy of them all, as stated in the said paper; my principal object in that essay was, to point out the *manner* in which mixed elastic fluids exist together, and to insist upon what I think a very important and fundamental position in the doctrine of such fluids:—namely, that the elastic or repulsive power of each particle is confined to those of its own kind; and consequently the force of such fluid, retained in a given vessel, or gravitating, is the same in a separate as in a mixed state, depending upon its proper density and temperature. This principle accords with all experience, and I have no doubt will soon be perceived and acknowledged by chemists and philosophers in general; and its application will elucidate a variety of facts, which are otherwise involved in obscurity.

[*Editor's Note:* Material has been omitted at this point.]

10B

Reprinted from *Manch. Philos. Soc. Mem.*, **1**, 259–262 (1805)

On the TENDENCY *of* ELASTIC FLUIDS *to* DIFFUSION *through each other.*

By JOHN DALTON.

Read Jan. 28, 1803.

IN an early period of pneumatic chemistry it was discovered that elastic fluids of different specific gravities being once diffused through each other, do not of themselves separate, by long standing, in such manner as that the heaviest is found in the lowest place; but on the contrary, remain in a state of uniform and equal diffusion.

Dr. Priestley has given us a section on this subject (vid. Experiments and Observations. &c. abridged. Vol. 2. page 441) in which he has proved the fact above-mentioned in a satisfactory manner; and every one's experience since, as far as I know, has coincided with his conclusions. He has not offered any conjecture concerning the cause of this deviation from the law observed by inelastic fluids; but he suggests that "if two kinds of air of very "different specific gravities, were put into the "same vessel, with very great care, without "the least agitation that might mix or blend "them together, they might continue separate, "as with the same care *wine* and *water* may "be made to do."

The determination of this point, which seems at first view but a trivial one, is of considerable importance; as from it we may obtain a striking trait, either of the agreement or disagreement of elastic and inelastic fluids in their mutual action on each other.

It is, therefore, the subject of the following experiments to ascertain whether two elastic fluids brought into contact, could intermix with each other, independently of agitation. The result seems to give it in the affirmative beyond a doubt, contrary to the suggestion of Dr. Priestley; and establishes this remarkable fact, *that a lighter elastic fluid cannot* REST *upon a heavier*, as is the case with liquids; but, they are constantly active in diffusing themselves through each other till an equilibrium is effected, and that without any regard to their specific gravity, except so far as it accelerates or retards the effect, according to circumstances.

The only apparatus found necessary was a few phials, and tubes with perforated corks; the tube mostly used was one 10 inches long, and of $\frac{1}{20}$ inch bore; in some cases a tube of 30 inches in length and $\frac{1}{3}$ inch bore was used; the phials held the gases that were subjects of experiment and the tube formed the connection. In all cases, the heavier gas was in the *under* phial, and the two were placed in a perpendicular position, and suffered to remain so during the experiment in a state of rest; thus circumstanced it is evident that the effect of agitation was sufficiently guarded against; for, a tube almost capillary and ten inches long, could not be instrumental in propagating an intermixture from a momentary commotion at the commencement of each Experiment.

FIRST CLASS.

CARBONIC ACID GAS,

with Atmospheric Air, Hydrogenous, Azotic and Nitrous Gases.

1. A pint phial filled with carbonic acid gas, the 30 inch tube and an ounce phial, the tube and small phial being filled with common air, were used at first. In one hour the small phial was removed, and had acquired no sen-

sible quantity of acid gas, as appeared from agitating lime water in it. In three hours it had the acid gas in great plenty, instantly making lime water milky. After this it was repeatedly removed in the space of half an hour, and never failed to exhibit signs of the acid gas. Things remaining just the same, the upper phial was filled with the different gases mentioned above repeatedly, and in half an hour there was always found acid sufficient to make the phial $\frac{1}{2}$ filled with lime water quite milky. There was not any perceptible difference whatever gas was in the upper phial.

[*Editor's Note:* Material has been omitted at this point.]

10C

Reprinted from *Manch. Philos. Soc. Mem.*, **1**, 282–284 (1805)

ON THE

ABSORPTION OF GASES

BY

Water and other Liquids.

By JOHN DALTON.

[*Editor's Note:* In the original, material precedes this excerpt.]

Theory of the Absorption of Gases by Water, &c.

From the facts developed in the preceding articles, the following theory of the absorption of gases by water seems deducible.

1. All gases that enter into water and other liquids by means of pressure, and are wholly disengaged again by the removal of that pressure, are *mechanically* mixed with the liquid, and not *chemically* combined with it.

2. Gases so mixed with water, &c. retain their elasticity or repulsive power amongst their own particles, just the same in the water as out of it, the intervening water having no other influence in this respect than a mere vacuum.

3. Each gas is retained in water by the pressure of gas of its own kind incumbent on its surface abstractedly considered, no other gas with which it may be mixed having any permanent influence in this respect.

4. When water has absorbed its bulk of carbonic acid gas, &c. the gas does not press on the water at all, but presses on the containing vessel just as if no water were in.— When water has absorbed its proper quantity of oxygenous gas, &c. that is, $\frac{1}{27}$ of its bulk, the exterior gas presses on the surface of the water with $\frac{26}{27}$ of its force, and on the internal gas with $\frac{1}{27}$ of its force, which force presses upon the containing vessel and not on the water. With azotic and hydrogenous gas the proportions are $\frac{63}{64}$ and $\frac{1}{64}$ respectively. When water contains no gas, its surface must support the whole pressure of any gas admitted to it, till the gas has, in part, forced its way into the water.

[*Editor's Note:* Material has been omitted at this point.]

11

Reprinted from *Barometric Pressure: Researches in Experimental Physiology* by Paul Bert, 1878, M. A. Hitchcock and F. A. Hitchcock, trans. College Book Company, Columbus, Ohio, 1943, pp. 980–984

BAROMETRIC PRESSURE: RESEARCHES IN EXPERIMENTAL PHYSIOLOGY

Paul Bert

[*Editor's Note:* In the original, material precedes this excerpt.]

Subchapter II

SUMMARY AND PRACTICAL APPLICATIONS

We have given, in our second part, with a superabundance which may perhaps have appeared excessive, the proofs of this truth that diminution in the barometric pressure acts on living beings only by diminishing the tension of the oxygen which they breathe, and if things are carried to the extreme, by asphyxiating them for lack of oxygen. Also that there exists a parallelism to the smallest details between two animals, one of which is subjected in normal air to a progressive diminution of pressure to the point of death, while the other breathes, also to the point of death, under normal pressure, an air that grows weaker and weaker in oxygen. Both will die after having presented the same symptoms; and at different moments of the experiment, at death even, one can observe in both the same proportion between the oxygen tension in the outer air and its proportion in their blood.

All the old theories about the mechanical action of decompression should have disappeared entirely, and it really should be enough to show their folly to recall the experiment in which I went down to the fatal pressure of 248 mm. without the least inconvenience, under the single condition of restoring the oxygen tension to its normal degree by breathing an artificial superoxygenated air.

The question then appears to have been reduced to a remarkable simplicity; but though the cause of the phenomena observed can thus be expressed in a word, its consequences are so diverse that they deserve to be studied in the different conditions in which the diminution of pressure can act.

1. *Aeronauts.*

Let us begin with the simplest case, and let us consider first the aeronaut, who, *without making any effort,* is lifted in the upward course of his balloon.

As he rises and the pressure diminishes, his blood loses its oxygen, as my experiments have shown: a very slight weakening at first, whose existence, nevertheless, my analyses have permitted me to prove as soon as the pressure is not more than 56 centimeters. Even then, the oxygen loss cannot have a very definite immediate effect; the difference is like those one observes between individuals who are in equally good health, like those which changes in respiratory rhythm or the different states of activity or of rest, of digestion or of abstinence bring in the same individual. The aeronaut cannot feel it.

If he rises higher, the loss of oxygen increases: at 2000 meters it was on the average 13%; at 3000, it becomes 21%; at 6500, 43%; at 8600 meters (26 centimeters pressure), the height at which Crocé-Spinelli and Sivel died, they must have lost half of the oxygen of their arterial blood. My animals at 17 centimeters pressure had lost 65%; their arterial blood then contained only 7 volumes instead of 20 per 100 volumes of blood, less than ordinary venous blood coming from a contracted muscle. This is the blood which, in the arteries, was given the task of nourishing and animating the muscles, the spinal cord, the sense organs, the brain! In considering these facts, we recall the celebrated experiment of Bichat, on dark blood injected into the vessels of the nervous centers.

We know that, in a general way, the effects of the rarefaction of the air began to be felt quite plainly about the height of 4000 meters, corresponding to a pressure of 46 cm. It is also at about this pressure that in our bells our animals ceased to move about and showed signs of discomfort. Now the graph of Figure 31 shows that at about this moment the proportion of oxygen in the blood diminishes more rapidly; there is a remarkable agreement here.

This decrease in the quantity of oxygen contained in the blood is the prime factor. From it are derived all the symptoms of decompression. Its cause, we have seen, is double: first, the proportion of oxygen which the blood can absorb grows proportionately less as the pressure lowers (See Part II, chapter II, subchapter V); in the second place, if we suppose that the respiratory rhythm has not changed, the quantity of oxygen which circulates in the lungs during a given time diminishes in the same proportion as the pressure. Now under normal pressure, the arterial blood, we have seen, is never completely saturated with oxygen, the agitation of the blood and the air not taking place with sufficient energy in the lungs.

The deviation must increase greatly when not only the coefficient of the oxygen absorption but also the intra-pulmonary circulation diminishes. Indeed, at a half-atmosphere, for example, to keep the conditions of intra-pulmonary mixing as they were at sea level, everything must be doubled: the respiratory movements must be double in amplitude and frequency; the heart beats must be double in strength and number. That is evidently impossible.

However, there is a tendency in this direction, as the accounts of all the aeronauts give witness, as I have observed in the animals and experienced myself in my apparatuses; at low pressures the respiration quickens, the heart beats are stronger and more rapid, and equilibrium can be nearly reestablished. We have seen, in fact, that if the pulmonary ventilation increases, the arterial blood may gain 3 or 4 volumes of oxygen per 100 volumes of blood.

But this can be only momentary, and such gymnastics cannot long continue without danger of emphysema and cardiac maladies; and so this increase does not last, and when the balloon becomes stationary, this dangerous acceleration does not continue in the aeronauts: the oxygen then decreases fatally in their blood.

Furthermore, when the pressure diminishes still more, the respiratory and circulatory acceleration not being able even for an instant to compensate for the insufficiency of the intra-pulmonary agitation of the air and the blood, the muscles of respiration, like those of the heart, lose their energy and grow weary, since they are receiving a blood that is insufficiently oxygenated, and yet are compelled to carry on continuous labor. The respirations, always numerous during activity, are shallow, so that the quantity of air inspired in a given time is hardly the same *in volume* as at normal pressure; in rest, they fall back to their ordinary number, while remaining very shallow, and it even seems, according to the remark of de Saussure, that one sometimes forgets to breathe. The heart movements give similar results; their frequency increases, it is true, but the cardiac tension drops considerably; in one of the sphygmographic graphs of M. Lortet, taken just as he arrived at the summit of Mont Blanc, it is hard to find indication of the pulse.

And so the organism, conquered in its struggle to compensate for the diminished density of the oxygen in the air by agitation of the air and the blood, returns to the regular routine of its movements, which the poverty of the blood soon weakens. At this time, the seriousness of the phenomena begins to increase rapidly; the blood's insufficient capacity for oxygen is complicated by a greater and greater imperfection in the intra-pulmonary ventilation and circulation caused by the insufficiency of the oxygen absorbed. That is why, as we have seen, the arterial blood of animals under decompression contains even less oxygen than it might absorb at that given pressure.

This rapid decrease in the oxygen content of the blood causes a profound disturbance in metabolism and consequently in the functioning of the organs. We have seen that in animals placed under bells with rarefied air, when the decompression is great enough, the quantity of carbonic acid exhaled and of urea excreted diminishes considerably; the temperature drops also, even when that of the outer air is average. The same thing must certainly happen to aeronauts, when they reach very great heights, where, in addition, the air is generally very cold. I recall that I showed experimentally that in cold air, resistance to decompression is less than at ordinary temperatures.

But under decompressions lower than those which we had to use to show experimentally, that is, roughly, the diminution of the inner workings of metabolism, it is revealed to the observer by the functioning of the organs. But here, as is always the case when we have to do with a cause capable of affecting the whole organism, it is the nervous system which reacts first, which is the first to complain, if I may use this expression. The sensation of fatigue, the weakening of the sense perceptions, the cerebral symptoms, vertigo, sleepiness, hallucinations, buzzing in the ears, dizziness, pricklings, reactions of the pneumogastric and sympathetic nerves, nausea, palpitation, dilation of the arterioles are the signs of insufficient oxygenation of central and peripheral nervous organs. After the nervous system comes the muscular system, which betrays weakness, is seized by convulsive contractions, and by shudders, in which the nervous system also certainly has its part. Finally, in the last stages, come paralysis, syncope, or to speak more exactly, loss of consciousness, and finally death without a last sigh and without convulsions, if the diminution of pressure has not been brought too suddenly to its fatal degree.

[*Editor's Note:* Material has been omitted at this point.]

II
MECHANICAL PROPERTIES OF THE LUNGS AND THORAX

Papers 12 Through 37

ELASTIC PROPERTIES OF LUNGS

12 **HOOKE**
Excerpts from *Lectures De Potentia Restitutiva, or Of Spring*

13 **ARON**
Excerpts from *The Intrapleural Pressure in Living Healthy Man*

14 **WIRZ**
Excerpts from *The Behavior of Pleural Pressure with Breathing and the Causes of Its Variability*

15 **NEERGAARD and WIRZ**
Excerpt from *A Method for Measuring Pulmonary Elasticity in Living Man, Especially in Emphysema*

16 **CHRISTIE**
Excerpt from *The Elastic Properties of the Emphysematous Lung and Their Clinical Significance*

17 **BUYTENDIJK**
Excerpts from *Esophageal Pressure and Lung Elasticity*

18 **DORNHORST and LEATHART**
A Method of Assessing the Mechanical Properties of Lungs and Air-Passages

19 **RAHN et al.**
The Pressure-Volume Diagram of the Thorax and Lung

20 **OTIS et al.**
Mechanics of Breathing in Man

21 **MEAD and WHITTENBERGER**
Excerpts from *Physical Properties of Human Lungs Measured During Spontaneous Respiration*

22 **OTIS et al.**
Mechanical Factors in Distribution of Pulmonary Ventilation

AIRWAY RESISTANCE

23 **POISEUILLE**
Excerpt from *Experimental Studies on the Movement of Fluids Through Tubes of Very Small Diameter*

24 **ROHRER**
Excerpts from *The Resistance to Flow in the Human Air Passages and the Influence of the Irregular Branching of the Bronchial System on the Course of Respiration in Different Regions of the Lungs*

25 **FLEISCH**
Excerpt from *The Pneumotachograph; an Apparatus for Determining the Velocity of Respired Air*

26 **DuBOIS et al.**
A New Method for Measuring Airway Resistance in Man Using a Body Plethysmograph: Values in Normal Subjects and in Patients with Respiratory Disease

27 **DAYMAN**
Excerpts from *Mechanics of Airflow in Health and in Emphysema*

28 **CAMPBELL et al.**
Mechanisms of Airway Obstruction

29 **HYATT et al.**
Relationship Between Maximum Expiratory Flow and Degree of Lung Inflation

SURFACE TENSION: PULMONARY SURFACTANT

30 **LAPLACE**
Excerpt from *Theory of Capillary Action*

31 **NEERGAARD**
New Notions on a Fundamental Principle of Respiratory Mechanics: The Retractile Force of the Lung, Dependent on the Surface Tension in the Alveoli

32 **MACKLIN**
Excerpts from *The Pulmonary Alveolar Mucoid Film and the Pneumonocytes*

33 PATTLE
Properties, Function and Origin of the Alveolar Lining Layer

34 CLEMENTS
Surface Tension of Lung Extracts

35 PATTLE
Excerpts from *Properties, Function, and Origin of the Alveolar Lining Layer*

36 AVERY and MEAD
Surface Properties in Relation to Atelectasis and Hyaline Membrane Disease

37 CLEMENTS
Excerpt from *Surface Phenomena in Relation to Pulmonary Function*

EDITOR'S COMMENTS

ELASTIC PROPERTIES OF LUNGS

In 1668, John Mayow (in *De Respiratione*) summed up what was then believed about the movements of the lungs and thorax by writing

> The lungs are placed in a recess so sacred and hidden that nature would seem to have specially withdrawn this part both from the eyes and from the intellect; for, beyond the wish, it has not as yet been granted to anyone to fit a window to the breast and redeem from darkness the profounder secrets of nature. For of all parts of the body, the lungs alone, as if shrinking from observation, cease from their movements and collapse at once on the first entrance of light and self-revelation. Hence, such an ignorance of respiration and a sort of holy wonder . . . . [*Editor's Note:* This, despite earlier work of Galen, da Vinci, Vesalius, and Borelli, either forgotten or disbelieved.]
>
> Everyone knows that when we inspire, air rushes into the expanded chest and inflates the lungs . . . . Some account for it by a vacuum and an attraction of I know not what imaginary sort.
>
> Others again suppose that the air about the chest, pushed forward by its expansion, propels that which is next it, and this again the next; and that so the propulsion goes on, and thus at last the air near the mouth is driven into the lungs.

Mayow then logically and systematically proved (with knowledge of Torricelli's experiments on the weight of air and Boyle's ongoing studies relating pressure and volume, and with the aid of clever models) that contraction of the diaphragm and inspiratory muscles enlarges the thorax, expands the air in the alveoli and airways, and permits the "superincumbent atmosphere," on account of its pressure and weight, to rush in and press against the lungs from within.

Ten years later, Robert Hooke published *The Theory of Springs* and provided the basis for later (much later) study of the physical properties of the elastic elements in the lungs and thorax (Paper 12).

From then until 1945, F. C. Donders (1849–1853), F. Rohrer (1915–21), and K. von Neergaard and K. Wirz (1923–1929) proposed most of the ideas and techniques used to study the mechanical properties of the lung, but actual measurements were few; Mead (1961) states that between 1896 and 1960 the total number of direct measurements of pleural pressure in healthy man was fewer than 10. E. Aron (1896, reported in 1900; Paper 13) appears to be the first to have inserted a trocar (2-mm diameter) into the pleural space of a healthy man. He states, "I was not brave enough to repeat it too often . . . ." In 36 measurements of pleural pressure (recorded on a kymogram in two subjects), the mean pressure at the peak of inspiration was −4.64 mm Hg and at the peak of expiration −3.02 mm Hg.

Between 1915 and 1921, Rohrer developed the first comprehensive, quantitative treatment of respiratory mechanics, derived in part from his painstaking measurements of the number, length, and diameter of the airways from mouth and nose to alveoli and calculations using aerodynamic principles (see Paper 24). He calculated the pressure required to overcome pulmonary elastic recoil, laminar flow, and turbulent flow, estimated airways resistance, and calculated the work of breathing. Equally important, he stimulated his pupil, Wirz, and his colleague, Neergaard, to provide direct experimental evidence. Wirz (Paper 14) recorded pressure–volume loops in experimental animals and from these, calculated the work of breathing. Neergaard and Wirz (Paper 15) recorded pleural pressure and velocity of air flow at different tidal volumes in man, and measured elastic recoil at points of no flow (at end-inspiration and end-expiration) when flow resistance must be zero.

An important extension of this work came from Christie's analysis (Paper 16) of changes in pleural pressure during respiration in patients with emphysema; in two cases, "ample evidence existed that there had been complete loss of pulmonary elasticity." But needle puncture of the pleura was too risky to use repeatedly or routinely, and a practical method for measuring static and dynamic pressure–volume relationships in man had to await Buytendijk's successful use of the esophageal balloon in 1949 (Paper 17) and the widespread acceptance of esophageal pressure (properly measured) as an index of pleural pressure. In 1952, Dornhorst and Leathart, unaware of Buytendijk's M.D. thesis in Dutch, published their technique for measuring esophageal pressure using a fine polythene tube, without a balloon, attached to a capacitance manometer (Paper 18); although soon supplanted by the esophageal balloon technique, it speeded acceptance of what is now a routine clinical test.

Buytendijk's new technique permitted physiologists and clinicians to gather vast amounts of data on the mechanical properties of lungs and thorax; it changed research in this field from the province of a few to an opportunity for many, and it permitted joining theory with fact in man. However, it is also another example of a very long lag between the initial idea and its clinical application: Luciani used an esophageal balloon to measure intrathoracic pressure in dogs in 1877; Wirz knew of it in 1923 but dismissed the indirect technique as "inadequate."

In the meantime, without benefit of direct measurement of esophageal pressure by puncture or indirect estimation from esophageal pressure, Fenn and his associates were making their classic contributions to measuring the pressure–volume diagram of the lungs and thorax of man (Papers 19 and 20). Fenn had worked with A. V. Hill on length–tension relationships in skeletal muscle and did fundamental studies on the heat of shortening of muscle and the viscoelastic properties of muscle; it was natural that, on request, he should turn his attention to respiratory muscles and to their maximal force during expiration. The request came during World War II, when physiologists became actively involved in problems of aviation physiology, chemical warfare, high pressures, and the like. Most of the work of the great team of W. O. Fenn, H. Rahn, and A. B. Otis was supported by the Wright-Patterson Air Force Base in Dayton, Ohio, because of its interest in pressure breathing. The first paper in their long series starts, "It is remarkable that physiologists have paid so little attention in the past to the mechanics of breathing that no accurate data are now on record concerning the pressure–volume characteristics of the chest and lungs in normal men" (Paper 19). The group decided that the flow of air through tubes should be analyzed from the point of view of an engineer who would require a stress–strain diagram (or, in terms of the measured quantities, a pressure–volume diagram), knowledge of maximal inspiratory and expiratory pressures, and calculation of the work of breathing and of the optimal frequency and stroke to produce adequate alveolar ventilation with minimal expenditure of energy. This they did. Their studies, coupled with new instruments (the esophageal balloon in 1949 and the body plethysmograph in 1956 to measure thoracic gas volume and airway resistance), provided the stimulus to thorough exploration of the mechanics of breathing in man.

Fenn, writing in 1964, noted that, until Rohrer's own experiments were completed in 1919, Rohrer was unaware of previous data obtained in 1907 by Jacquet and in 1911 by Bernoulli (even though all three worked in Basel); even more ironic, Rohrer's own studies attracted so little attention (they were never referred to in standard textbooks of physiology) that Fenn and his associates in 1946 completed their studies of pressure and volume with no knowledge of *Rohrer's* previous work.

Other important contributions were those of Mead and his associates. Mead's classic paper (1961) deserves to be read in full. It is too long (50 pages) to be reproduced in full and too important to be excerpted. Included here (Paper 21) is an important technical advance by Mead and Whittenberger that by electrical subtraction of lung compliance, permitted instantaneous measurement of the resistive component of total change in pressure. Paper 22 is an analysis of mechanical factors responsible for uniform and nonuniform distribution of ventilation in terms of time constants (compliance × resistance) of separate pathways in the lungs.

AIRWAY RESISTANCE

The first quantitative approach to measuring resistance to flow through tubes was made by J. L. M. Poiseuille, a French physician and physicist (Paper 23). Poiseuille had made blood pressure easy to measure in 1828 by converting the straight tube into a U-tube and partly filling the two arms with mercury (19 years later Ludwig added a float and pen to one column and a kymograph for recording). Convinced that the then current concept that arterial blood pressure fell linearly from the aortic valves to the veins was incorrect, Poiseuille used his manometer to record blood pressure directly along arteries; he found little decrease from that in a large artery to that in an artery 2 mm in diameter. Because he could not make direct measurements in smaller arteries, he used narrow glass tubes, some as narrow as 0.014 mm. He measured pressure difference, flow, length and radius of tubes, viscosity and temperature of the fluid, and in 1840 formulated Poiseuille's equation. Neglected by physiologists for 80 years, the equation then became widely used by both cardiovascular and pulmonary physiologists interested in streamline flow of blood or gas.

Rohrer (Paper 24) estimated airway resistance by measuring the number, length, and diameter of all the conducting airways in a cadaver (all his work was done on one excised, undistended lung) and then calculating the resistance of airflow through such a system of tubes. He developed the equation $P = K_1(\dot{V}) + K_2(\dot{V})^2$, where P is alveolar pressure in centimeters of water, and $\dot{V}$ is flow of air in liters/s; the first part of the equation deals with streamline flow (bronchi and brochioles), the second part with eddies, turbulent flow, and orifice flow (trachea, larynx, nose).

Fleisch (Paper 25) devised his pneumotachograph in 1925 and it was immediately used by his Swiss colleagues, Rohrer, Wirz, and Neergaard, in their studies of the mechanics of breathing.

In 1927, Neergaard and Wirz, following upon Rohrer's anatomical measurements and calculations, attempted to determine airway resistance to flow using simultaneous measurements of pleural pressure and instantaneous air flow; they made use of Fleisch's pneumotachograph, Poiseuille's law for laminar flow, and Rohrer's equations. They realized the need to know *alveolar* pressure (not *pleural* pressure) and attempted to measure it by momentary occlusion of the airway—to make pressures equal throughout the respiratory tract [the "interruption method" later used by Vuilleumier (1944) and Otis (1948)].

The first acceptable and clinically useful measurements of alveolar pressure were made by DuBois and associates using a whole-body plethysmograph and Boyle's law (Paper 26). Pflüger had attempted to use such a plethysmograph in 1882 to measure lung volume, but without success.

In the 1950s, Botelho and Comroe designed a twin-chambered, walk-in body box; the subject, seated in one closed chamber, breathed in and out through a flow meter from the other. During inspiration, air flow from one chamber lagged behind enlargement of the subject's thorax in the other; change in alveolar pressure could be calculated from the difference at any moment, and by knowing alveolar pressure and flow, airway resistance could be calculated. However, changes in the temperature and humidity of air during a respiratory cycle prevented accurate measurements. One solution, to keep the air at body temperature and saturated with water vapor, is wholly impractical for routine clinical use. DuBois hit upon an ingenious and simple solution—to have the subject pant during the measurement, at volumes considerably less than the dead space of the flow meter—and so confine the temperature and humidity interface to the zone of the flow meter. This led to a rapid and easy way to calculate alveolar pressure and *airway* (not *pulmonary*) resistance.

In the meantime, physiologists were using maximal breathing capacity and then forced expirations to learn why patients with disorders of the alveoli and airways had difficulties during forced expiration. Dayman (Paper 27) was the first to state clearly that "the operation of an expiratory check valve mechanism is subject to the interrelated factors of lung tension, pulmonary pressure, rate of airflow and intrinsic disease of the airways, in such a way as to minimize the obstruction in health and render it virtually absolute in certain forms of emphysema." Campbell, Martin, and Riley (Paper 28) analyzed in greater detail the mechanisms involved, and by equations and schematic diagrams proposed the concept of airway segments critically vulnerable to narrowing and obstruction. Hyatt, Schilder, and Fry (Paper 29) took a major step forward in measuring isovolume pressure–flow curves. Reasoning that airway diameter is a function of lung volume (other things being equal), and that in tests using forced expirations the patient's lung volume changes at every moment during the expiration, they decided to measure maximal flow rates at known lung volumes and known driving pressures. Their work has led to a more precise way of evaluating airway mechanics; it has also led to the currently used flow–volume curves and resistance–volume curves, all of which take into account the lung volume at which measurements are made.

Physiologists have concerned themselves largely with the physical factors that influence air flow and little with the physiological regulation of bronchioles and alveolar ducts. The first major study of the bronchial muscles was by Dixon and Brodie in 1903. In 1929, Macklin reviewed the then modern concept of the airways and urged his readers to apply "a steadily increasing wealth of technical maneuvers" to the study of the airway. That this has at last begun is shown by the neurophysiological studies of the airway by Widdicombe (1964, 1974), studies of alveolar ducts by Nadel et al. (1964), the use by Nadel et al. (1968) of tantalum dust to outline living airways and measure their responses radiologically, and detailed examination of a variety of cell types by transmission and scanning electron microscopy. A limit to the size of this volume prevents reprinting articles in these areas.

SURFACE TENSION, PULMONARY SURFACTANT, AND RESPIRATORY DISTRESS SYNDROME

Until the late 1950s, most pulmonary physiologists believed that recoil of the lung in expiration originated in elastic fibers that had been stretched during inspiration. Then came the awareness that lungs consist of hundreds of millions of alveoli with moist surfaces, and that the surface tension of each tends to make it recoil; if unchecked, surface tension recoil added to elastic recoil could lead to collapse of alveoli. Fortunately, healthy lungs contain an anticollapse factor, a unique surfactant that lowers surface tension to near zero as alveolar volume decreases.

The papers in this section tell of the initial considerations of surface tension by Laplace (1812), the first physiological experiments by Neergaard in 1929, and studies by Macklin, Pattle, Clements, Avery, and Mead in the 1950s that led to the discovery of pulmonary surfactant and of its role in atelectasis of the newborn. Probably the most fascinating chapter in the surfactant story is just unfolding. It is now known that surfactant is synthesized by specific cells of the lungs, that it is present in type II alveolar cells in late fetal life and moves onto alveolar surface before birth, and that its synthesis or release is subject to hormonal regulation. Cell biologists are now busy learning more about the structure and function of each of the cell types that make up the airways, alveoli, and pulmonary vessels.

The Marquis de Laplace, French mathematician and physicist, is usually credited with formulating the equation pressure = 2 × tension/radius, although Tenney has noted that Thomas Young's work (1805) preceded Laplace's (1807). (Laplace does, in fact, mention Young's earlier work.) Laplace published his law in his profound analysis of the solar system, *Mécanique Céleste;* the law is in a supplement to Volume 4 entitled "Théorie de l'Action Capillaire" (see Paper 30).

An American, Nathaniel Bowditch, devoted much of his life to translating Laplace's huge work into English and, more important, to annotating it, explaining it, and correcting errors—this by a man who had no schooling beyond the age of 10 and signed as a clerk on a sailing vessel between the ages of 21 and 31. Americans also remember Bowditch as the father of a professor of medicine at Harvard and the grandfather of Henry Pickering Bowditch, who established the first physiological laboratory in the United States and was one of the three founders of the American Physiological Society. John Clements's 1961 Bowditch lecture (Paper 37) honors both Nathaniel and Henry Bowditch.

In 1929, Neergaard (Paper 31) discovered much of what we know about surface phenomena and the lung, but his work was either forgotten or unappreciated until 1953 (six years after his death) when pulmonary surface tension was "rediscovered" and Neergaard's paper was unearthed. Neergaard's classic experiment consisted of measuring the pressure–volume curve of lungs when they were filled with air (and the alveoli had a liquid–air interface) and again when filled with isotonic salt solution (when they did not have this interface). He recognized that unrestrained surface forces could cause alveoli to collapse, and stated his belief that surface tension in alveoli is of vital importance in the expansion or collapse of lungs of newborn animals.

In 1954, Macklin (Paper 32) suggested that granular pneumonocytes manufacture a mucoid film that covers the alveolar surfaces and may be responsible for maintaining constant surface tension; he also suggested it may be causally related to myelin figures seen to emerge from alveolar walls in sections of fresh lungs mounted in water. That same year, Radford (1954) calculated the surface area of the lungs available for gas exchange from elastic energy stored in the lungs and alveolar surface tension. His calculated area, 5–10 m^2, was one tenth that estimated by others from histologic methods; Radford stated, "None of the assumptions on which the surface energy method depends could account for this difference unless the lung surface were a semisolid phase or consisted of a highly surface active substance. Neither of these possibilities is at all likely." Radford's analysis was of great importance; it renewed interest in the forgotten subject of surface tension and stimulated Clements (Paper 34) to make his crucial observations that surface tension, high at high lung volumes, decreased to very low values when lung volume decreased, and that this phenomenon was due to a unique surfactant, later found to be synthesized and secreted by alveolar type II cells.

In 1955, Pattle (Papers 33 and 35) observed that pulmonary edema foam is stable, whereas froth from serum is not; he concluded that the surface tension of lung bubbles is zero, and that a layer of some form of mucus, secreted in the depths of the lungs, is the source of the alveolar lining layer. He squeezed bubbles from the inflated lung of a mature fetal rabbit; since these too were stable, he deduced that the layer was present in fetal lung, although it probably matured further during the first few hours after birth.

In 1959, Avery and Mead (Paper 36), using a Clements surface balance, observed that this unique surfactant was present in the lungs of mature newborn babies but deficient in the lungs of very small premature infants and infants dying of hyaline membrane disease.

The march of research outlined here demonstrates the hazards in predicting the direction in which science will advance. Studies on a *biophysical* problem (the elastic recoil of the lung) led on the one hand to learning the cause, diagnosis, and effective treatment of a serious and common disorder of the newborn and, on the other hand, to a surge of interest in the *biochemistry* of the lungs and cell structure and function. A most unlikely course, but true.

ADDITIONAL READING

Bayliss, L. E., and Robertson, G. W. The visco-elastic properties of the lungs. *Q. J. Exp. Physiol.,* **29**:27–47, 1939.

Dean, R. B., and M. B. Visscher. The kinetics of lung ventilation. An evaluation of the viscous and elastic resistance to lung ventilation with particular reference to the effects of turbulence and the therapeutic use of helium. *Am. J. Physiol.,* **134**:450–468, 1941.

Dixon, W. E., and Brodie, T. G. Contributions to the physiology of the lungs: Part I. The bronchial muscles, their innervation, and the action of drugs upon them. *J. Physiol (Lond.),* **29**:97–173, 1903.

Donders, F. C. Beiträge zum Mechanismus der Respiration und Circulation im gesunden und kranken Zustande. *Z. Rat. Med. N. F.,* **3**:287–319, 1853.

Einthoven, W. Ueber die Wirkung der Bronchialmuskeln, nach einer neuen Methode untersucht, und über Asthma nervosum. *Pfluegers Arch.* **51**:367–445, 1892.

Fenn, W. O. A quantitative comparison between the energy liberated and the work performed by the isolated sartorius muscle of the frog. *J. Physiol. (Lond.),* **58**:175–203, 1923.

Hutchinson, J. Thorax. In *Todd's Cyclopedia of Anatomy and Physiology,* **4**(Pt. 2), p. 1016, London, 1849–1852.

Macklin, C. C. The musculature of the bronchi and lungs. *Physiol. Rev.* **9**:1–60, 1929.

Mead, J. Mechanical properties of lungs. *Physiol. Rev.,* **41**:281–330, 1961.

Mead, J., Takishima, T., and Leith, D. Stress distribution in lungs: a model of pulmonary elasticity. *J. Appl. Physiol.,* **28**:596–608, 1970.

Nadel, J. A., Colebatch, H. J. H., and Olsen, C. R. Location and mechanism of airway constriction after barium sulfate microembolism. *J. Appl. Physiol.,* **19**:387–394, 1964.

Nadel, J. A., Wolfe, W. G., and Graf, P. D. Powdered tantalum as a medium for bronchography in canine and human lungs. *Invest. Radiol.,* **3**:229–238, 1968.

Neergaard, K. von, and Wirz, K. Die Messung der Strömungswiderstände in den Atemwegen des Menschen, insbesondere bei Asthma und Emphysem. *Z. Klin. Med.,* **105**:51–82, 1927. (English translation by Rattenborg and Kain in *Cardiopulmonary Facts,* **2**:1–13, Sept. 1961, Instrumentation Assoc., New York.

Otis, A. B., and D. F. Proctor. Measurement of Alveolar Pressure in Human Subjects. Am. J. Physiol., **152**:106, 1948.

Radford, E. P., Jr. Method for estimating respiratory surface area of mammalian lungs from their physical characteristics. *Proc. Soc. Exp. Biol. Med.,* **87**:58–63, 1954.

Vuilleumier, P. Über eine Methode zur Messung des intraalveolären Druckes und der Strömungswiderstände in den Atemwegen des Menschen. Z. Klin. Med., **143**:698, 1944.

Widdicombe, J. G. Respiratory Reflexes. In: *Handbook of Physiology.* Section 3. Respiration. Fenn, W. O., and Rahn, H., Eds. Washington: American Physiological Society, 1964, pp. 585–630.

Widdicombe, J. G. Reflex Control of Breathing. In: *Respiratory Physiology.* Widdicombe, J. G., Ed. London, Butterworths, 1974, pp. 273–301.

12

LECTURES

De Potentia Restitutiva,

OR OF

SPRING

Explaining the Power of Springing Bodies.

To which are added some

COLLECTIONS

Viz.

A Description of Dr. Pappins *Wind-Fountain and Force-Pump.*
Mr. Young's *Observation concerning natural Fountains.*
Some other Considerations concerning that Subject.
Captain Sturmy's *remarks of a Subterraneous Cave and Cistern.*
Mr. G. T. *Observations made on the* Pike *of* Teneriff, 1674.
Some Reflections and Conjectures occasioned thereupon.
A Relation of a late Eruption in the Isle of Palma.

By *ROBERT HOOKE*. S.R.S.

LONDON,
Printed for *John Martyn* Printer to the *Royal Society*, at the Bell in St. *Pauls* Church-Yard, 1678.

Reprinted from *Early Science in Oxford*, Vol. 8, R. T. Gunther, Oxford, 1931, pp. 333–335

Potentia Reſtitutiva,
OR
SPRING.

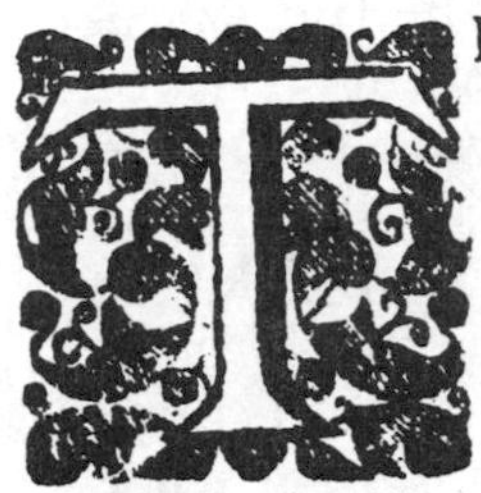

He Theory of Springs, though attempted by divers eminent Mathematicians of this Age has hitherto not been Publiſhed by any. It it now about eighteen years ſince I firſt found it out, but deſigning to apply it to ſome particular uſe, I omitted the publiſhing thereof.

About three years ſince His Majeſty was pleaſed to ſee the Experiment that made out this Theory tried at *White-Hall*, as alſo my Spring Watch.

About two years ſince I printed this Theory in an Anagram at the end of my Book of the Deſcriptions of Helioſcopes, *viz. c e i i i n o s s s t t u u, id eſt, Ut tenſio ſic vis*; That is, The Power of any Spring is in the ſame proportion with the Tenſion thereof: That is, if one power ſtretch or bend it one ſpace, two will bend it two, and three will bend it three, and ſo forward. Now as the Theory is very ſhort, ſo the way of trying it is very eaſie.

Take then a quantity of even-drawn Wire, either Steel, Iron, or Braſs, and coyl it on an even Cylinder into a Helix of what length or number of turns you pleaſe, then turn the ends of the Wire into Loops, by one of which ſuſpend this coyl upon a nail, and by the other ſuſtain the weight that you would have to extend it, and hanging on ſeveral Weights obſerve exactly to what length each of the weights do extend it beyond the length that its own weight doth ſtretch it to, and you ſhall find that if one ounce, or one pound, or one certain weight doth lengthen it one line, or one inch, or one certain length, then two ounces, two pounds, or two weights will extend it two lines, two inches, or two lengths; and three ounces, pounds, or weights, three lines, inches, or lengths; and ſo forwards. And this is the Rule or Law of Nature, upon which all manner of Reſtituent or Springing motion doth proceed, whether it be of Rarefaction, or Extenſion, or Condenſation and Compreſſion.

Or take a Watch Spring, and coyl it into a Spiral, ſo as no part thereof may touch another, then provide a very light wheel of Braſs, or the like, and fix it on an arbor that hath two ſmall Pivots of Steel, upon which Pivot turn the edge of the ſaid Wheel very even and ſmooth, ſo that a ſmall ſilk may be coyled upon it; then put this Wheel into a Frame, ſo that the Wheel may move very freely on its Pivots; faſten the central end of the aforeſaid Spring cloſe to the Pivot hole or center of the frame in which the Arbor of the Wheel doth move, and the other end thereof to the Rim of the Wheel, then coyling a fine limber thread of ſilk upon the edge of the Wheel hang a ſmall light ſcale at the end thereof fit to receive the weight that ſhall be put thereinto; then ſuffering the Wheel to ſtand in its own poſition by a little index faſtned to the frame, and pointing to the Rim of the Wheel, make a mark with Ink, or the like, on that part of the Rim that the Index pointeth at; then put in a drachm weight into the ſcale, and ſuffer the Wheel to ſettle, and make another mark on the Rim where the Index doth point; then add a drachm more, and let the Wheel ſettle again, and note with Ink, as before, the place of the Rim pointed at by the Index; then add a third drachm, and do as before, and ſo a fourth, fifth, ſixth, ſeventh, eighth, &c. ſuffering the Wheel to ſettle, and marking the ſeveral places pointed at by the Index, then examine the

Diſtances of all thoſe marks, and comparing them together you ſhall find that they will all be equal the one to the other, ſo that if a drachm doth move the Wheel ten degrees, two drachms will move it twenty, and three thirty, and four forty, and five fifty, and ſo forwards.

Or take a Wire ſtring of twenty, or thirty, or forty foot long, and faſten the upper part thereof to a nail, and to the other end faſten a Scale to receive the weights: Then with a pair of Compaſſes take the diſtance of the bottom of the ſcale from the ground or floor underneath, and ſet down the ſaid diſtance, then put in weights into the ſaid ſcale in the ſame manner as in the former trials, and meaſure the ſeveral ſtretchings of the ſaid ſtring, and ſet them down. Then compare the ſeveral ſtretchings of the ſaid ſtring, and you will find that they will always bear the ſame proportions one to the other that the weights do that made them.

The ſame will be found, if trial be made, with a piece of dry wood that will bend and return, if one end thereof be fi x; in a horizontal poſture, and to the other end be hanged weights to make it bend downwards.

The manner of trying the ſame thing upon a body of Air, whether it be for the rarefaction or for the compreſſion thereof I did about fourteen years ſince publiſh in my *Micrographia*, and therefore I ſhall not need to add any further deſcription thereof.

Each of theſe ways will be more plainly underſtood by the explanations of the annexed figures.

The firſt whereof doth repreſent by A B the coyl or helix of Wire, C the end of it, by which it is ſuſpended, D the other end thereof, by which a ſmall Scale E is hanged, into which putting Weights as F G H I K L M N, ſingly and ſeparately they being in proportion to one another as 1 2 3 4 5 6 7 8, the Spring will be thereby equally ſtretcht to *o,p,q,r,s,t,u,w.*

[*Editor's Note:* See Figures 1–5, p. 72. Material has been omitted at this point.]

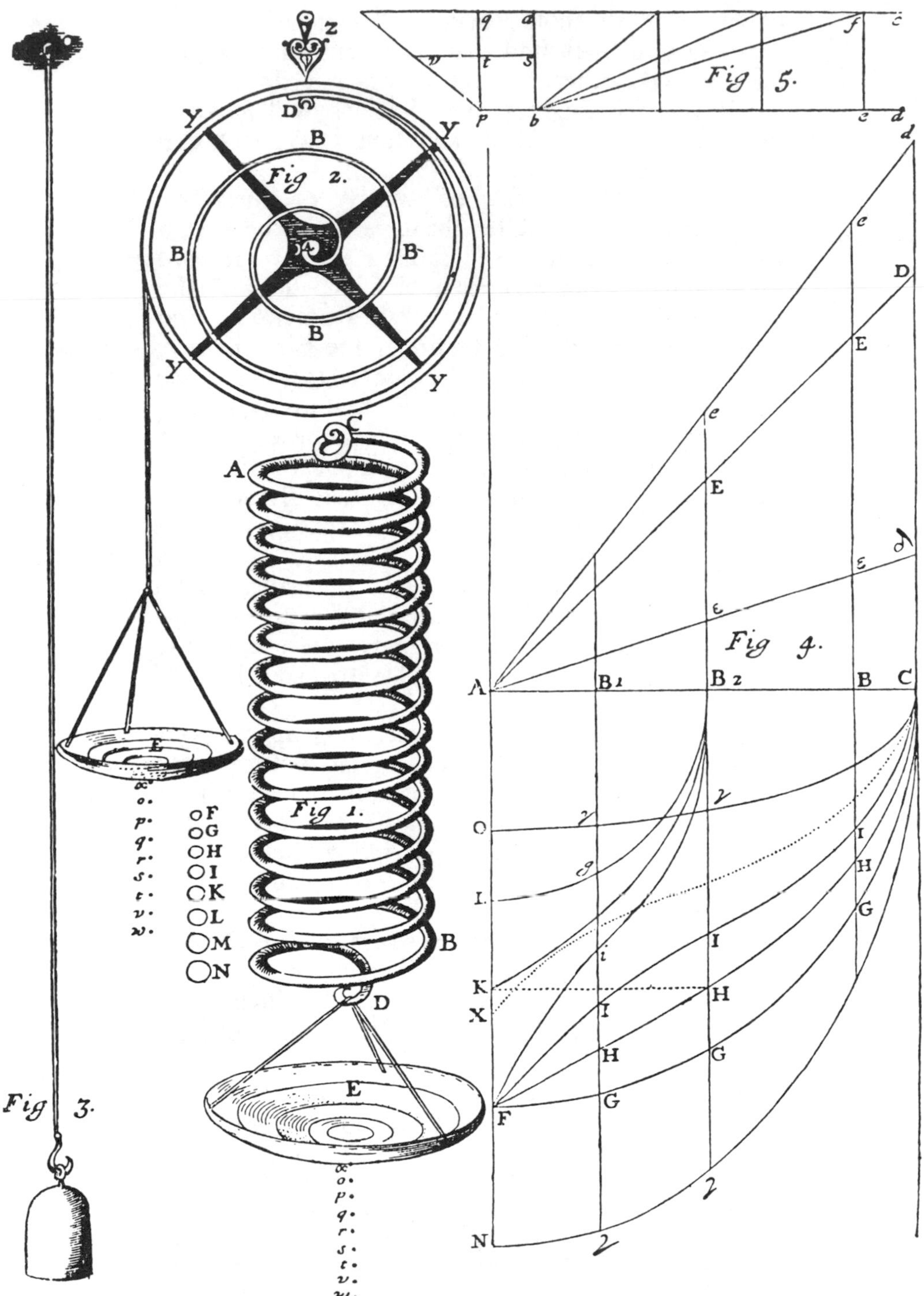
Fig 1.
Fig 2.
Fig 3.
Fig 4.
Fig 5.
A
B
C
D
E
F
G
H
I
K
L
M
N
Y
Z
o
p
q
r
s
t
v
w
O
X
B 1
B 2

13

THE INTRAPLEURAL PRESSURE IN LIVING HEALTHY MAN

E. Aron

These excerpts were prepared expressly for this Benchmark volume by Hans Hahn, North Senior Fellow, Cardiovascular Research Institute, University of California, San Francisco, from "Der Intrapleurale Druck beim lebenden gesunden Menschen," Arch. Pathol. Anat. Physiol. Klin. Med., ***160,*** *228, 230, 231 (1900)*

It is perhaps debatable whether an experiment of this kind on a living, healthy human being is justified. Nevertheless, trusting the reliability of today's asepsis and antisepsis, I decided to risk it as soon as I found a suitable individual, to whom I explained what I had in mind. To remove pain as far as possible and also because pain might alter breathing, I injected 0.02 g of cocaine into the spot where I was going to make the puncture. Then I pushed an airtight, well-sterilized Fräntzel-type trocar of 2 mm diameter into the pleural space in the 6th interspace and in the anterior axillary line. The instrument was tightly connected to a glycerine manometer equipped with a float and marker pen. When the stylet of the trocar was removed, the manometer immediately recorded a negative pressure, and it was easy to record, on a rotating paper strip, a curve showing the pressure changes in the pleural space with breathing.

[*Editor's Note:* Material has been omitted at this point.]

It is self-evident that extreme care must be taken when doing such an experiment and I was not brave enough to repeat it too often.

[*Editor's Note:* Material has been omitted at this point.]

On June 6, 1896, I performed a similar puncture on a 34-year-old, tall (165 cm), healthy, and moderately strong man. His chest circumference was 89 cm on inspiration, 85 cm on expiration, and he had a vital capacity of 3950 cc. The operation was tolerated without any consequences. I followed this man for some time and was unable to find any objective evidence of a harmful consequence of the procedure nor did he have any subjective complaints related to it. As soon as the stylet had been taken out of the trocar and the opening of the cannula had been cleared, the glycerine manometer showed a negative pressure. When we now started our kymograph drum, we obtained a curve which was a faithful representation of the pressure changes that were taking place in this man's right pleural space during breathing.

[*Editor's Note:* Material has been omitted at this point.]

In 36 measurements of pleural pressure, we obtained a mean value of −4.64 mm Hg at the peak of inspiration and −3.02 mm Hg at peak expiration during quiet breathing.

14

THE BEHAVIOR OF PLEURAL PRESSURE WITH BREATHING AND THE CAUSES OF ITS VARIABILITY

Karl Wirz

These excerpts were prepared expressly for this Benchmark volume by Hans Hahn, North Senior Fellow, Cardiovascular Research Institute, University of California, San Francisco, from "Das Verhalten des Druckes im Pleuraraum bei der Atmung und die Ursachen seiner Veränderlichkeit," Pfluegers Arch., ***199,** 47, 52 (1923)*

[*Editor's Note:* In the original, material precedes this excerpt.]

5. Diagrams of Work of Breathing

As mentioned, we recorded diagrams of pleural pressure, tracheal pressure, and the pressure difference between the two against tidal volume, also marking time (see Figure 13).

Experimental conditions were varied as before; thus we obtained diagrams in the following conditions: normal breathing, dyspnea (rebreathing), breathing with increased resistance (both distal and central to tracheal pressure tap), also in combination with rebreathing, and finally vagotomy.

a. *Quantitation* The area of the diagrams gives the work done during a breath (inspiration and expiration), expressed in g/cm, that is, in physical units.

1. The diagram of the pleural pressure represents the total work done by the forces acting on the pleural surface during a breath. As indicated in the introduction, that part of the total work which serves merely to alter lung volume equals zero, because whatever energy has to be put in during one phase of respiration (inspiration) to expand the lung is regained in its entirety in the other phase (expiration). The same holds for mass forces if these play a part during this volume change, except that energy lost through these forces is regained within the same phase of respiration.

Therefore, the major part of the energy loss demonstrated in the pleural pressure diagram is due to flow work, which we can subdivide into a central part, due to flow between alveoli and trachea, and a peripheral part, due to the peripheral flow area (trachea and volume recording setup). Another source of energy loss contained in the diagram is frictional forces, which have to be overcome to alter lung volume and shape.

2. The tracheal pressure diagram represents energy consumption due to flow between trachea and volume-recording apparatus.

3. The differential pressure diagram gives the energy loss due to flow between alveoli and trachea (= flow part) and energy loss in parenchymal tissue (= deformation resistance).

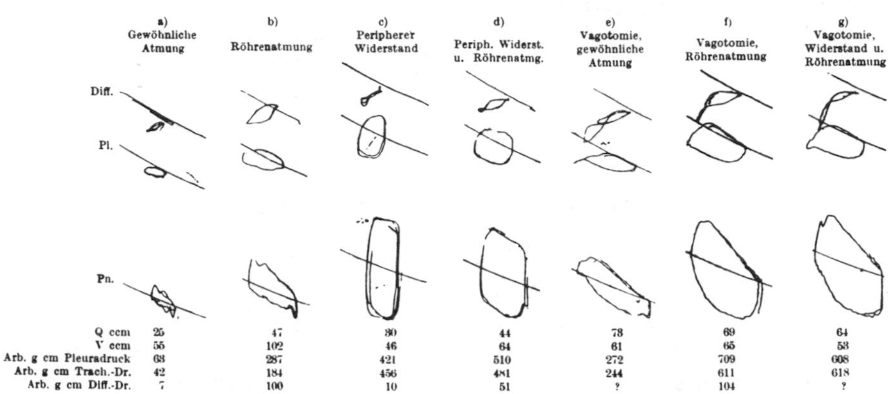

	a)	b)	c)	d)	e)	f)	g)
Q ccm	25	47	80	44	78	69	64
V ccm	55	102	46	64	61	65	53
Arb. g cm Pleuradruck	63	287	421	510	272	709	608
Arb. g cm Trach.-Dr.	42	184	456	481	244	611	618
Arb. g cm Diff.-Dr.	7	100	10	51	?	104	?

Figure 13 Diagram of work of breathing. (a) Normal breathing; (b) Rebreathing; (c) Peripheral resistance; (d) Peripheral resistance during rebreathing; (e) Vagotomy, normal breathing; (f) Vagotomy, rebreathing; (g) Vagotomy, peripheral resistance and rebreathing. Diff., transpleural pressure; Pl., pleural pressure; Pn., lateral tracheal pressure. Qccm, tidal volume in ml; Vccm, flow in ml/sec. Work g/cm, pleural pressure; Work g/cm, tracheal pressure; Work g/cm, transpleural pressure. (Reproduced from *Pfluegers Arch.*, **199,** 52 (1923); copyright © 1923 by Springer-Verlag, Berlin.)

15

A METHOD FOR MEASURING PULMONARY ELASTICITY IN LIVING MAN, ESPECIALLY IN EMPHYSEMA

K. v. Neergaard and K. Wirz

This excerpt was prepared expressly for this Benchmark volume by Hans Hahn, North Senior Fellow, Cardiovascular Research Institute, University of California, San Francisco, *from Über eine Methode zur Messung der Lungenelastizität am lebenden Menschen, insbesondere beim Emphysem,"* Z. Klin. Med., 105, 43 (1927)

[*Editor's Note:* In the original, material precedes this excerpt.]

The patient C. was a 52-year-old man with isolated exudative pulmonary tuberculosis of the right upper lobe, the rest of the lung and pleura being clear on physical and radiological examination. Only in the region of the upper lobe did he have partial adhesions, shown radiologically.

In the course of our measurements we induced a pneumothorax in this patient for therapeutic reasons. The pleural cannula was introduced in the 8th intercostal space in the right posterior axillary line. Measurements were made with the patient sitting, but we waited until his breathing had become calm and steady again after the puncture. Curves were registered before introducing any gas into the pleural space and again after putting in 100, 300, 600, 900, and 1100 ml of gas (the first 100 ml were CO_2, the rest N_2). Simultaneously, we measured pressure with an aperiodic water manometer and an integrating manometer from a side tap that was closed during the photographic recordings.

The special shapes of the dynamic pleural pressure curve and its quantitative aspects will be dealt with in more detail in another publication. In the present paper we will only discuss the static pleural pressure curve (Figure 2).

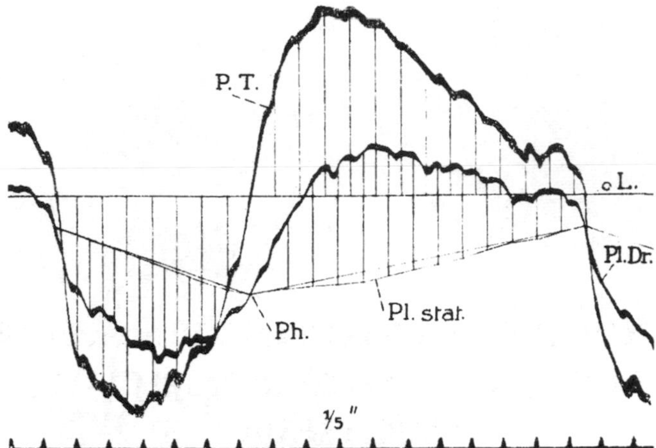

Figure 2 P.T., pneumotachogram; Pl. Dr., pleural pressure; oL., zero line; Pl. stat., static pleural pressure; Ph., phase reversal point. (Reproduced from *Z. Klin. Med.*, 105 (1927); copyright © 1927 by Springer-Verlag, Berlin.)

16

Reprinted from *J. Clin. Invest.*, **13**(2), 295–299 (1934)

THE ELASTIC PROPERTIES OF THE EMPHYSEMATOUS LUNG AND THEIR CLINICAL SIGNIFICANCE[1]

By RONALD V. CHRISTIE

(*From the Department of Medicine, McGill University Clinic, Royal Victoria Hospital, Montreal*)

(Received for publication November 17, 1933)

In spite of much dogmatism in the literature, the etiology of pulmonary emphysema remains largely a matter for conjecture. It is clear that what is apparently true emphysema can be produced experimentally by several simple procedures, but their very simplicity and difference makes for scepticism in ascribing etiological significance to any one factor.

Respiratory resistance has long been suspected to be a factor in the production of emphysema. Although the etiological significance of glass blowing and the playing of wind instruments is not so certain as the text-books perhaps imply (Becker (1911), Tendeloo (1925), Jagić and Spengler (1924), Loeschcke (1928)), there is no doubt that experimental obstruction of the trachea or bronchi can occasion a lesion which is indistinguishable from the variety of emphysema which follows bronchial asthma (Sudsuki (1899), Nissen (1927) and Loeschcke (1928); Kountz, Alexander and Dowell (1929)). The anatomical changes are presumably due to overdistension of the alveoli, from the resistance to expiration, a factor probably of supreme importance in emphysema following bronchial asthma. Over the controversy whether there is atrophy of the elastic fibres or whether they are merely overstretched, it suffices to say that, in this type of emphysema, there is histological evidence of functional impairment of the elastic fibres of the lungs (Eppinger and Schauenstein (1904), Orsós (1907)), and that this impairment is secondary to overstretching of the alveoli. Similarly the loss of elasticity of the pleura and costal cartilages and immobilisation of the chest wall are probably secondary to increase in lung volume, and no clinical improvement follows mobilisation of the chest wall by surgical means (Hofbauer (1925), Nissen (1927)). There are several forms of emphysema which are, however, not preceded by bronchial asthma or any other demonstrable form of bronchial obstruction such as: so-called senile emphysema, emphysema of middle age, which is associated with kyphosis and other changes of the bony thorax (Loeschcke (1911), Tendeloo (1925), Loeschcke (1928), Kountz and Alexander (1933)), emphysema of those acclimatized to high altitudes (Campbell (1928 and 1929), Hofbauer (1925)), and patchy emphysema following heart failure with congestion, lobar pneumonia, pulmonary atelectasis, and pneumothorax. These conditions are not usually associated with obstruction to respiration. Although numerous theories have been advanced, it is difficult to draw any conclusion as to etiology from

[1] Read before the American Society for Clinical Investigation at Washington, D. C., May 8, 1933.

the experimental production of emphysema by acclimatization to high altitudes, by removal of one lung, or by any procedure which lessens the amount of functioning pulmonary tissue. A priori it would seem reasonable to expect a "compensatory emphysema," either where a whole lung or portions of a lung are called upon to hyperventilate for a considerable period of time. This assumption does not bear careful analysis, and, in a subsequent communication, we will give evidence that the etiological factor in these forms of emphysema may well be circulatory rather than respiratory.

There may or may not be an etiological factor common to all types of emphysema but, both from a histological and functional point of view, certain features seem to be invariably present. Without going into controversial details as to the nature of the changes in the alveolar walls, it can be said that the walls are thin, stretched and torn, the respiratory bronchioles enlarged and distorted, and many of the capillaries torn and obliterated. The lungs do not collapse when the thorax is opened at autopsy and their appearance is one suggestive of impairment of their elastic properties. Considerable differences of opinion exist, however, as to whether there is a true loss of elasticity in emphysema. Measurements of the pulmonary elasticity at autopsy have yielded conflicting results in the hands of various observers, and few or no conclusions can be drawn from them (Tendeloo (1925), Loeschcke (1928), Thies (1932)). The significance of postmortem measurements of pulmonary elasticity has already been questioned (Christie and McIntosh (1934)).

During life there is evidence, although mostly indirect, that a loss of pulmonary elasticity exists in emphysema. From the somewhat dubious method of measuring the elastic recoil of the lungs from the intratracheal pressure recorded during complete obstruction to a passive expiration, Rohrer (1916) suggests that there is some such loss. The pleural pressure during respiration may fluctuate around that of the atmosphere (Kountz, Pearson and Koenig (1932), and the same changes have been shown to occur in experimental obstructive emphysema (Nissen and Cokkalis (1925–26), Kountz, Alexander and Dowell (1929)).[2] These changes would naturally follow loss of elasticity but we have been unable to find a quantitative measurement, or even proof of such a loss. The functional significance of impairment of pulmonary elasticity in emphysema seems, indeed, to have been ignored.

METHODS

The measurement of pulmonary elasticity and distensibility involves the simultaneous registration of the intrapleural pressure and of the volume of tidal air (Christie and McIntosh (1934)). *The measurement of the lung volume and its subdivisions* has also been described in a previous communication (Christie (1932)).

Samples of alveolar air were collected by the standard Haldane-Priestley procedure and also, in most cases, by the Henderson-Haggard automatic sampler (1925), modified in the following respects. The capacity of the sampling tube is reduced to 25 cc., so that if from 3 to 5 cc. of air be trapped at the end of each expiration, 20 breaths are sufficient to flush the tube with alveolar air. The

[2] We would not include the cases of v. Neergaard and Wirz (1927), since from the protocols they were evidently asthmatic while the measurements were being made.

pressure fluctuation in the mouthpiece between the inspiratory and expiratory valves is conducted to a recording tambour so that any respiratory irregularities will be revealed. It is obvious that a single shallow breath results in a fallacious alveolar sample. The tambour tracing reveals such irregularities; it has been our custom to accept only those samples the average tidal air of which is over 400 cc. and when 20 regular breaths precede the removal of the sample. The *expired air* is collected in a Douglas bag while the sampler is operating so that, by dividing the volume of expired air by the number of respirations recorded by the tambour, the average *tidal air* can be calculated with considerable accuracy. The calculation of the *dead space* is rendered more accurate, or rather less inaccurate.

In patients who suffer an impairment of respiratory function, we have found the Haldane-Priestley method unsatisfactory and often obviously fallacious. In many cases, and this refers more especially to those of circulatory failure and those conditions such as artificial pneumothorax in which there is a reduction of the reserve air, this modification of the Henderson-Haggard automatic sampler is of definite use. In normal individuals this sampler yields results which are very slightly lower than those obtained by the Haldane-Priestley method (Table I).

TABLE I

The alveolar air of two normal subjects, measured by the automatic sampler and by the Haldane-Priestley method

Case	Automatic sampler					Haldane-Priestley				
	Number of obser-vations	pCO_2			Average respira-tory quotient	Number of obser-vations	pCO_2			Average respira-tory quotient
		Maxi-mum	Mini-mum	Aver-age			Maxi-mum	Mini-mum	Aver-age	
		mm. Hg	*mm. Hg*	*mm. Hg*			*mm. Hg*	*mm. Hg*	*mm. Hg*	
L.O.	16	41.7	37.7	39.1	0.79	22	42.9	36.4	39.7	0.76
W.D.P. . .	7	37.6	43.2	40.3	0.83	5	44.0	39.5	40.9	0.87

In many cases of circulatory failure and in cases of pneumothorax and thoracoplasty (Christie and McIntosh, unpublished data), in which the use of the Haldane-Priestley method is either inaccurate or impossible, this sampler yields results which correspond closely to the gas tension of the arterial blood. In emphysema neither method yields true samples of alveolar air and the use of the sampler is especially unsatisfactory on account of shallow breathing, but gives information on the gas pressure gradient between the alveolar and expired air.

The *arterial blood* is analysed for CO_2 and O_2 content and capacity by the method of Van Slyke (Peters and Van Slyke (1932)), each estimation being done in duplicate. The pH is measured by the colorimetric method of Cullen (Peters and Van Slyke (1932)), each estimation being checked with a sample of plasma of known CO_2 content and tension. The CO_2 tension is calculated from the CO_2 content and pH by the Henderson-Hasselbach equation.

RESULTS

I. Intrapleural pressure

We have shown that, with simultaneous tracings of the volume of the tidal air and of the level of intrapleural pressure, it is possible to measure both the elasticity and distensibility of the lungs. Demonstration shows, at least within the limits of experimental error, that the elasticity of the normal lung is perfect. The bases for this statement are first, that the degree of distension is proportional to the change in intrapleural pressure; second, if distension of the lungs be maintained, the intrapleural pressure remains at a constant level; and, third, there is no "set" when the lungs are allowed to deflate. In emphysematous lungs these criteria are lacking and, in the later stages of emphysema at least, there is evidently almost complete loss of elasticity. The degree of distension is not proportional to the change in intrapleural pressure. This is well illustrated in Figure I where the total increase in lung volume is plotted against the change in intrapleural pressure per 100 cc. volume increase. (Only the negative pressure generated is measured, since, at the beginning of inspiration, the intrapleural pressure is atmospheric.) It has previously been shown that, in healthy lungs, the points fall on a horizontal line, the stress being proportional to the strain (Christie and McIntosh (1934), Figure IV), but in emphysema a logarithmic curve is obtained, characteristic of a non-elastic body in which the same force can produce different degrees of distension, the duration of application of the force being the variant. So long as the intrapleural pressure remains negative, the lungs keep on distending (Figures II, III and IV); when distension is complete, the intrapleural pressure returns to that of the atmosphere (Figure II), (c.f. Christie and McIntosh, 1934, Figures V and VI). It follows that, with respiration, the intrapleural pressure fluctuates around that of the atmosphere (Figures II, III, IV and VIII). Another necessary consequence of complete loss of elasticity is that collapse of a lung due to creating a pneumothorax leads to no change in mean intrapleural pressure. In other words, the pressure still fluctuates around that of the atmosphere (S. H. and I. H., Figures III and IV).

Such a complete analysis of the intrapleural pressure was attempted only in two cases, but in these ample evidence existed that there had been complete loss of pulmonary elasticity. With loss of elasticity, distension of the lungs becomes a function of the duration of application as well as of the magnitude of the force, and the "Distensibility" varies with the depth of the breath. It is clear (Figure I) that with ordinary breathing the distensibility of the lung is much decreased, although with a deep breath it may be actually increased. The significance of decrease in distensibility with normal breathing will be discussed later.

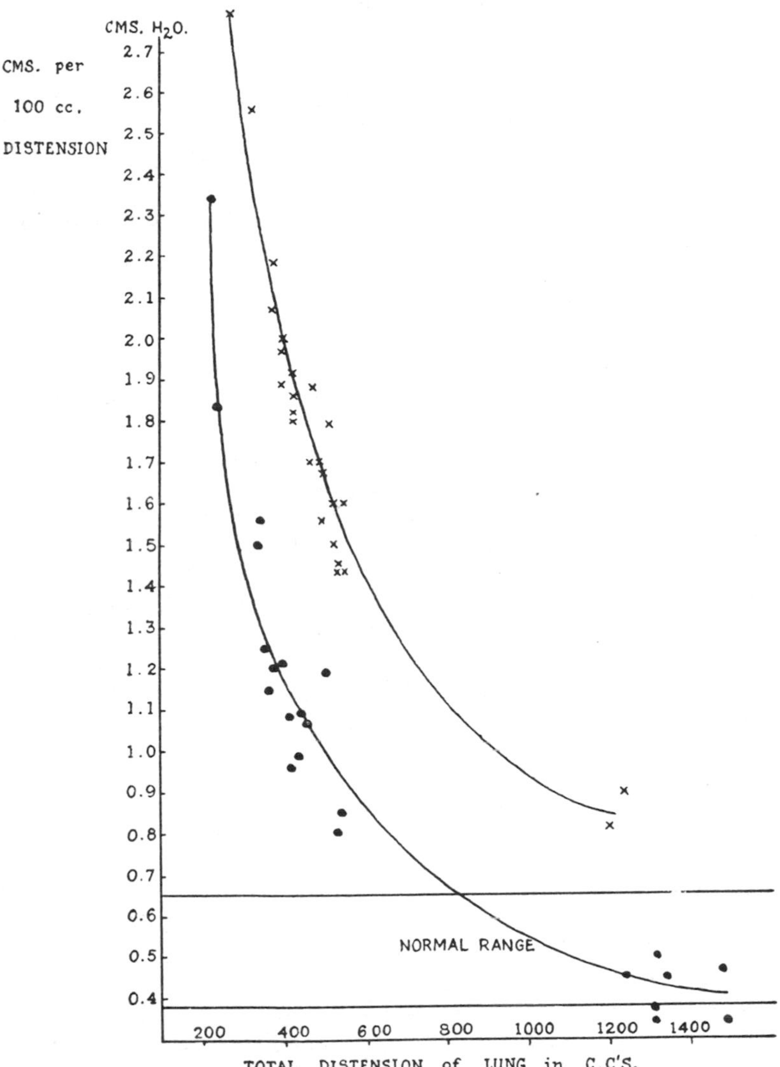

FIGURE I. PULMONARY DISTENSIBILITY IN EMPHYSEMA

Case I. H. Depth of inspiration is plotted against

$$\frac{\text{Total negative pressure change in intrapleural pressure}}{\text{Depth of breath in cc.}} \times 100.$$

Normal range calculated by assuming normal range of coefficient of elasticity between 3.5 and 6.0. Dots represent measurements taken from a right-sided pneumothorax. Crosses are measurements taken before a refill 6 days later. (To compare with normal see Christie and McIntosh (1934), Figure IV.)

[*Editor's Note:* Material has been omitted at this point.]

Bibliography

Becker, E., Führt die funktionelle Beanspruchung der Lungen beim Spielen von Blasinstrumenten zu Emphysem? Beitr. z. klin. d. Tuberk., 1911, **19,** 337.

Campbell, J. A., Concerning the problems of Mount Everest. Lancet, 1928, **2,** 84.

Comparison of the pathological effects of prolonged exposure to carbon monoxide with those produced by very low oxygen pressure. Brit. J. Exper. Path., 1929, **10,** 304.

Christie, R. V., The lung volume and its subdivisions. I. Methods of measurement. J. Clin. Invest., 1932, **11,** 1099.

Christie, R. V., and McIntosh, C. A., The measurement of the intrapleural pressure in man and its significance. J. Clin. Invest., 1934, **13,** 279.

Eppinger, H., and Schauenstein, W., Krankheiten der Lungen. Ergebn. d. allg. Path. u. path. Anat., 1904, **8,** 267.

Henderson, Y., and Haggard, H. W., The circulation and its measurement. Am. J. Physiol., 1925, **73,** 193.

Hofbauer, L., Pathologische Physiologie der Atmung: h) Lungenemphysem. Handb. d. norm. u. path. physiol., 1925, **2,** 399.

Jagić, N., and Spengler, G., Emphysem und Emphysemherz. Springer, Berlin, 1924.

Kountz, W. B., Alexander, H. L., and Dowell, D., Emphysema simulating cardiac decompensation. J. A. M. A., 1929, **93,** 1369.

Kountz, W. B., Pearson, E. F., and Koenig, K. F., Observations on intrapleural pressure and its influence on the relative circulation rate in emphysema. J. Clin. Invest., 1932, **11,** 1281.

Kountz, W. B., and Alexander, H. L., Nonobstructive emphysema. J. A. M. A., 1933, **100,** 551.

Loeschcke, H., Ueber Wechselbeziehungen zwischen Lunge und Thorax bei Emphysem. Deutsche med. Wchnschr., 1911, **37,** 916.

Loeschcke, H., Das Lungenemphysem. Hand. d. spez. path. Anat. u. Histol. Berlin, 1928, **111**/i, 612.

v. Neegaard, K., and Wirz, K., Über eine Methode zur Messung der Lungenelastizität am lebenden Menschen, insbesondere beim Emphysem. Ztschr. f. klin. Med., 1927, **105,** 35.

Nissen, R., Experimentelle Untersuchungen zur Theorie der Entstehung des Lungenemphysems. Deutsche Ztschr. f. Chir., 1927, **200,** 177.

Nissen, R., and Cokkalis, P., Experimentelle Untersuchungen über Mechanische Atmungsstörungen und einige Folgezustände. Deutsche Ztschr. f. Chir., 1925–26, **194,** 50.

Orsós. F., Über das elastische Gerüst der normalen und der emphysematösen Lunge. Beitr. z. path. Anat. u. z. Allg. Path., 1907, **41,** 95.

Peters, J. P., and Van Slyke, D. D., Quantitative Clinical Chemistry. II. Methods. Baltimore, 1932.

Rohrer. F., Der Zusammenhang der Atemkräfte und ihre Abhangigkeit vom Dehnungszustand der Atmungsorgane. Arch. f. d. ges. physiol., 1916, **165,** 419.

Sudsuki, K., Ueber Lungen-Emphysem. Virchow's Arch. f. path. Anat., 1899, **157,** 438.

Tendeloo, N. Ph., Allegemeine Pathologie. J. Springer, Berlin, 1925.

Thies, O., Beiträge zur Atemmechanik auf Grund von Leichenversuchen. II. Untersuchungen über die Retraktionskraft und die sog. Elastizität der Lunge. Virchow's Arch. f. path. Anat., 1932, **284,** 796.

17

ESOPHAGEAL PRESSURE AND LUNG ELASTICITY

Hermanus Johannes Buytendijk

These excerpts were translated by B. Van't Riet, from Oesophagusdruk en Longelasticiteit, *Drukkerij I. Oppenheim N. V., 1949, pp. 13–14, 24–25, 34–37, 48, 55, 126*

[*Editor's Note:* In the original, material precedes this excerpt.]

The static component of the retractive power of the lungs can be measured by pleural pressure measurements at different degrees of expansion of the lungs, and the dynamic component by measurements made at different velocity of volume change. In either case, however, measurement of the pleural pressure is necessary. The importance of pleural pressure and the factors that influence it have been mentioned here briefly; it has also been indicated that measurement of pleural pressure can make possible quantitative detection of pathological changes in these factors. The expectation that this would be possible was the reason for searching for a method that could be carried out without great inconvenience. The most direct method, pleural puncture, should not be used until all possibilities offered by measurement of pressure in the intrathoracic esophagus have been investigated because pressure measurement in the esophagus is a much less traumatic procedure than pleural puncture and so is preferable for routine investigation in patients. That is why this thesis gives a report of investigations done with the purpose of finding a method for measuring the esophageal pressure and of investigating how far this method is capable of recording changes in the retractive force. A number of patients have been examined with this method in whom clinical or pathological changes of the lungs have been proved by different methods or in whom such changes were suspected.

[*Editor's Note:* Material has been omitted at this point.]

Efforts to measure the pressure outside the pleura were made quite early. Luciani and Rosenthal (1878–1880) placed cannulas in the esophagus, and pressure measurements using the same idea were made by Adamkiewicz, Jacobson, Meltzer, Waldenburg, Ewald, Valentin, Cohn, Ganter, Daniélopolu, Langley, Dahmann, and others.

The best investigations carried out with an extrapleural method were published in 1937 by Nordenfelt. In these studies, the subject after a deep inspiration had to bring a mercury manometer to a certain level during expiration. He accomplished this by expiring into a tube connected to the manometer. At the same time, the intraesophageal pressure in a rubber balloon in the esophagus was transferred to a second mercury manometer. The difference between the intrapulmonary pressure and the intraesophageal pressure in mm Hg was called the elastic power of the lungs. The tonus of the esophageal wall was not considered and no measurements of lung volume were made. Furthermore, the mercury manometer method was much too coarse. Nordenfelt observed a difference of 10 mm Hg of pressure with various subjects.

[*Editor's Note:* Material has been omitted at this point.]

OUR OWN EXPERIMENTS

Movements of the Esophagus

Method Balloons have been used to record exactly the movements of the esophagus by registering the pressure variations in the lumen of the esophagus. Before proceeding with experiments in man, the method was first tried in rabbits narcotized with urethane (1 g/kg); the esophagus was exposed in the neck for the insertion of the balloon. These experiments served to define the problem, to accustom us to the apparatus, and also, of importance, to prepare us for the investigations in man. As concerns the study of the motility of the esophagus, the results did not differ from those found in man.

The method used in the test animals and that used in man was based upon a simple principle: a balloon is connected by a catheter and a three-way stopcock with a membrane manometer. To the free arm of the stopcock, a syringe and a water manometer are attached. A picture of this apparatus as used in rabbits is given in Figure 2A. The syringe makes it possible to vary the volume and pressure in the balloon and the manometer to read the pressure variations.

The esophageal balloon (Figure 2B) consists of a small part of a very thin walled rubber tube of 1.5-cm diameter, which is secured around the end of the much narrower catheter (0.5-cm diameter) by means of a short, very thin, copper tube (e). The balloon must be wide in relation to the catheter and must lie around it as a loose sack; otherwise, the rubber wall may be so stretched that the elasticity of the balloon will exert its own influence upon the measurements of esophageal pressure. The connection of the balloon with the catheter must be airtight to prevent leakage. The method of fixing the balloon to the tube with a wire, as used by other investigators, has the disadvantage of requiring the use of wax or glue to make the balloon air-tight; at the location of the knot, there is an irregularity that can cause local irritation of the very

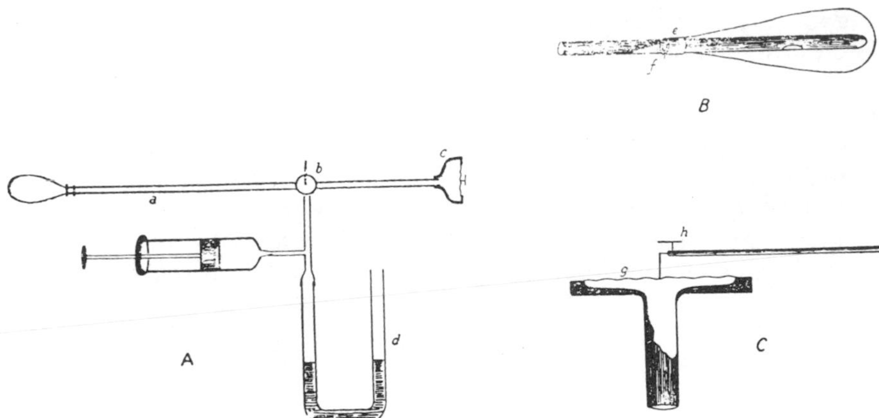

Figure 2 A, apparatus used to record intraesophageal pressure in the rabbit; B, catheter with rubber balloon in place, held by metal ring e; C, copper membrane manometer; a, catheter; b, three-way stopcock; c, membrane manometer; d, water manometer; e, copper ring; f, supporting inner metal tube; g, copper membrane; h, optical recorder. (Reproduced from *Oesophagusdruk en Longeslasticiteit,* by Hermanus Johannes Buytendijk, Drukkerij I, Oppenheim N. V., The Netherlands, 1949, p. 35.)

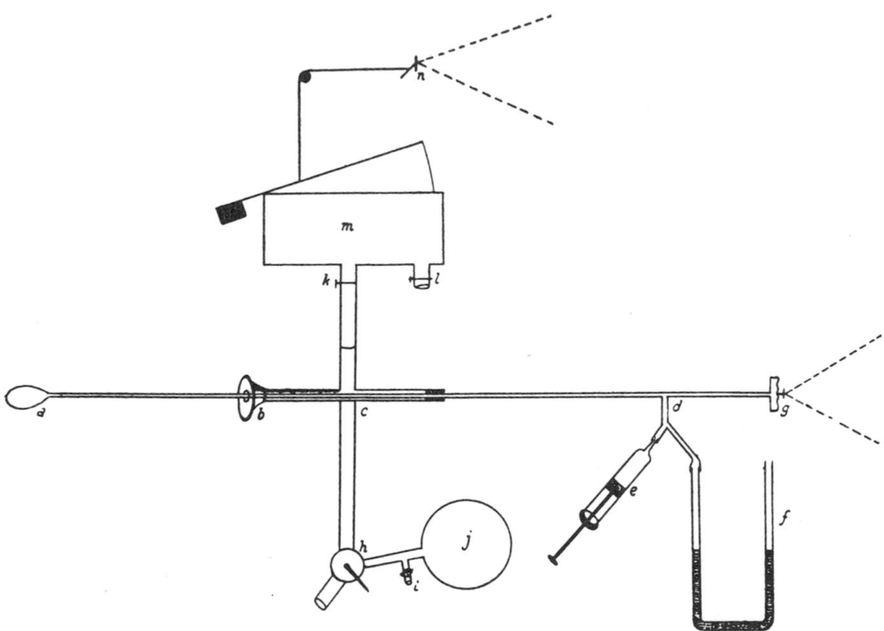

Figure 10 Diagram of the recording method. a, balloon with catheter; b, rubber mouthpiece; c, crosspiece; d, place for clamp; e, syringe; f, water manometer; g, membrane manometer; h, three-way value; i, side tube; j, breathing bag; k, tap; l, filling tube; m, spirometer; n, small mirror of the spirometer. (Reproduced from *Oesophagusdruk en Longelasticiteit,* by Hermanus Johannes Buytendijk, Drukkerij I, Oppenheim, N. V., The Netherlands, 1949, p. 48.)

sensitive esophageal wall. The condom rubber tube of 1.5-cm diameter that was used to make my balloon had to be stretched forcefully to diminish its diameter to one third and so fit the catheter closely. Then a short (0.4 cm), thin copper ringlet, which fits the catheter exactly, was placed around the stretched balloon at a distance of 4.3 cm from the end of the catheter. Because the balloon grows thinner with stretching, the copper tube will automatically fix the rubber against the catheter without causing folds at this spot when it relaxes. Although the seal is perfect then, the copper ringlet is pinched together a bit, but without involving the hazard of narrowing the catheter lumen because a piece of stronger tubing inside the catheter for support. In this manner a smooth, well-covered connection between the catheter and the balloon can be obtained.

The catheter used is a regular urethral catheter (a) of 0.5-cm diameter and of sufficient length to reach the correct spot in the esophagus. At the end of the catheter is placed a smooth side hole, which must not be too large (otherwise the end becomes too flaccid to permit easy insertion). The point of the catheter must be blunt to make it easier for the subject to swallow. The diameter used (0.5 cm) is best suited for this purpose because the tube must have a certain stiffness to be inserted easily and rapidly and so to shorten the disagreeable experience for the subject as much as possible. And the wall must not be too thin or its own elasticity may influence the measurement of the pressure. Wide tubes have the disadvantage of having too great a volume and of being too irritating to the esophageal wall. The usual duodenal tube is too flexible, especially with a balloon attached to it. After some experience with inserting this type of catheter, one almost always succeeds and, if there are no movements, the wall will not be irritated. Furthermore, the volume is small enough to avoid disturbing the measurements.

Besides the balloon and the catheter, the apparatus for the measurement of the pressure is an important part of our equipment. The volume variation, that is, the rise or fall in the manometer per unit of pressure increase or decrease, is the standard for the choice of a pressure recorder. The volume changes should be kept small; otherwise the balloon may be stretched because of its small volume (4 ml), and this may cause variations in tone and influence the recording. For comparable values the volume of the balloon in the esophagus should vary as little as possible during the measurements; for this reason, a water manometer could not be used. And trying rubber membranes with and without carbon-black writers, we changed to the copper membrane manometer illustrated in Figure 2C, with optical registration (h). The wavy membrane (g) has a diameter of 3 cm and is 0.1 mm thick. A deflection of 50 mm for 20-mm water pressure was achieved on the screen by optical magnification. The volume of our manometer amounted to about 350 mm^3 and the maximum volume variation was about 250 mm^3. The deflection of our manometer did not prove to be

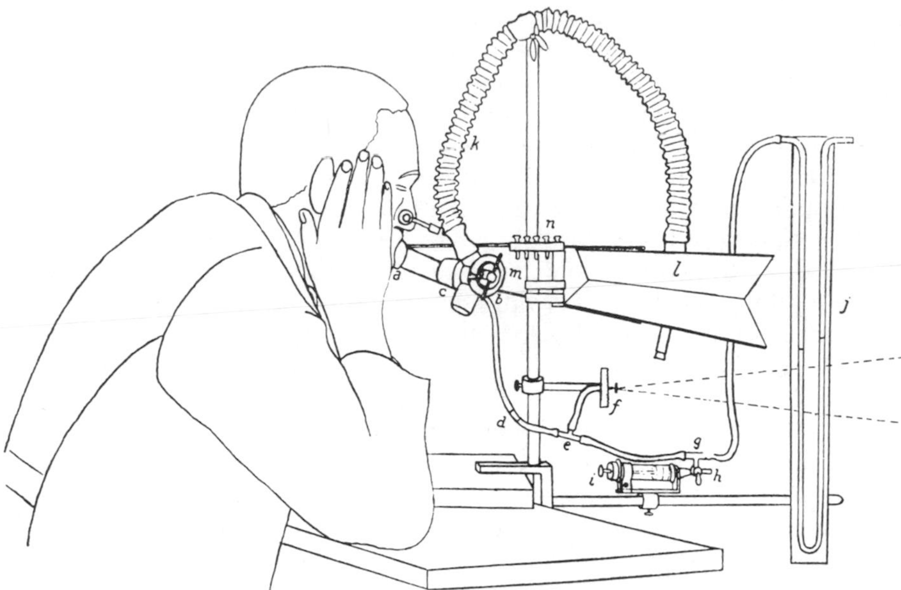

Figure 14 Diagram of the clinical method. a, mouthpiece; b, three-way valve; c, T-piece; d, capillary tube; e, T-tube (small); f, membrane manometer; g, T-tube (small); h, three-way stopcock; i, syringe; j, water manometer; k, rubber accordion tube; l, spirometer; m, switch. (Reproduced from *Oesophagusdruk en Longelasticiteit,* by Hermanus Johannes Buytendijk, Drukkerij I, Oppenheim, N. V., The Netherlands, 1949, p. 55.)

exactly proportional to the pressure, so it was necessary to make a calibration curve; this was done repeatedly because of the possible variation of the distance from the manometer to the screen. This calibration was done with the syringe and the water manometer and, at the same time, before each experiment an excess pressure was created in the system to detect any possible leak. In addition, the volume and pressure in the system can be regulated with the syringe. The balloon is inserted in an empty state and the manometers are closed by a plug. The distance from the teeth must be 35 cm in men and 31 cm in women. The balloon then lies in the lower third of the esophagus. It must not lie in the cervical or middle part because here increases in tonus and contractions occur and are felt subjectively as a "feeling that something sticks." Furthermore, the pulsations of the vessels are important considerations in these areas, and they make good pressure tracings impossible.

[*Editor's Note:* Material has been omitted at this point.]

In summary, examination by the routine method (as described here) is quite possible in the clinic, but it still has to be determined in which groups of patients the measurement of the retractive force will be of greatest value. In particular, the progress of pulmonary surgery, bronchoscopy, and research in pulmonary tuberculosis requires further data on lung physiology. This investigation must, therefore, be considered as one of the many building blocks that still must be contributed in order to erect a structure of investigation of pulmonary function to enable us to obtain a good insight into the functions of human lung tissue.

18

Reprinted from *Lancet,* **2,** 109–111 (1952)

A METHOD OF ASSESSING THE MECHANICAL PROPERTIES OF LUNGS AND AIR-PASSAGES

A. C. DORNHORST — M.D. Lond., M.R.C.P. — READER IN MEDICINE

G. L. LEATHART — M.B. Camb., M.R.C.P. — LECTURER IN MEDICINE

ST. THOMAS'S HOSPITAL MEDICAL SCHOOL, LONDON

THIS paper describes a method of estimating the force needed to ventilate the lungs. When this force is increased, the method helps to define its cause; it also provides an objective test for bronchodilator drugs.

METHOD

Principle

The respiratory muscles have to overcome two types of force: elastic force due to the stretching of the lungs and therefore depending on the depth of inspiration; and viscous force due mainly to the resistance offered by the air-passages to the flow of air and therefore depending on the rate of air movement.

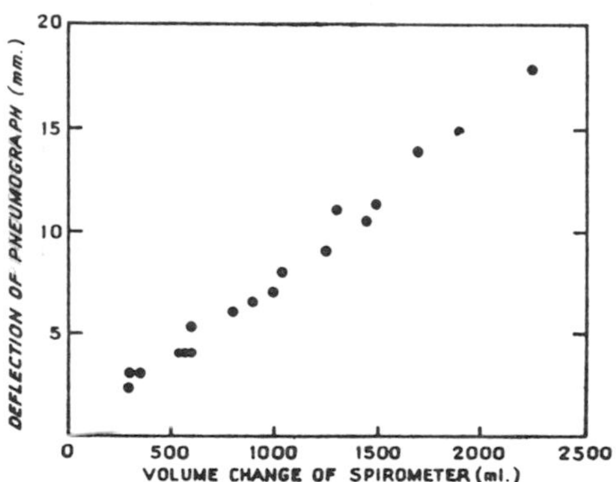

Fig. 1—The approximate linear relationship between expansion of trunk and tidal air measured with a spirometer.

Fibrosis renders the lungs less distensible and increases the first type of force: bronchiolar narrowing, or other impediment to airflow, increases the second. Simultaneous records of the total force applied to the lungs and of the resulting movement allow an assessment of the contributions of the elastic and viscous components. The total force is proportional to the pressure round the lungs—i.e., the intrathoracic pressure. To estimate this we have measured the pressure in the œsophagus. Lung expansion has been estimated from records of increase in the girth of the chest and abdomen.

Procedure

A 'Polythene' tube of about 1 mm. external and 0·5 mm. internal diameter is prepared by cutting two or three lateral holes near one end. This end is passed through the nose into the œsophagus. The free end is attached to a capacitance manometer, and the system is filled with water. The fine plastic tube disturbs the patient less than does a tube of the Ryle type.

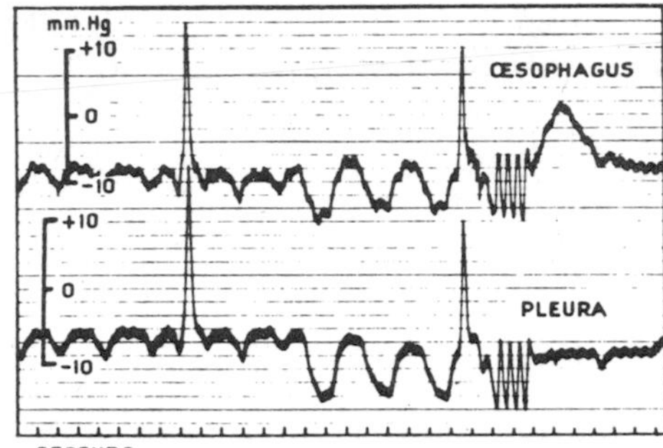

Fig. 2—Dynamic agreement of œsophageal and pleural pressures in a case of spontaneous pneumothorax. The spikes are due to small coughs. At the right of the tracing the œsophageal pressure rises in a characteristic way due to a swallow. Time is marked in seconds.

To record trunk expansion a length of "elephant" tubing is lightly strapped round the chest and another round the abdomen. The two lengths are joined by a Y connection to a second manometer, which records the

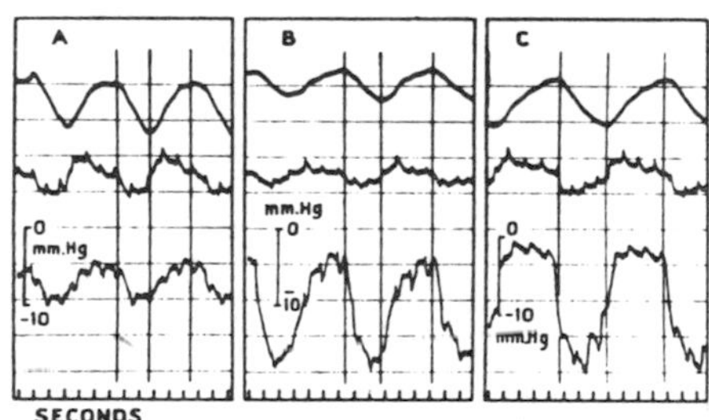

Fig. 3—Pneumograph, pneumotachygraph, and œsophageal pressure from a normal person: A, unimpeded breathing; B, breathing from a closed tank, simulating increased elastic forces; C, breathing through a narrow tube, simulating increased viscous forces. Note different form and timing of enhanced intrathoracic pressure swing in the last two sections.

decrease in pressure produced by stretching the tubing. The output of this manometer may be passed through a circuit that gives the rate of change of expansion as an additional record.

Validation

Fig. 1 shows that the deflection produced by the pneumograph agrees well with the amount of air inspired.

When a person blows (or sucks) against a mercury column, the applied pressure is found to be transmitted to the œsophagus and fully maintained there. Fig. 2 shows that changes in intrapleural pressure are duplicated in the œsophageal.

ILLUSTRATIVE RESULTS

Fig. 3 is from the record of a normal person and shows the differing effects of factitious increases in elastic and viscous forces.

Fig. 4 illustrates the corresponding patterns in pathological states.

Fig. 5 illustrates an unequivocal bronchodilator response to a drug.

DISCUSSION

The method here described relates the pressure applied to the lungs to their consequent movement, and thus defines their mechanical impedance. An increase in this is one factor in the production of dyspnœa. When it is increased, it is of interest whether the viscous or the elastic component is chiefly responsible. An inspection of the records will usually answer this question ; or, if necessary, the magnitude of the components may be estimated by a method due to von Neergaard and Wirz (1927). The analysis depends on the fact that at the end of an inspiration, when there is no air movement, the recorded pressure is due to elastic forces only. By comparing a series of respirations of differing depth it is possible to construct an elastic (depth-pressure) characteristic for the subject. One may then subtract from the observed pressure at any point of a respiratory cycle that part due to lung stretch. What remains must be due to viscous forces and is related to the rate of airflow at that moment. The viscous characteristic may thus be constructed.

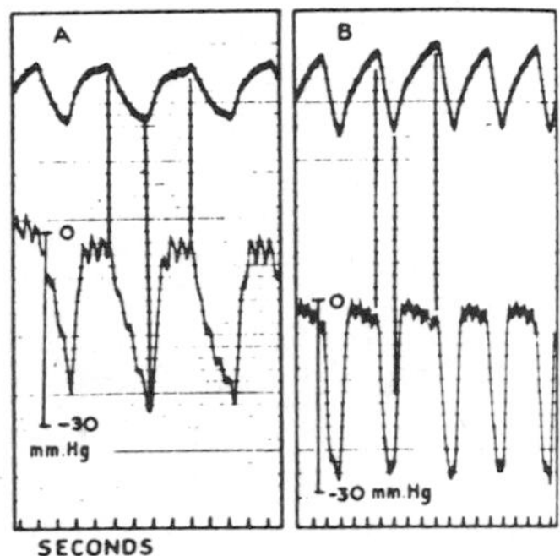

Fig. 4—Pneumograph and intra-œsophageal pressure : A, from a case of pulmonary fibrosis, illustrating increased elastic forces (cf. fig. 3B); B, from a case of severe asthma, illustrating increased viscous forces (cf. fig. 3C).

Previous workers have measured the intrapleural pressure in patients with pneumothorax, but this technique is not generally applicable. We are satisfied that the intra-œsophageal pressure, which can be measured in any patient with very little disturbance, is an adequate substitute.

We have measured trunk expansion, rather than air movement, for greater comfort to the patient and for greater ease of recording. We consider this, and the "pneumotachygraph" obtained by electrical differentiation, adequate for visual analysis, but for the quantitative treatment outlined above a direct record of airflow would be preferred.

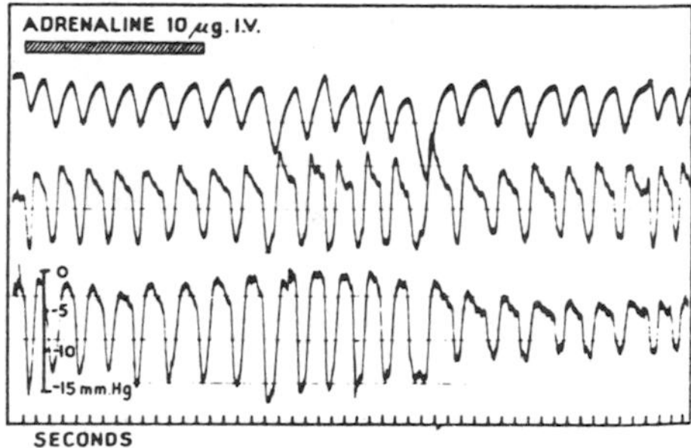

Fig. 5—Pneumograph, pneumotachygraph, and intra-œsophageal pressure in moderate asthma, showing effect of adrenaline. After brief stimulation of respiration adrenaline dilates bronchioles and decreases intrathoracic pressure swing.

When applying the method to the assessment of bronchodilator drugs one selects from the record, before and after treatment, respiratory cycles which agree in their volume patterns. One thus eliminates any action of the drug on respiratory drive ; any change in the pressure pattern may then be attributed to an effect on the bronchioles.

SUMMARY

The pressure in the œsophagus is readily measured, and is a satisfactory index of the general intrathoracic pressure.

By simultaneous measurement of œsophageal pressure and trunk expansion it is possible to estimate and analyse the force needed to expand the lungs.

Some applications are described and illustrated.

REFERENCE

von Neergaard, K., Wirz, K. (1927) *Z. klin. Med.* **105**, 35, 51.

19

Reprinted by permission of the American Physiological Society from *Am. J. Physiol.*, **146**(6), 161–178 (1946)

THE PRESSURE-VOLUME DIAGRAM OF THE THORAX AND LUNG[1]

HERMANN RAHN, ARTHUR B. OTIS, LEIGH E. CHADWICK AND WALLACE O. FENN

From the Department of Physiology, School of Medicine and Dentistry, The University of Rochester, Rochester, N. Y.

Received for publication December 13, 1945

It is remarkable that physiologists have paid so little attention in the past to the mechanics of breathing that no adequate data are now on record concerning the pressure-volume characteristics of the chest and lungs in normal men. The literature contains innumerable investigations of the various fractions of the lung volume and the vital capacity and also a number of observations concerning the positive and negative pressures that can be exerted but these two sets of data have not been correlated. There is little indication of how the vital capacity or other lung volumes vary with pressures nor, conversely, of how the pressures vary with the volume at which they are developed. Likewise there is little information concerning the relaxation pressures at different lung volumes and the relation between these data and the venous pressure. In this paper data are presented concerning the positive and negative pressures which can be produced by voluntary effort, and a diagram which gives a comprehensive picture of all these mechanical factors. Since completing this work we have discovered similar diagrams from papers by Rohrer (1916) and Senner (1921) each based upon measurements on a single individual as well as a partially similar effort by Jacquet (1908) and Bernouilli (1911).

Three types of measurement were used for the pressure-volume diagram of the lung: (1) maximum expiratory and inspiratory pressures at different lung volumes, (2) relaxation pressures at different lung volumes, (3) vital capacities, tidal air, and inspiratory and expiratory reserves at different lung pressures.

METHODS. (1) *Maximum inspiratory and expiratory pressures.* Measurements were made with a recording mercury manometer connected to a one hole rubber stopper cut to fit one nostril. The other nostril was held closed while the subject expired or inspired with maximum force. The nose was used in preference to the mouth in order to avoid all possibility of using the cheeks. It was found to be important to keep the subject from bending over in his effort to

[1] Based on work done under contract recommended by the Committee on Medical Research between the Office of Scientific Research and Development and the University of Rochester.

exert pressure since this gives him added mechanical pressure against the thoracic cage. The pressure was developed slowly in order to avoid overshoot of the mercury and was maintained at the final level for some three seconds in order to give time for oscillations to cease before the reading was taken. This measurement was repeated three times each at different lung volumes which were determined by first exhaling to the maximum possible, then inserting in the mouth a tube to a spirometer and inhaling any desired percentage (Vo) of the vital capacity. Finally without changing the volume of air in the lungs the mouth was closed and the tube was inserted in the nostril for the recording of pressure. The lung volume read from the spirometer was corrected for the decrease resulting from the development of pressure assuming a residual air of 28 per cent of the vital capacity. Correction was made according to the formula

$$Vc = \frac{(B - 47)\,Vo - pR}{B - 47 + p} \qquad \text{(Equation 1)}$$

where Vo and Vc are the uncorrected and corrected expirable volumes respectively in per cent of vital capacity, R is the residual air, and p the extra pressure developed (either positive or negative) by active effort.

(2) *Relaxation pressures.* This measurement was carried out exactly like that described for the maximum and minimum pressures except that after the desired lung volume was obtained the subject relaxed completely with one nostril connected with a water manometer the position of which was read directly. Because the relaxation pressures were so low the corrections for pressure change were omitted as insignificant. Some subjects are unable to keep the glottis open during the measurement of the relaxation pressures and a few others are unable to relax completely especially when negative relaxation pressures are being measured. This may be due to air hunger or to involuntary spasms of the diaphragm. All such subjects were eliminated from our series.

(3) *Vital capacity and lung volumes at different lung pressures.* In this series of experiments the subject was placed either supine or sitting in a body box with the head projecting through an air tight sponge rubber collar fitted around the neck. For the supine position we used a Drinker respirator set for the maintenance of constant positive or negative pressures. For the sitting position a special "body-box" was built. The subject entered through a door on the front, pushed his head through the rubber collar and seated himself on a stool underneath. The nose was occluded and the subject breathed through a mouth piece in a closed circuit which included a recording spirometer, a CO_2 absorber, and suitable check valves to keep the air circulating. The pressure in the body box was maintained at any desired level from -30 to $+40$ cm. of water by an electrically operated valve. At intervals the subject was asked to give a maximum exhalation followed by a maximum inhalation. From the graphic record measurements were made of the vital capacity, the expiratory reserve (supplemental air or the amount which could be exhaled after the end of a normal expiration) and inspiratory reserve (complemental air or the amount which could be inhaled after the end of a normal inspiration).

In these measurements there is of course a continual change of the base line on the recording drum due to the consumption of oxygen. If it could be assumed that the oxygen consumption remains constant at different pressures it should be possible to measure from the record the immediate change in volume which results from a given change of pressure. In practice it was found that the errors involved in this assumption were too large so that we decided to measure only relative volumes. The estimate of the absolute volume change in the residual air at different pressures must depend therefore upon measurements of maximum pressures voluntarily developed at different volumes as described under (1).

Since all measurements of lung volumes were expressed as percentages of the vital capacity and were corrected for pressures above or below ambient pressures the results represent relative, actual anatomical volumes.

TABLE 1

Average maximum expiratory and inspiratory and average relaxation pressures at different lung volumes with standard deviations

MAXIMUM EXPIRATORY PRESSURES		MAXIMUM INSPIRATORY PRESSURES		RELAXATION PRESSURES	
12 male subjects		11 male subjects		14 male subjects	
Volume	Positive Pressures	Volume	Negative Pressures	Volume	Pressures
per cent	*mm. Hg*	*per cent*	*mm. Hg*	*per cent*	*mm. Hg*
9.7	41.5 ± 13.4	3.9	86.0 ± 19.5	0	−19.2 ± 6.3
25.0	52.5 ± 20.8	21.7	74.6 ± 14.1	13.9	−8.5 ± 3.5
43.8	69.6 ± 19.7	34.8	63.3 ± 18.7	31.0	−1.3 ± 4.3
60.0	90.0 ± 21.5	55.6	56.8 ± 15.6	51.0	+4.1 ± 3.0
75.0	95.3 ± 17.6	75.7	44.8 ± 14.0	72.0	+10.5 ± 4.3
83.0	107.0 ± 16.3	91.0	23.6 ± 12.9	87.0	+14.9 ± 7.3
				100.0	+20.6 ± 5.2

Observations were grouped according to lung volumes and the actual volumes within each group were averaged to give the recorded values. The groups chosen were as follows: 0%, 1–20%, 21–40%, 41–60%, 61–80%, 81–99% and 100%. All volumes are expressed in percent of the vital capacity at ambient pressure. All measurements were made in the seated position.

RESULTS. (1) *Maximum expiratory and inspiratory pressures.* All the figures obtained on 11 or 12 subjects were arbitrarily divided into class groups according to the lung volumes. The figures in table 1 represent the average pressures and volumes of all the observations within each of these groups. Individual figures are not given because it is felt that the variations in any one subject from one time to another are as great as the variations between individuals so that individual differences would not be significant unless many more measurements were made.

These average figures are plotted in figure 1 as curves *Pe* (expiratory pressures) and *Pi* (inspiratory pressures). It is evident from these curves that the expiratory pressures are larger when the chest is inflated and inspiratory pressures are larger when it is deflated. This depends upon many mechanical factors but is partly dependent upon the fact that muscles in general can exert greater pressures when they are at greater lengths; the expiratory muscles are of course stretched on inflation and vice versa. The dotted portions of these curves indicate lack of experimental basis because of the somewhat hazardous nature of the experiments required to fill these gaps.

In table 2 the data available in the literature relative to maximum pulmonary pressures are summarized for comparison with our own values. Presumably these measurements were made at a lung volume close to the optimum, i.e., at maximum inspiration for expiratory pressures and at full expiration for inspira-

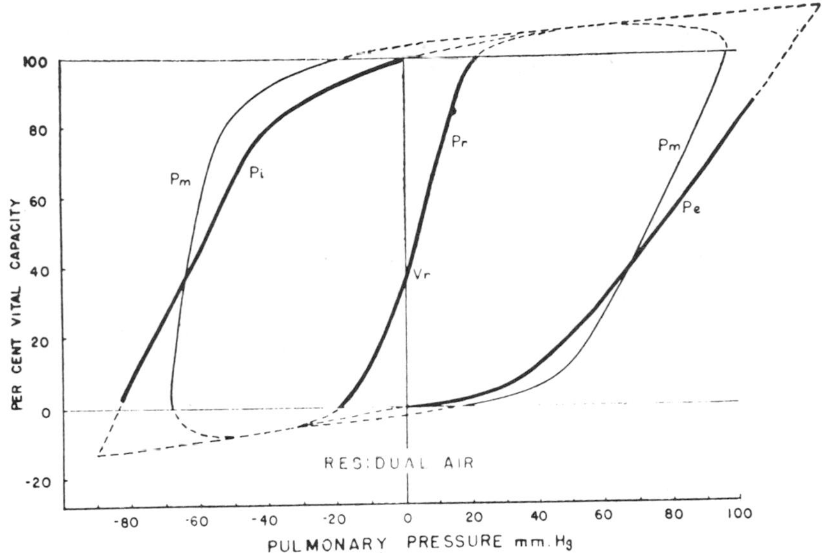

Fig. 1. Pressure-volume diagram of breathing. *Pi* and *Pe*, maximal inspiratory and expiratory pressures respectively; *Pm*, maximal pressure exerted by muscles; *Pr*, relaxation pressure; and *Vr*, relaxation volume.

tory pressures. There is apparently a paucity of data for inspiratory pressures but our values for expiratory pressures agree closely with the average.

The curve *Pr* in figure 1 represents the average relaxation pressures. Actual figures and standard errors are given in table 1 from data obtained on 14 subjects. The differences between the relaxation pressure and the active inspiratory and expiratory pressures are shown by the *Pm* curves which represent the net effect of the active contraction of the respiratory muscles.

$$Pm = Pe - Pr \text{ or } Pi - Pr \qquad \text{(Equation 2)}$$

Pr intersects the zero pressure line at the relaxation volume, *Vr*. At volumes $> Vr$, *Pr* assists the expiratory and opposes the inspiratory muscles, while at lower volumes the reverse is true. Even after making this correction for passive forces it is still true that the muscles exert more pressure when they are more stretched although this relationship is obscured in extreme inspiration and expiration by the mechanical limitations of the chest.

The pressure volume diagram of the lungs is useful in representing any of the mechanical events of breathing. The right side of the diagram represents the field of positive pressure breathing as it is used in the clinical treatment of pulmonary edema, in thoracic surgery, and in aviation. The negative side of the diagram is less commonly experienced in daily life. Small relative negative pressures can be attained by merely standing in water up to the neck. Higher negative pressures are attained by submerging with a tube in the mouth connected to the surface. The experience reported by Stigler (1911) in attempting an experiment of this sort indicates that it is likely to lead to dilatation of the heart. One of us (W. O. F.), however, tried the same experiment years ago for a short period at a depth which was close to the limit of the breathing capacity and experienced no ill affects.

TABLE 2

Maximum pulmonary pressures in normal males

AUTHORITY	NO. OF CASES	MAX. EXP. PRESSURE	MAX. INSP. PRESSURE	VITAL CAPACITY
		mm. Hg	*mm. Hg*	*liters*
Hutchinson, 1852	1061	95.5	65.3	
Schneider, 1921	123	123.0		4.33
Cripps, 1924	950	133.1		4.60
Shilling, 1933	419	114.2		
Gross, 1943	30	119.0		4.60
Our data	31	116.0	80.0	4.84
Weighted average or total	2614	114.0	65.7	4.58

The safe range of the pressure volume diagram may be taken arbitrarily as that between 30 mm. Hg positive and 20 mm. Hg negative, although higher pressures in both directions can be endured safely for short periods. Katz (1909) and Kronecker (1909) found in rabbits that air passed into the abdominal cavity from the lungs at pressures of 30 and 40 mm. Hg. Other references are given by Haldane (p. 360, 1935). Polack and Adams (1932) observed air coming out the carotid cannula when the pulmonary pressure reached 60 mm. Hg. With excessive positive pressures there is therefore danger of pneumothorax and interstitial emphysema.

When an attempt is made to measure maximum inspiratory and expiratory pressures at altitude by the method described above very different results are obtained. For example, when the lungs are completely inflated at 40,000 feet and pressure is then exerted against a manometer the increased pressure is nearly as large as the ambient pressure so that the gases in the lungs are compressed to nearly half the vital capacity. At this lower volume the force which can be exerted is much less than when the chest is fully inflated. No systematic attempt has been made to make measurements of this sort at altitude but the

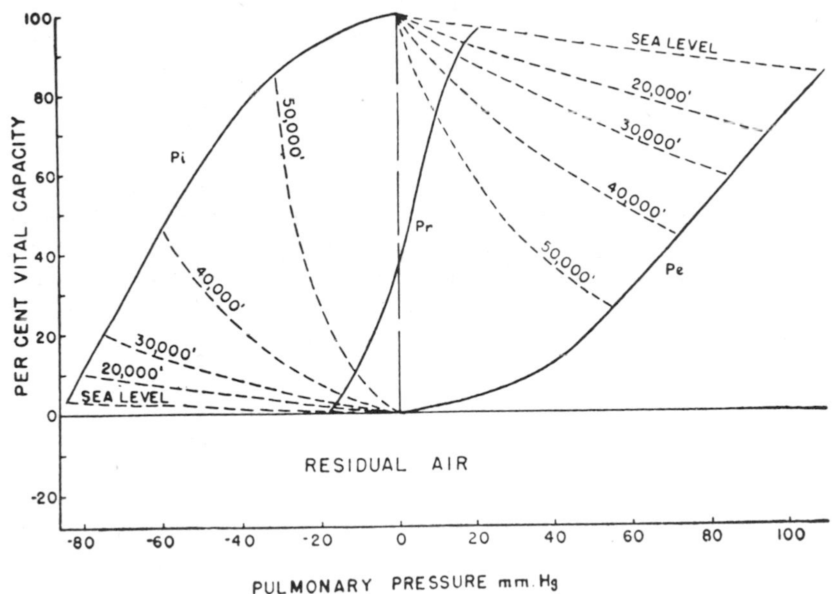

Fig. 2. The effect of altitude on the expiratory and inspiratory pressures which can be exerted starting respectively at maximum inspiration and maximum expiration.

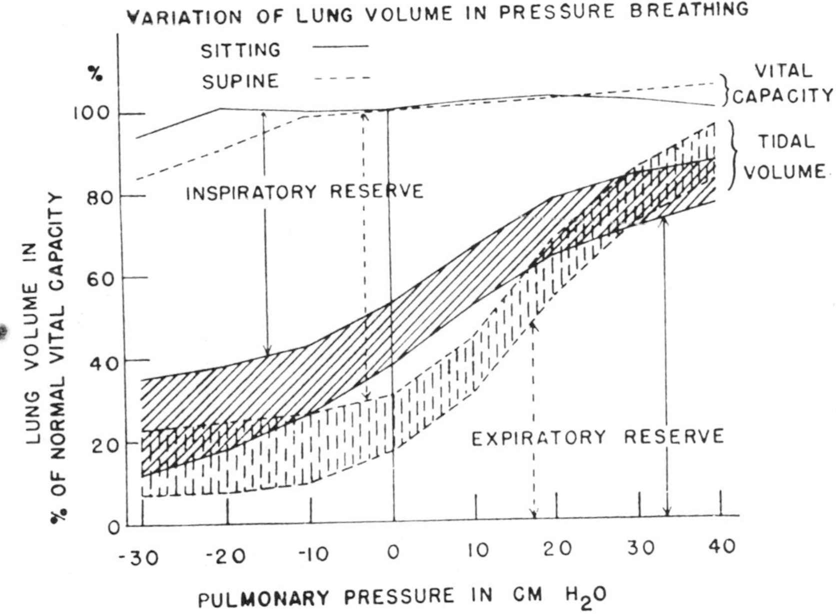

Fig. 3. Variation of lung volume in pressure breathing. The effects of intrapulmonary pressure on vital capacity, tidal volumes and expiratory and inspiratory reserves.

expected pressures have been calculated according to equation 1 (above) and the results are shown in figure 2. The solid lines are the same as those in figure 1 but the dotted lines represent the course which the oxygen or air would take as the subject developed pressure, starting at maximum expiration or maximum inspiration. The relaxation pressures for a given initial volume would likewise be different at altitude and the values obtained by relaxing at maximum inspiration and maximum expiration are given for each altitude by the intersection of the dotted lines with the relaxation pressure curve. At 50,000 feet the whole diagram would be very much curtailed although of course the actual mechanics of the chest are not changed at all. If additional oxygen could be added to or subtracted from the lungs as the pressure was being developed in order to prevent any change in the volume of the lung, the diagram would

TABLE 3

Average lung volumes and standard deviations, seated and supine at different pressures in per cent of vital capacity (in the seated position) at ambient pressure

LUNG PRESSURE	9–10 SUBJECTS (ONE ♀) SEATED				4 SUBJECTS (ALL ♂) SUPINE			
	Vital Cap.	Expir. Res.	Tidal	Insp. Res.	Vit Cap.	Exp. Res.	Tidal	Insp. Res.
cm. H_2O	*per cent*	*per cent*	*per cent*	*per cent*	*per cent*	*per cent*	*per cent*	*per cent*
−30	95 ± 5	12 ± 5	23 ± 7	58 ± 12	83	7	16	60
−20	101 ± 6	19 ± 7	20 ± 5	61 ± 12	92	7	17	68
−10	100 ± 4	26 ± 4	17 ± 3	55 ± 10	99	10	17	72
0	100	38 ± 8	15 ± 3	52 ± 11	100	17	14	75
+10	102 ± 4	52 ± 9	14 ± 4	37 ± 9	102	31	13	58
+20	103 ± 5	64 ± 8	14 ± 4	25 ± 8	103	54	14	35
+30	102 ± 6	71 ± 6	13 ± 4	17 ± 5	104	72	13	19
+40	100 ± 8	77 ± 3	11 ± 6	11 ± 4	106	83	13	10

Average vital capacity at atmospheric pressure seated = 4188 cc. Exp. Res. = the volume which can be exhaled at the end of a normal expiration and Insp. Res. = the volume which can be inhaled after the end of a normal inspiration.

presumably be identical with that obtained at sea level. The corollary of this statement is that the sea level pressure-volume diagram is applicable to pressure breathing where the pressure is obtained passively rather than by voluntary effort.

(2) *Lung volumes.* The results of the measurements of the lung volumes at different pressures are summarized in table 3 where average values and standard deviations are given. The results are also plotted in figure 3. In this graph the point of maximum expiration is considered arbitrarily as zero volume at all pressures. The changes in the residual air are not therefore portrayed in the figure. It is evident that there is little change in the vital capacity in either position except for a slight decrease at the extreme negative pressures. With positive pressures up to 40 cm. H_2O it may be said that the greater expansion of the chest on inspiration is balanced by the diminished deflation on expiration so that the vital capacity remains substantially unaltered. At still higher positive

pressures the vital capacity would eventually decrease. The diminution of the expiratory reserve at zero or low pressures in the supine position as compared to the seated position is evident. A similar effect of posture is seen in the relaxation pressure curves to be described below (see fig. 6).

The data of figure 3 for the seated position have been combined with those of figure 1 in figure 4. At positive pressures the lung volumes have been added to the curve *Pe* while at negative pressures the lung volumes have been subtracted from curve *Pi*. This makes it possible to extend *Pe* (as a solid line) for a short distance into the negative pressure range and to extend *Pi* for a

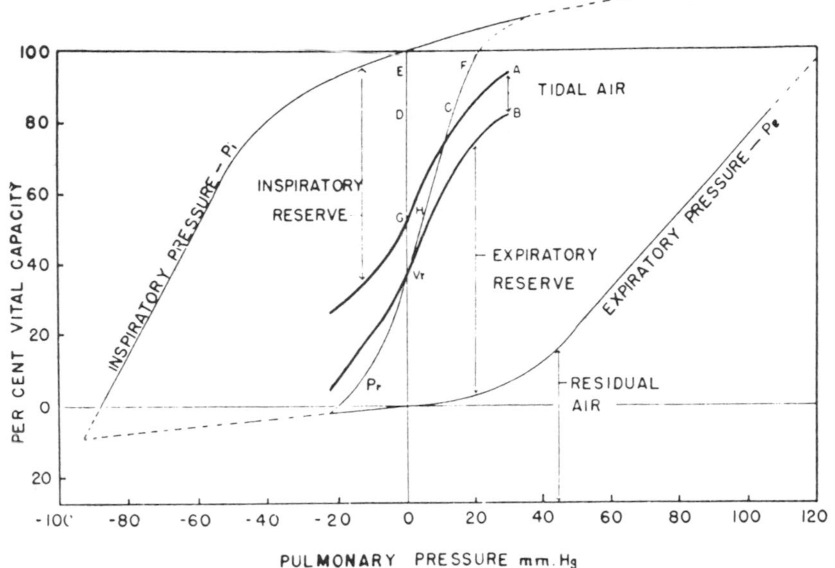

Fig. 4. Pressure-volume diagram of the lung with tidal air and relaxation pressure (*Pr* curves added. Areas *GHVr* and *FABC* represent the elastic work of breathing at norma and 30 mm. Hg positive pressure respectively.

short distance into the positive pressure range. The actual position of the breathing range or tidal air band can be seen in relation to the relaxation pressure curve. The relaxation pressure curve is found to cut the zero pressure line at the same volume as the lower edge of the tidal air band. This is to be expected if the two sets of data are derived from the same or comparable subjects. As the pressure increases the tidal air band is found to fall below the relaxation pressure curve and as the pressures become more negative the tidal air is found to fall above the relaxation pressure curve. This means that the respiratory reflexes do not permit the subject to relax completely on inspiration when breathing against positive pressures nor to relax completely on expiration when breathing against negative pressures. This tendency of the body to resist the pressures or to fight against them considerably increases the work of breathing.

It is also evident from figure 4 that positive pressure causes an increase in the volume of the residual air even though the vital capacity remains substantially unchanged. This has not been verified directly but the change is large enough so that further verification is hardly necessary. Many of the features of figure 4 have been confirmed in reports from the Mayo Aero-medical Laboratory under Doctor Boothby and from the Aviation Research Laboratory at Columbia University under Doctor Barach.

In 22 subjects during these experiments with the body-box, measurements were made of the frequency and depth of breathing at normal pressure and at a positive pulmonary pressure of 30 cm. of water. The average values so obtained are given in table 4 together with the rates of oxygen consumption obtained from the graphical record of the movements of the kymograph. It is evident that during the first 5 minutes of positive pressure breathing there is some hyper-

TABLE 4

Effect of positive pressure breathing on the ventilation and metabolic rate. Average values on 22 male subjects seated in a body box for five minutes at 30 cm. of water negative (relative positive pulmonary) pressure

PULMONARY PRESSURE	BREATHS PER MIN.	TIDAL VOL.	VENTILATION	O_2 CONSUMPTION
cm. H_2O		*cc*	*lit/min.*	*cc/min.*
0	14	657	9.2	341
+30	16	855	13.7	356

Volumes were measured wet at room temperature and pressure.

ventilation without much change in frequency and only a small change in the rate of oxygen consumption which may or may not be significant. A small increase in metabolic rate would be expected because of the increased work of breathing.

Of the 22 men examined seven showed increases in minute volume amounting to more than 50 per cent One of these subjects claimed to feel no discomfort and seemed otherwise normal; three felt considerable discomfort and were near the limit of endurance; three others collapsed after 5 minutes' exposure or less. All other subjects (15 men) were in good condition throughout and felt that they could have continued positive pressure breathing more or less indefinitely, though nearly all stated that they found it more fatiguing than normal breathing.

The hyperventilation shown here for pressure breathing is only an initial effect. The average subject soon adjusts himself to the new condition and his alveolar carbon dioxide tension returns to normal. The detailed evidence for this statement need not be presented here but it depends upon the fact that the average alveolar carbon dioxide tension is not changed by pressure breathing.

(3) *The relaxation pressure, Pr,* can readily be analyzed into two fractions, the lung elasticity Pl and the chest elasticity Pc where the latter includes all the elastic or gravitational factors other than those of the lungs themselves.

Then: $Pr = Pl + Pc$ (Equation 3)

The approximate relation between these quantities at different lung volumes is shown in figure 5. The evidence for this figure is indirect and requires some explanation. The lung pressures, *Pl*, will always be positive so long as the lung is not collapsed and to judge from animal experiments (Cloetta, 1913) it increases linearly over normal tidal ranges. It is assumed to be zero after all but the minimal air is expelled. The magnitude of the *Pl* may be estimated from the intrapleural pressure but care must be taken to avoid a dynamic measure which includes the head of pressure necessary to cause the air to move from the nose to

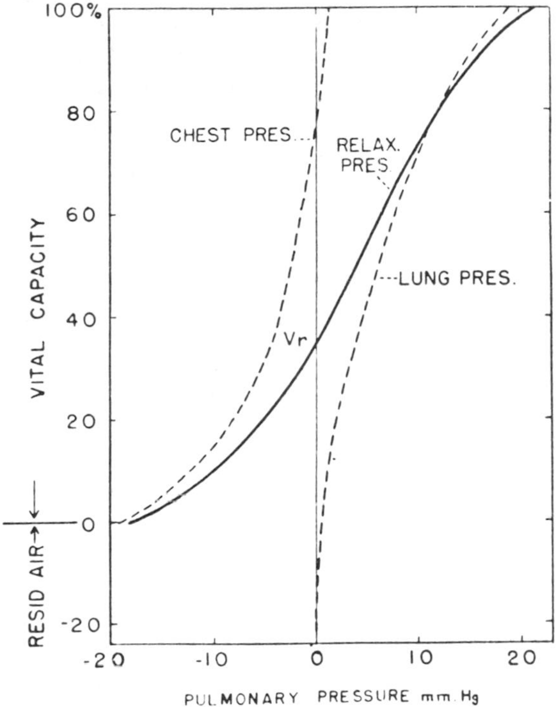

Fig. 5. The relaxation pressure curve (solid) and its two fractions (dotted), that due to the elasticity of the lungs and that due to the chest, diaphragm etc.

the alveoli (Neergaard and Wirz, 1927). From evidence of this sort the value of *Pl* at the end of a normal expiration may be taken as 4 mm. Hg.[2] Since *Pr* is zero at this point *Pc* must be −4 mm. Hg. In other words, at the end of a normal expiration the lungs are tending to collapse and the chest is tending to expand, each with a pressure of 4 mm. Hg. This is confirmed by the fact that the thoracic cage expands when the animal is given a pneumothorax (Bunta, 1936). It has been observed in patients with emphysema that the chest tends to expand due to atrophy of the elastic fibers of the lung from 40 per cent to about 72 per cent of

[2] This value has been estimated for the slightly different conditions of our experiments from the data of Bunta (1936) who recorded a value of −6 cm H_2O at the end of a normal inspiration in the recumbent position with a water manometer.

the vital capacity (Christie, 1934; Hurtado, Kaltreider, Fray, Brooks and McCann, 1934). If in these patients the *Pc* is normal while *Pl* is zero then in normal persons also the chest pressure, *Pc*, is zero at 72 per cent of the vital capacity. In figure 5 the chest pressure curve is drawn through this point and the lung pressure curve must then intersect the relaxation pressure curve at 72 per cent of the vital capacity. The position of this point is largely a matter of guesswork although some experimental evidence can be obtained from measurements of the venous pressure at different pulmonary pressures which will be presented elsewhere. This concept is qualitatively supported by the observation of Gerhardt (1908) that in dogs the intrapleural injection of fluids caused an expansion of the chest and a progressive fall in the intrapleural pressure until 1 liter had been injected. At this point the chest was in its neutral position and the lung was

TABLE 5

Effect of posture on the relaxation pressures at different lung volumes

LUNG VOL.	STANDING	SUPINE	DIFFERENCE
per cent	*mm. Hg*	*mm. Hg*	*mm. Hg*
		13 men	
100	21.2 ± 5.6	27.2 ± 5.9	6.0 ± 1.7
Vr = 38	0	7.5 ± 2.2	7.5 ± 2.2
0	−21.6 ± 5.9	−13.4 ± 4.3	8.2 ± 1.5
		4 women	
100	17.8	24.1	6.3
Vr	0	6.0	6.0
0*	−10.4	−3.0	7.4

* One subject only.

Vr = relaxation volume. The average value for men was 38% of the vital capacity but was not determined for the women.

Individual data for all the subjects are found in Appendix E of Committee of Aviation Medicine report No. 430 of the O.S.R.D.

nearly collapsed. In a dog one liter must represent a large fraction of the vital capacity indicating that 72 per cent for man is perhaps an underestimate.

(4) *The effect of posture* was first determined in acute experiments in which the subject was suddenly tilted from a nearly erect position into the supine position while his relaxation pressure at a given lung volume was recording on a manometer connecting to one nostril. Measurements of this sort have been made on 13 subjects at three different lung volumes: maximum inspiration, normal expiration, and maximum expiration. Upon tilting to the supine position the relaxation pressures for these three positions increased on the average 6.0 mm., 7.5 mm. and 8.2 mm. Hg respectively. The figures are given in table 5. The indications from the use of this method are that the change from the standing to the supine position merely moves the curve over to the right. A similar change was reported by Rohrer on a single subject (1916).

This change in the relaxation pressure curve is attributed to the weight of the viscera which press against the diaphragm in the supine but not in the standing position, thus increasing the pressure in the lungs. If the abdominal contents are thought of as behaving like so much fluid then the observed effect can be quantitatively predicted with reasonable accuracy. For the purpose of this calculation the abdomen can be regarded as a cylinder with an elastic membrane, the diaphragm, tied over one end. In the vertical position the pressure against this membrane is zero or negative but in the supine position the contained fluid presses against the rubber membrane, the pressure being greatest at the bottom and least at the top. If the diameter is 20 cm., which is the average figure given by Hitzenberger (1929) for the diameter of the abdomen, then the average pressure against the membrane is 10 cm. of water or 7.4 mm. Hg. This is obviously close to the value found experimentally. This pressure could, of course, be absorbed by an increased tonus of the diaphragm without change in its position. If, however, the escape of air from the lung were prevented and the chest were kept fixed in position, then this increased abdominal pressure might force the diaphragm upward, thus raising the pulmonary pressure to equal the increased abdominal pressure. The volume of the lungs and diameter of the diaphragm is such that a movement upward of only about 1 mm. would be required. It is reasonable, therefore, that the increased relaxation pressure should be about equal to the theoretical increase in abdominal pressure. If the chest expanded much with the increased pressure, the required movement of the diaphragm would be greater than 1 mm., but probably not enough greater to change its tension so as to vitiate this comparison.

At the end of a normal expiration in the sitting position the lungs come to rest at point Vr where the relaxation pressure curve crosses the Y axis in figure 5. If the subject is tilted to the supine position with the nostrils connected to a manometer so that the lung volume remains constant the pressure increases as already explained. If on the other hand the lungs are connected to a spirometer so that the pressure remains constant at the ambinent value then the spirometer rises and the lung volume decreases as illustrated in figure 6. This experiment with the spirometer has been done on 29 subjects. The average displacement was 637 ± 240 cc. which represents 13.3 per cent of the average vital capacity of 4800 cc.

A similar volume change due to posture in 8 subjects is illustrated in table 6 for the positions of maximum inspiration and maximum expiration. When a subject in the standing position expires maximally into a spirometer and is then tilted into the supine position (while his expiratory efforts continue) an additional 144 cc. on the average is forced out into the recording spirometer (column A). Conversely when a subject in the supine position inhales to the limit and is then rapidly tilted into the standing position (while his inspiratory efforts continue) he finds it possible to inhale an additional 225 cc. on the average (column B). All of these observations show that in the supine position the relaxation pressure curve in figure 5 is moved downward and to the right.

In another series of experiments, an effort was made to confirm this effect of

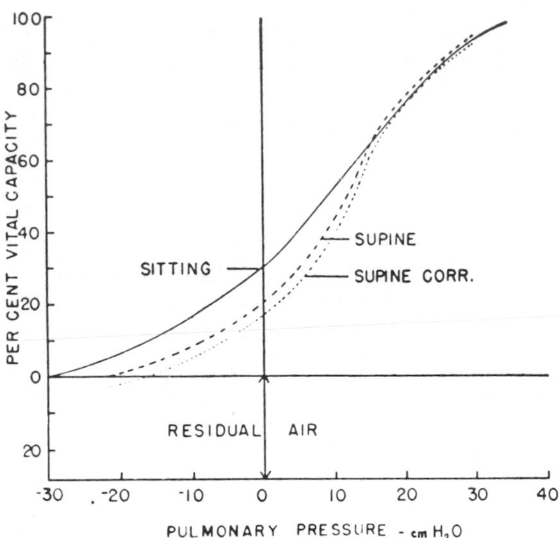

Fig. 6. Effect of posture on the relaxation pressure curve. The corrected supine curve is 3% lower than the "supine" curve at all pressures.

TABLE 6

Difference in lung volume at maximum expiration (A) and maximum inspiration (B) due to change in posture from standing to supine or the reverse

SUBJECT	POSTURAL VOLUME CHANGE		VITAL CAPACITY
	A	B	
	cc	*cc*	*liters*
1	253	260	5.68
2	170	293	4.55
3	132	120	4.81
4	90	260	5.10
5	174	226	4.40
6	193	253	4.39
7	53	80	3.79
8	86	313	4.01
Mean	144	225	4.59
% of V.C.	3.1%	4.9%	100%

Each figure presents the average of three measurements. Column A represents the additional volume expired in the supine position after tilting from the standing position at the end of a complete expiration. It is the volume decrease of the standing residual air.

Column B represents the additional volume inspired in the standing position after tilting from the supine position at the end of a complete inspiration.

posture by a different method. In these experiments, each of 10 subjects recorded his relaxation pressure in the sitting position in the usual way. Later, in the supine position, usually on the same day, the determinations were repeated.

The same posture was therefore maintained throughout the determinations of each curve and no attempt was made to tilt the subject rapidly "from a point on one curve to the corresponding point on the other".

The results of these experiments are presented in tables 7 and 8, and the averages for each of the two positions are plotted in figure 6. All of the results in the graph are expressed in per cent of the vital capacity for the sitting position. In 8 out of the 10 individuals, the vital capacity was larger in the sitting than in the supine position, but the average figures were so nearly equal (4690 cc. sitting and 4610, supine) that it makes little difference which value is used. In these experiments the fixed point arbitrarily selected for the measurement of the lung

TABLE 7

Lung volumes of 10 subjects in the sitting position at different relaxation pressures

SUBJECT	CM. H_2O																VIT. CAP.
	−35	−30	−25	−20	−15	−10	−5	0	5	10	15	20	25	30	35	40	
	Lung volumes in per cent of vital capacity																*cc.*
J. F.			3	7	12	19	25	30	38	48	62	74	85	90	95	99	6000
M. H.								20	32	48	60	72	84	92	100		3600
R. S.	0	3	7	10	14	19	26	36	54	68	82	91	96	100			4300
L. E. C.			0	5	11	18	26	33	46	64	78	86	93	99			4500
M. E.				2	5	8	14	21	30	39	50	63	76	85	96		5500
J. M.								34	46	57	70	86	100				4100
A. O.		3	8	12	18	24	30	36	43	50	60	73	86	96			5000
J. H.						20	23	27	31	39	50	66	82	92	100		4400
H. R.				9	16	22	28	36	47	57	66	74	83	91	98		5600
C. B.				1	8	13	17	22	34	51	68	80	88	94	100		3900
Averages	0	3	4.5	6.6	12	17.9	23.6	29.5	40.1	52.1	64.6	76.5	87.3	93.2	98.1	99	4690

Values at the particular pressures indicated were obtained by graphical interpolation.

volume in each position is the point of maximum expiration in that position. Since according to data of table 6 the residual air is less in the supine than in the erect (standing) position by 3.1 per cent of the vital capacity, the supine (dotted) curve in figure 6 has been corrected by subtracting 3 per cent from all of the values. This does not appreciably change the relative positions of the two curves. As in the comparison with the standing position the assumption of the supine position from the sitting position moves the relaxation pressure curve downward and to the right. In this case the change in volume is particularly great at the lower volumes. Attention is called to the close resemblance between these curves and the curves for the sitting and supine positions in figure 3 where the expiratory reserve varies in a similar manner. The curves of figure 6 suggest that there would be little change in relaxation pressure on going from the sitting to the supine position at maximum inspiration whereas an increase of 6 mm. Hg was found in table 5 for the change from the standing to the supine position. This has not been verified experimentally. On the other hand the curves of figure 6 confirm the figures quoted above which show a greater volume change at *Vr* than at either maximum inspiration or maximum expiration on changing from the standing to the supine position (i.e., 637 cc. compared to 144 and 225 cc). Note that the vertical difference between the solid and dotted (corrected) curves in figure 6 at zero pressure is very nearly equal to 637 cc.

(5) *Work of breathing.* The slope of the relaxation pressure curve at small positive pressures just above the relaxation volume is a value of some interest from

TABLE 8

Lung volumes of 10 subjects in the supine position at different relaxation pressures

SUBJECT	CM H_2O														VIT. CAP.
	−25	−20	−15	−10	−5	0	5	10	15	20	25	30	35	40	
	Lung volumes in per cent of vital capacity														
															cc.
J. F.	2	5	8	12	16	20	24	32	44	60	74	86	92	100	6000
M. H.	0	2	4	8	11	16	22	38	60	76	87	97			3400
R. S.	2	5	8	11	15	20	33	48	62	76	88	97			4200
L. C.		0	4	9	16	22	30	48	70	84	97				4300
M. E.				1	8	14	26	44	64	76	85	94			5800
J. M.				2	8	22	36	59	75	86	98				4000
A. O.	0	4	10	14	20	25	30	40	60	76	90	99			4900
J. H.			5	12	16	20	28	44	64	80	94				4200
H. R.		0	4	10	17	26	38	50	66	82	91	98			5500
C. B.			2	6	10	15	24	44	60	75	86	96			3800
Averages	1	2.7	5.6	8.5	13.7	20.0	29.1	44.7	62.5	77.1	89.0	95.3	100		4610
Av. in % of sitting Vit. Cap.	1	2.7	5.5	8.3	13.5	19.7	28.6	44.0	61.5	75.9	87.5	93.5	100		4690

Values at the particular pressures indicated were obtained by graphic interpolation.

the point of view of the mechanics of normal breathing. From this may be deduced the elastic work of breathing as well as the mechanical characteristics which are needed to simulate a normal chest for purposes of experimentation such as the testing of artificial respiration apparatus. This slope can be deduced from the data of tables 7 and 8 by averaging the increments of volume recorded for a change in pressure from 0 to +5 mm. Hg. For the seated position (table 7) this slope turns out to be 94 ± 35 cc. per mm. Hg. For the supine position (table 8) the corresponding value is 85 ± 31 cc. per mm. Hg. These figures correspond well with similar figures given for individual subjects by Rohrer (1916) and Senner (1921). Their values were, respectively, 107 and 97 cc. per mm. Hg.

Using our values of 94 cc. per mm. Hg for the seated position the elastic work required for an intake of 500 cc. of tidal air would be

$$500 \times \frac{500}{94} \times \frac{13.54}{10} \times \frac{1}{2} = 1800 \text{ gm. cm.}$$

This figure is in the same range as the values 1424 to 2460 gm. cm. per breath measured on dogs by Dean and Visscher (1941). This elastic work is represented by the small triangular area *GHVr* in figure 4. The error in determining these slopes between two successive points on the curve is fairly large and the value obtained from the data on relaxation pressures given in table 1 is 180 cc. per mm. Hg. Nevertheless these data as a whole give curves very similar to those plotted from tables 7 and 8. The latter data are probably more reliable because they give lung volumes graphically determined at given pressures while in table 1 average pressures were given at average volumes within an arbitrarily selected range.

The elastic work of pressure breathing can also be calculated from the graphs of figure 4. Thus at the maximum positive pressure for which data are available (30 mm. Hg), the tidal air is represented by the line *AB* and the work of expira

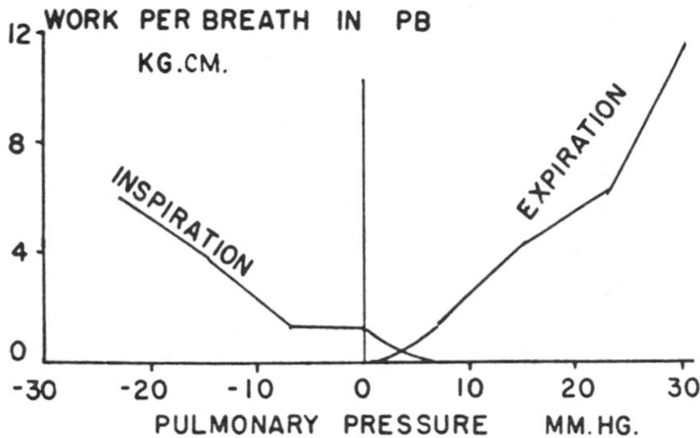

Fig. 7. The increase in the elastic work of breathing at increasing negative and positive pulmonary pressures. Figures determined graphically from areas on a diagram similar to but not identical with figure 4.

tion is given by the area *ABDE*. However, the relaxation pressure curve indicates that a part of this work could be done by elastic potential energy stored in the thoracic wall and lungs, this fraction being represented by the area *FCDE*. The net work done by active contraction of the expiratory muscles is therefore the difference between these two areas or *ABCF*. The values of these areas for different pressures have been calculated from another graph similar to that in figure 4 but differing in details, and the results are plotted in figure 7. Two curves are shown, one for inspiration and one for expiration. At zero pressure all the elastic work is inspiratory. At more negative pressures the inspiratory work increases because the chest is not allowed to relax completely on expiration.

At positive pressures the inspiratory work falls off to zero at 7.5 mm. Hg. (In fig. 4 this occurs at 10 mm. Hg where the inspiratory side of the tidal air band crosses the relaxation pressure curve.) As the pressure becomes positive however expiration becomes more and more active and the work of expiration increases, as already explained. It is an interesting point that at a pressure of about 3.5 mm. Hg half the work is inspiratory and half is expiratory and the sum of the two is less than the inspiratory work at zero pressure. The work of breathing is therefore slightly but inconsequentially diminished by increasing the pulmonary pressure a few millimeters of Hg.

To obtain an artificial lung which will have the same elastic characteristics it is only necessary to use a rigid container having a capacity of 760 x 94 = 71 liters. We have found an ordinary kitchen hot water tank very satisfactory for the purpose.

SUMMARY

1. Average data from 10 or more individuals are presented for the construction of a pressure-volume diagram of the lung and thorax. The data consist of measurements of maximum expiratory and inspiratory pressures at different lung volumes and relaxation pressures.

2. Calculations are made to show the changes in this diagram which would result from an increase in altitude.

3. Measurements are made of the vital capacity, expiratory reserve, tidal air and inspiratory reserve in 14 individuals at 8 different pulmonary pressures ranging from 30 cm. of water negative to 40 cm. of water positive. It is shown that with positive pressures the expiratory reserve (and residual air) increase, the inspiratory reserve decreases, while the tidal air and vital capacity remain approximately unaltered.

4. During pressure breathing the chest does not relax completely to the position indicated by the relaxation pressure curve so that the work of breathing is considerably increased.

5. When positive pressure breathing begins there is usually a temporary hyperventilation which disappears after 5 or 10 minutes or less. The rate of oxygen consumption is not appreciably increased.

6. The relaxation pressure curve is resolved into two components, the lung elasticity proper and the other factors (chest and diaphragm). Data are presented to indicate how these components vary with lung volume.

7. When the subject is tilted from the standing to the supine position air is expelled from the lungs amounting to 637 ± 240 cc. (if respiratory muscles are relaxed) or, if this is prevented, the pressure in the lungs rises 6 to 8 mm. Hg due to the weight of the viscera against the diaphragm. There are other factors also which modify the shape of the relaxation pressure curve in the supine as compared to the sitting position.

8. The slope of the relaxation pressure curve is such that an increase of 1 mm. Hg in the pulmonary pressure increases the lung volume by 94 ± 35 cc. The elastic work of breathing calculated from this slope is 1800 gm. cm. for a tidal volume of 500 cc.

9. In pressure breathing it is shown that a slight increase of pulmonary pressure of 3 to 5 mm. Hg results in a decrease in the work of breathing half of it being inspiratory work and half being expiratory work. With larger positive pressures or increasing negative pressures, the work of breathing increases as much as ten-fold.

REFERENCES

BERNOULLI, E. Arch. f. exper. Path **66**: 313, 1911.
BUNTA, E. Am. Rev. Tuberc. **33**: 203, 1936.
CHRISTIE, R. V. J. Clin. Investigation **13**: 295, 1934.
CLOETTA, M. Pflüger's Arch. **152**: 339, 1913.
CRIPPS, L. D. Med. Res. Council, Sp. Rep. Ser. **84**: 1, 1924.
DEAN, R. B. AND M. B. VISSCHER. This Journal **134**: 450, 1941.
GERHARDT, D. Arch f. exper. Path. Suppl. **108**: 228, 1908.
GROSS, D. Am. Heart J. **25**: 335, 1943.
HALDANE, J. S. AND J. G. PRIESTLEY. Respiration. p. 360, New Haven University Press, 1935.
HITZENBERGER, K. Klin. Wchnschr. **8**: 961, 1929.
HURTADO, A., N. L. KALTREIDER, W. W. FRAY, W. B. BROOKS AND W. S. McCANN. J. Clin. Investigation **13**: 1027, 1934.
HUTCHINSON, T. Todd's cyclopaedia of anatomy and physiology. Vol. IV, pp. 1016–1087, 1852.
JAQUET, A. Arch f. exper. Path. u. Pharmakol. Suppl. p. 309, 1908.
KATZ, S. Ztschr. Biol. **52**: 236, 1909.
KRONECKER, H. J. Physiol. **38**: 75P, 1909.
NEERGAARD, K. AND K. WIRZ, Ztschr. klin. Med. **105**: 35, 1927.
POLACK, B. AND H. ADAMS. Nav. Med. Bull., Washington **30**: 165, 1932.
ROHRER, F. Pflüger's Arch. **165**: 419, 1916.
SCHNEIDER, E. C. Am. J. Med. Sci. **161**: 395, 1921.
SENNER, W. Pflüger's Arch. **190**: 97, 1921.
SHILLING, C. W. U. S. Naval Med. Bull. **31**: 1, 1933.
STIGLER, R. Pflüger's Arch. **139**: 234, 1911.

20

Reprinted by permission of the American Physiological Society from *J. Appl. Physiol.*, 2(11), 592–607 (1950)

Mechanics of Breathing in Man[1]

ARTHUR B. OTIS, WALLACE O. FENN AND HERMANN RAHN. *From the Department of Physiology and Vital Economics, University of Rochester School of Medicine and Dentistry, Rochester, New York*

THE MECHANICAL WORK done by the respiratory muscles in producing the movements of breathing has been studied relatively little by physiologists. Although most text-books of physiology give values for the work done by the heart, similar estimates for the work of breathing are lacking. The classic contributions of Rohrer (1–3) lay the foundation for this subject, but only a few pertinent papers, notably those of Neergaard and Wirz (4), Vuilleumier (5), Bayliss and Robertson (6), and Dean and Visscher (7), have since appeared.

The material presented below, although based on data which are neither sufficiently precise nor extensive enough to furnish an exact description of the mechanics of breathing, constitutes an approximate analysis, which we have found valuable as a way of thinking about certain respiratory problems.

FORCES INVOLVED IN BREATHING

From the work of previous investigators and on the basis of *a priori* reasoning, we should expect that the respiratory muscles in carrying out the breathing movements would have to overcome several types of resisting forces. These forces will be mentioned briefly now and considered later in more detail. The chest and lungs are elastic in nature and must be stretched during inspiration to accommodate an increased volume. The air in moving through the respiratory tract encounters viscous and turbulent resistance, and there is probably some additional non-elastic resistance associated with deformation of tissues, and with the sliding of organs over one another when they are displaced. Finally, since the system is almost continuously accelerating or decelerating, inertia should be mentioned as a possible factor. The calculations of Rohrer (3), however, indicate that the force required for acceleration must be ordinarily very small, and we shall, in general, consider it negligible. Another factor of relatively inconsequential magnitude is the kinetic energy imparted to the air.

Received for publication March 31, 1950.

[1] This work was completed under contract between the University of Rochester and the Air Materiel Command, Wright-Patterson Air Force Base, Dayton, Ohio. Some of our earlier work was reported in C.M.R. Report No. 430, May 10, 1945 and in *Federation Proc.* 6: 173, 1947. An abstract of a preliminary report, presented before the National Academy of Sciences, appears in *Science* 110: 443, 1949.

Elastic Forces. If a person relaxes his respiratory muscles completely, the lungs assume a volume close to that which is customary at the end of a normal expiration, the mid-capacity or *relaxation volume.* At this volume the elastic forces of the chest must be equal and opposite to those of the lung. When the chest-lung system is displaced to any other volume, elastic forces which oppose the displacing force are developed. The method of measuring these elastic forces as *relaxation pressures* and a curve showing the relationship between relaxation pressure and lung volume have been presented in a previous paper from this laboratory (8). The reciprocal slope, $\Delta P/\Delta V$, of the relaxation pressure curve is the elastic resistance or 'elastance' (pressure required to produce unit change in volume (6, 7)). Although the relaxation pressure curve is not linear, it is approximately so over a considerable part of its range, and as a first approximation the elastance may be expressed by the following equation:

$$P_{el.} = KV \qquad (1)$$

where K is the elastance and $P_{el.}$ is the pressure developed when the displacement from the relaxation volume is V.

Air Viscance and Turbulence. A method for estimating the magnitude of the viscous and turbulent forces that must be overcome in moving air through the respiratory tract has been described previously (9, 10), and data have been presented which indicate that the relationship between these forces and the velocity of air flow may be described approximately by the following equation:

$$P_{alv.} = k_1\left(\frac{dV}{dt}\right) + k_2\left(\frac{dV}{dt}\right)^2 \qquad (2)$$

where $P_{alv.}$ is the pressure gradient between alveoli and mouth that is required to move the air with a velocity (dV/dt). The constants k_1 and k_2 are the air *viscance*[2] and the *turbulent resistance*, respectively.

An example of the sort of record from which data were obtained for purposes of the present investigation is shown in figure 1, and the points obtained from measurement of records made on *subject R* are shown in figure 3. The parabola was fitted to these points by the method of residuals.

Resistance Associated with Tissue Deformation. It does not seem feasible to measure directly the non-elastic resistance associated with tissue deformation, but an estimate may be obtained in the following fashion. A trained subject is placed in a Drinker respirator and is instructed to relax as completely as

[2] Our usage of the word 'viscance' in this paper is implicit in *equation 2* and may be used synonomously with 'viscous resistance'; it is expressed in dimensions of pressure per unit flow of respired gas. 'Viscance' was defined by Bayliss and Robertson (6) as "the viscous force per unit deformation" or "viscous pressure per unit of tidal air volume." Dean and Visscher (7), however, use the same term to mean "viscous resistance to a unit velocity of flow." Although the definition of Bayliss and Robertson was stated to make 'viscance' analagous to 'electrical resistance,' we believe that our usage of the term is a better analogy.

possible so that his breathing movements are produced by the alternating pressure within the respirator instead of by the action of his respiratory muscles. The pressure gradient between the respirator and the mouth of the subject and the velocity of air flow are simultaneously recorded. The pressure recorded at any moment is, of course, that required to overcome the total resistance, and since the elastance and air viscance and turbulent resistance can be obtained as described above, the non-elastic tissue resistance can be estimated by difference. Figure 2 shows a sample record obtained in this type of experiment.

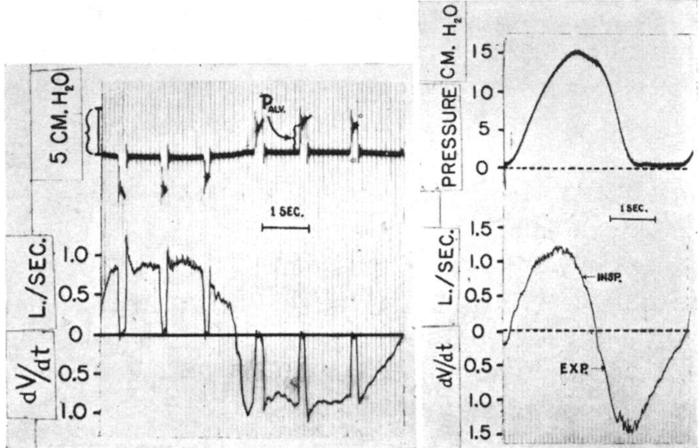

Fig. 1 (*left*). SIMULTANEOUS RECORDS of pressure at mouth (*upper tracing*) and pneumotachogram (*lower tracing*). In pneumotachogram, inspiration is above and expiration below baseline. Sudden changes in pressure at mouth and simultaneous interruptions of air flow were produced by brief closure of solenoid valve located in airway between mouth and pneumotachograph. Method of estimating alveolar pressure ($P_{alv.}$) is indicated.

Fig. 2 (*right*). SIMULTANEOUS RECORDS of pressure gradient between mouth and inside of Drinker respirator (*upper tracing*) and pneumotachogram (*lower tracing*). *Subject R.*

A useful way of representing some of the data that can be obtained from such a record is shown in figure 4 in which pressure is plotted against accumulated volume for one breathing cycle. The method of constructing such a diagram will now be described.

The velocity of flow and the simultaneous pressure were measured and tabulated for each 0.1-second interval of the record of the respiratory cycle shown in figure 3. Then starting at the beginning of inspiration each 0.1-second interval of the flow curve was integrated by multiplying the mean velocity of flow during each period by 0.1 second. This gave the volume that flowed during each 0.1-second period. These volumes were then added in a cumulative fashion and the total volume at the end of each time interval was plotted against the corresponding pressure gradient that existed at the end of that interval. The plotted points determine the solid lines that form the large loop in figure 4.

This closed curve represents the relationship between the changes in the volume of the lung during the respiratory cycle and the external forces (as represented by the pressure gradient between the respirator and mouth) acting to produce this change. At two moments (when the cycle reverses from in-

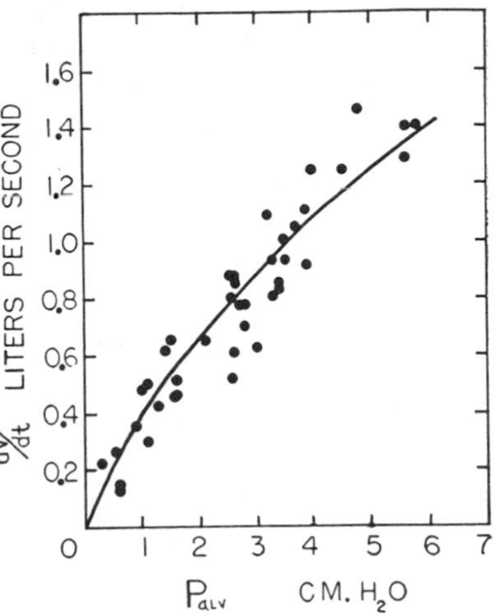

Fig. 3. Relationship between instantaneous rate of flow of respired gas and pressure gradient between alveoli and mouth for *subject R*. Curve drawn through points represents equation:

$$P_{alv.} = 1.7\left(\frac{dV}{dt}\right) + 1.9\left(\frac{dV}{dt}\right)^2.$$

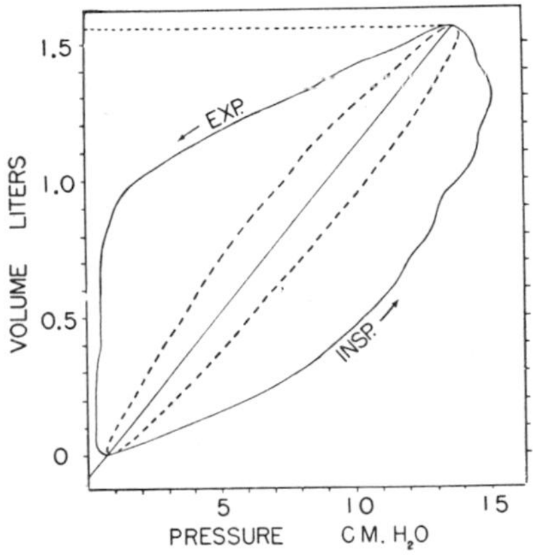

Fig. 4. Relationship between volume of respired gas and pressure gradient during one respiratory cycle for *Subject R*. For explanation, see text.

spiration to expiration and vice versa) no air is being moved in either direction. At these instants, therefore, the total force acting is being used to maintain elastic tension that has been developed, inertia being assumed to be negligible. If we assume a linear relationship between elastic pressure and lung volume, then the diagonal in figure 4 represents this relationship. Approximately, it is a segment of the relaxation pressure curve.

Some of the information represented by figure 4 may be summarized as follows. As the lung volume is increased during inspiration, the total pressure gradient between the mouth and the inside of the respirator is represented by the abscissal distance from the axis of ordinates to the inspiratory loop. Of this total inspiratory pressure ($P_{in.}$) at any given lung volume, a certain amount ($P_{el.}$), represented by the abscissal distance from the axis of ordinates to the diagonal, is required to overcome elastance; the remainder ($P_{in.} - P_{el.}$) is the pressure required to overcome air and tissue viscance and turbulent resistance.

Expiration is produced by the elastic forces that were developed in the chest and lung during inspiration. However, the total elastic force is not available, in this case, for overcoming the viscous and turbulent resistances of expiration, because the pressure within the respirator continues to be negative especially during the first part of expiration. The pressure actually used in overcoming viscance and turbulence at any moment during expiration is of course ($P_{el.} - P_{ex.}$) where $P_{ex.}$ is the abscissal distance from the axis of ordinates to the expiratory loop, i.e. the pressure gradient between the mouth and the inside of the respirator during expiration. Under the conditions of the particular experiment illustrated in figure 4, the lung volume does not quite get back to the relaxation volume by the end of expiration; the respirator starts an inspiratory movement before expiration is as complete as it would be if more time were allowed.

The relationship between numerous values of ($P_{in.} - P_{el.}$) or ($P_{el.} - P_{ex.}$) and the corresponding velocities of flow is represented by the points plotted in figure 5. These data were obtained from figures 2 and 4 and other similarly plotted cycles measured on *subject R*. The parabolic curve drawn through the point S was fitted by the method of residuals and may be generally represented by

$$P_n = K'\left(\frac{dV}{dt}\right) + K''\left(\frac{dV}{dt}\right)^2 \tag{3}$$

the slope of which represents the total viscous and turbulent resistance of breathing.

By subtracting the curve of figure 3 from that of figure 5 a relationship of the following form is obtained

$$P_t = k_3\left(\frac{dV}{dt}\right) + k_4\left(\frac{dV}{dt}\right)^2 \tag{4}$$

Its slope represents the resistance associated with the non-elastic component of tissue deformation.

By means of *equation 4*, P_t was calculated for each 0.1-second interval of figure 2 and the resulting values were added to the corresponding values of $P_{el.}$ during inspiration and subtracted during expiration. These sums or differences were plotted against the cumulative volume for the corresponding time interval to form the loop indicated by the broken line in figure 4. The abscissal distance from the diagonal to this loop is the pressure required to overcome non-elastic resistance of tissue.

Constants for *equations 1, 2, 3* and *4* evaluated as outlined above are recorded in table 1 for *subject R* and for two other subjects who were similarly studied. The values shown for each subject are based on measurements of several cycles.

Total Force Required for Breathing. The total force required for breathing is the sum of *equations 1* and *3* or

$$P_\Sigma = KV + K'\left(\frac{dV}{dt}\right) + K''\left(\frac{dV}{dt}\right)^2 \tag{5}$$

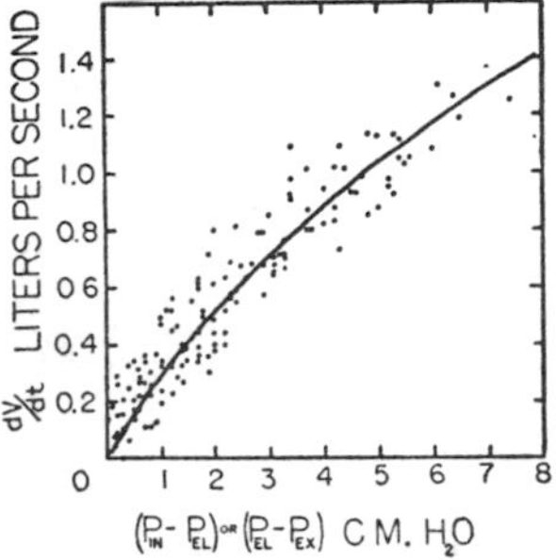

Fig. 5. RELATIONSHIP between instantaneous rate of flow of respired gas and pressure required to overcome non-elastic resistance to breathing. *Subject R.* Curve drawn through points represents equation:

$$P_n = 2.7\left(\frac{dV}{dt}\right) + 2.1\left(\frac{dV}{dt}\right)^2.$$

TABLE 1. VALUES OF RESISTANCE CONSTANTS ESTIMATED FOR THREE SUBJECTS

SUBJECT	ELASTIC RESISTANCE	ADDITIONAL RESISTANCE OF AIR		ADDITIONAL RESISTANCE OF TISSUE		TOTAL ADDITIONAL RESISTANCE	
	K	k_1	k_2	k_3	k_4	K'	K''
	$cm.H_2O/l.$	$cm.H_2O/(l/sec.)$	$cm.H_2O/(l/sec.)^2$	$cm.H_2O/(l/sec.)$	$cm.H_2O/(l/sec.)^2$	$cm.H_2O/(l/sec.)$	$cm.H_2O/(l/sec.)^2$
R	8.00	1.7	1.9	1.0	0.2	2.7	2.1
B	9.38	3.2	0.8	1.0	0	4.2	0.8
D	8.19	2.9	1.4	0.6	0.1	3.5	1.5
Mean.........	8.52	2.6	1.4	.9	.1	3.5	1.5

THE WORK OF BREATHING

Another useful feature of the method shown in figure 4 of representing a breathing cycle is that area on such a diagram has the dimensions of work. For example, the area of the triangle formed by the diagonal, the horizontal broken line and the axis of ordinates in figure 4 represents the amount of work done during inspiration in overcoming elastic resistance. The area bounded by the diagonal and the curved line labeled *inspiration* is the additional work required to overcome the viscous and turbulent resistance of inspiration. This area may be subdivided into work done on non-elastic resistance of tissue (area between diagonal and broken line) and work done in overcoming air viscance and turbulent resistance.

The elastic energy stored during inspiration and represented by the triangle is available as a power supply for expiration. However, only that portion bounded by the diagonal and the curve labeled *expiration* is actually used in this instance to overcome viscous and turbulent forces; the remainder is expended in working against the continued action of the respirator which opposes expiration during the first part of this phase of the breathing cycle.

Table 2 summarizes measurements of the work of breathing and its fractions obtained by planimetric integration of diagrams such as that illustrated by figure 4. These data indicate that on the average 63 per cent of the total work done in inspiration was used in overcoming elastic forces, 29 per cent in

TABLE 2. WORK OF BREATHING IN DRINKER RESPIRATOR AT FREQUENCY OF 15 PER MINUTE

SUBJECT	TIDAL VOLUME	TOTAL WORK OF INSPIRATION	ELASTIC WORK OF INSPIRATION	WORK ON AIR DURING INSPIRATION	WORK ON TISSUES DURING INSPIRATION
	cm.^{3}	*gm. cm.*	*% of total*	*% of total*	*% of total*
R	1550	17,295	63.0	27.4	9.5
	1340	13,170	59.7	31.5	8.8
	950	6,265	61.5	27.8	10.7
	500	2,091	63.6	28.8	7.6
B	2275	47,660	66.8	25.8	7.4
	1620	23,665	69.2	22.7	8.1
	840	6,220	60.1	32.1	7.8
D	995	7,462	59.6	34.9	5.5
	1365	9,225	65.8	25.0	9.2
	1095	7,720	64.0	28.7	7.3
Mean Values.............			63.3	28.5	8.2

overcoming resistance associated with the movement of air, and 8 per cent in deforming tissues. These percentages apply, of course, only to the particular pattern of breathing employed in this experiment. As will be pointed out later, both the absolute and relative magnitudes of these factors depend to some extent on the particular pattern of breathing employed.

If one assumes that *equation 5* is reasonably valid, the information contained in it makes possible the estimation of the work of breathing for any breathing cycle for which the velocity pattern (pneumotachogram) is known. One method would be to calculate the corresponding pressures for numerous points along the velocity curve and then to follow the procedure described above that was used in getting the data of table 2. This empirical method is very tedious, however, and if one can describe the velocity curve by a simple mathematical expression, the work of breathing may be calculated in a more direct fashion.

For example, assume as a first approximation that the velocity pattern of inspiration is a sine wave (fig. 6). Then

$$\frac{dV}{dt} = a \sin bt \tag{6}$$

where dV/dt is the velocity of air flow, a is the maximal velocity, and $b/2\pi = f$ is the frequency of breathing.

The tidal volume, V_T, is given by

$$V_T = \int_0^{\pi/b} a \sin bt\, dt = \frac{2a}{b} = \frac{a}{\pi f} \tag{7}$$

The differential expression for work is $dW = PdV$ which by substitution from *equations 5* and *6* becomes

$$dW = KV\,dV + K'a^2 \sin^2 bt\,dt + K''a^3 \sin^3 bt\,dt \tag{8}$$

In this expression for the differential of work, the first term represents elastic work, the second viscous work, and the third work done in overcoming

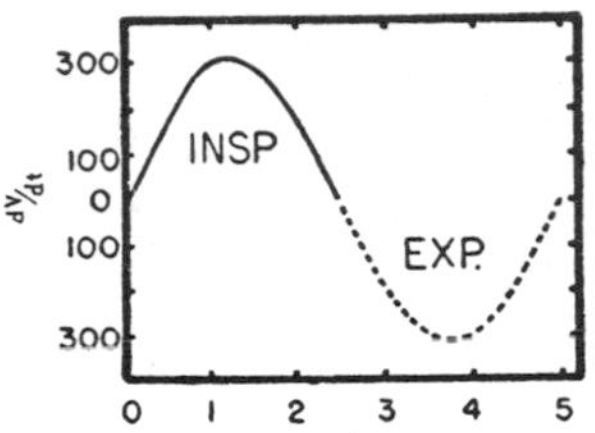

Fig. 6. IDEALIZED REPRESENTATION of pneumotachogram as sine wave. *Ordinates:* Flow of respired gas in cc/sec. *Abscissae:* Time in sec. In this example a mean ventilation of 6 l/min. with tidals of 500 cc. and frequency of 12 breaths/min. is assumed. Constants of *equation 6* in this case are, therefore: $a = 314$ cc/sec. and $b = .0.4\,\pi$ reciprocal seconds.

turbulent resistance. The total work done during a single inspiration of volume V_T and duration π/b may be obtained by integration of *equation 8* as indicated below

$$W = \int_0^{V_T} KV\,dV + \int_0^{\pi/b} (K'\,a^2 \sin^2 bt + K''\,a^3 \sin^3 bt)\,dt \tag{9}$$

$$W = \tfrac{1}{2}KV_T^2 + \tfrac{1}{4}K'\,\pi^2 f\,V_T^2 + \tfrac{2}{3}K''\,\pi^2 f^2\,V_T^3 \tag{10}$$

The mean rate of doing work is the work per breath times the frequency of breathing.
Mean rate of work =

$$\tfrac{1}{2}Kf\,V_T^2 + \tfrac{1}{4}K'\,\pi^2(f\,V_T)^2 + \tfrac{2}{3}K''\,\pi^2(f\,V_T)^3 \tag{11}$$

This is the inspiratory work per unit time but if it is assumed that expiration is passive, it is of course an expression of the total work of breathing per unit time as a function of tidal volume and frequency. If the tidal volume is divided into an effective or alveolar portion, V_A, and a dead space portion, V_D, *equation 11* becomes

Work per unit time =

$$\tfrac{1}{2}Kf\left(\frac{\dot{V}_A}{f} + V_D\right)^2 + \tfrac{1}{4}K'\pi^2(\dot{V}_A + fV_D)^2 + \tfrac{2}{3}K''\pi^2(\dot{V}_A + fV_D)^3 \qquad (12)$$

where $V_A f = \dot{V}_A$ = alveolar ventilation.

By *equation 12* the rate of work of breathing can be calculated for any given alveolar ventilation, frequency and dead space. Figure 7 shows the calculated work per minute at various breathing frequencies when the alveolar ventilation is 6 liters per minute and the dead space is assumed to be constant at 200 cc., values which are reasonably typical for a resting subject.

In making these calculations the mean values for K, K' and K'' given in table 1 were converted to appropriate units so that $\dot{V}_A$ could be expressed in liters per minute and f in breaths per minute and rounded off for ease of computation. The equation as used was gm. cm. of work per minute =

$$5000\, f\left(\frac{\dot{V}_A}{f} + 0.2\right)^2 + 150(\dot{V}_A + 0.2f)^2 + 3(\dot{V}_A + 0.2f)^3 \quad (13)$$

Of special interest is the fact, illustrated by this graph, that for a constant alveolar ventilation there is a frequency which is optimal (in the sense of minimal work). This minimum occurs because when the frequency is too low, much elastic work is required to produce the large tidal volumes and when the frequency is too high, much work is uselessly done in ventilating the dead space with each breath.

The fact that the optimal frequency in this case is in the range ordinarily observed in the breathing of resting subjects suggests itself as an example of the principle of minimal effort according to which so many of the body functions seem to be regulated.

By differentiating *equation 12* with respect to f, setting the result equal to 0, and solving for V_A we have the general solution for the conditions of minimal rate of doing work.

$$V_A = \frac{KDf + K'\pi^2 Df^2 + 4K''\pi^2 D^2 f^3}{K - 4K''\pi^2 Df^2} \qquad (14)$$

Various values of f have been substituted in *equation 14* and the resulting curve is shown in figure 8 (curve labeled $W_{min.}$). This curve predicts that the greater the alveolar ventilation, the higher will be the frequency for the condition of minimal work. Since this curve actually applies to the condition of minimal inspiratory work, it can not be accepted for minimal total work unless expiration is completely passive. The curve labeled $W_V + W_T = W_E$ in figure 8 shows the frequency at which the work required for expiration (assuming this is the same as that required to overcome viscous and turbulent resistance of inspiration) becomes equal to the elastic energy stored during inspiration. Conditions represented by the area above this curve will, therefore, require the active participation of the expiratory muscles. For alveolar ventilations greater than about 15 liters per minute, the curve $W_{min.}$, while defining conditions for minimal inspiratory work, will predict frequencies that are too high for minimal work of inspiration plus expiration. The curve $W_V + W_T = W_E$ defines, in a sense, conditions for minimal expiratory work in that it indicates conditions such that the elastic energy stored in inspiration is just enough to meet the needs of expiration. At the higher alveolar ventilations, however, the conditions demanded by this curve become absurd, because the required tidal volume becomes impossibly large. The conditions for a tidal volume of 4 liters are indicated for purposes of illustration, by the line $V_T = 4$.

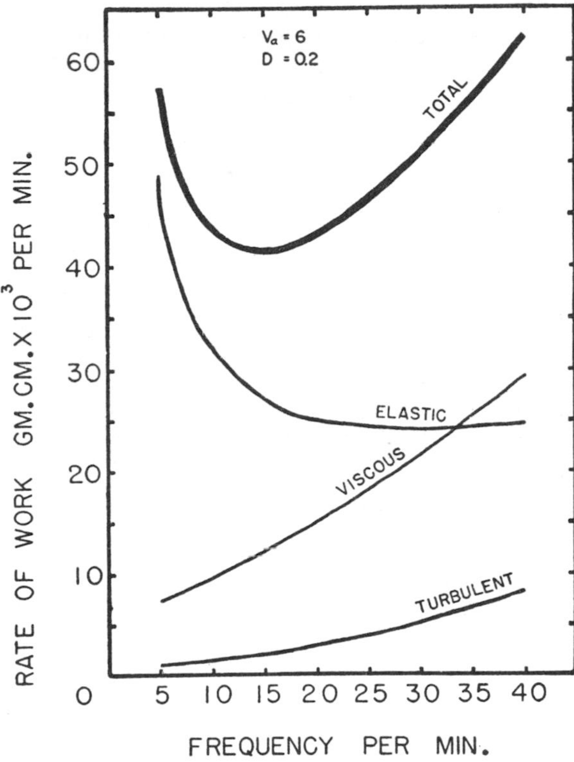

Fig. 7. RELATIONSHIP of elastic, viscous, turbulent, and total work of breathing/min. to frequency of breathing when alveolar ventilation is 6 l/min., and dead space is 200 cc. Curves calculated according to *equation 13*.

One might expect then that for the lower range of ventilations the optimal frequency would be defined by curve $W_{min.}$, but at the higher ventilations the optimal frequencies would lie between the curve $W_V + W_T = W_E$ and the dotted section of curve W_{min}.

Several sets of data from the literature showing frequencies voluntarily chosen by subjects whose breathing was stimulated by added dead space, by CO_2 added to the inspired air, or by exercise bear out this expectation in a general way, as indicated by the plotted points in figure 8.

Although these considerations yield no exact description they do perhaps indicate roughly how various factors may interact to determine the frequency at which we breathe under various ventilatory requirements. It would be desirable, of course, to determine what the exact velocity patterns of inspiration and of expiration should be for optimal conditions. To do this would require a much more involved treatment which is probably not justified without more exact data as a basis.

The above discussion has been predicated on the principle of minimal effort but we do not wish to imply that this is the only principle involved. Another important consideration, especially in unusual situations, might be called the 'principle of maximal comfort.' If a patient with pleurisy, for example, finds that one pattern of breathing is less painful than another, it is likely that he will sacrifice a few calories for the sake of comfort.

Mechanical Efficiency of Breathing. Several investigators (11–13) have estimated the total energy required for breathing at various depths and frequencies by measuring the extra oxygen consumption during hyperpnea either voluntarily produced or stimulated by CO_2 added to the inspired air. The most comprehensive series of such measurements is that of Liljestrand (11), whose data are represented in part by the solid lines in figure 9.

On the same graph are plotted dotted lines representing the mechanical work (calculated by *equation 11*) required for the corresponding conditions of

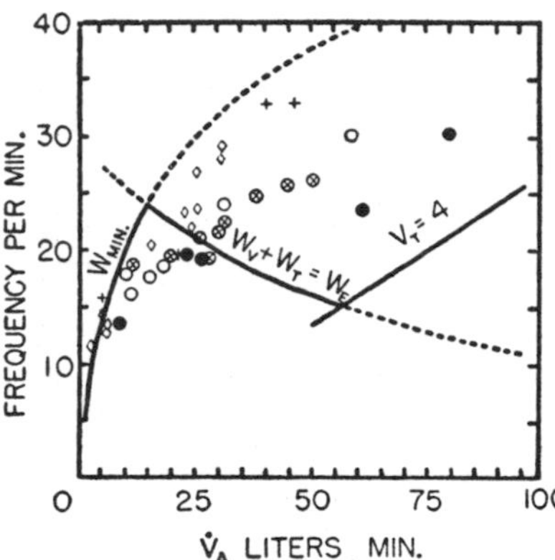

Fig. 8. FACTORS DETERMINING OPTIMAL BREATHING FREQUENCIES for various alveolar ventilations. For explanation of curves, see text. Plotted points represent data from literature as follows: *open circles, subject R.M.*, Barcroft and Margaria (21); *solid circles, subject J.B.*, Barcroft and Margaria (21); *circles with X, subject J.J.*, Lindhard (22); *diamonds, subject I.B.*, Hansen (23); *crosses, subject G.L.*, Liljestrand (11). Alveolar ventilations calculated from recorded total ventilations by assuming dead space of 200 cc.

ventilation and frequency. The scale of ordinates for the calculated mechanical work has been adjusted so that it is equal to 5.4 per cent of that for the extra oxygen consumption. This figure is the average of 19 values obtained by dividing each of Liljestrand's measurements into the mechanical work calculated for the corresponding condition. The individual values for mechanical efficiency obtained in this fashion varied from 3.0 per cent for a frequency of 5 and a ventilation of 20 liters per minute to 7.6 per cent for a frequency of 20 and a ventilation of 30 liters per minute.

This variation in the calculated efficiency is reflected, of course, in the discrepancies between the curves for total energy and those for mechanical work in figure 9, because exact agreement between these two families of curves would require that the calculated efficiency be constant for all conditions.

Part of this apparent variability in efficiency under different conditions can, of course, be attributed to the inexactness of our equation for calculating mechanical work, but part is probably real, since it is well known that the efficiency of muscular work varies with muscle length and load.

In Liljestrand's experiments the breathing was voluntarily regulated and for the most part the tidal-frequency combinations employed were not those that the body naturally chooses (cf. figs. 8 and 9). It is perhaps of significance that the highest calculated efficiency appears for the condition (30 l/min. at a frequency of 20) that most closely corresponds to a naturally occurring one. This suggests that the respiratory apparatus may be so designed that the

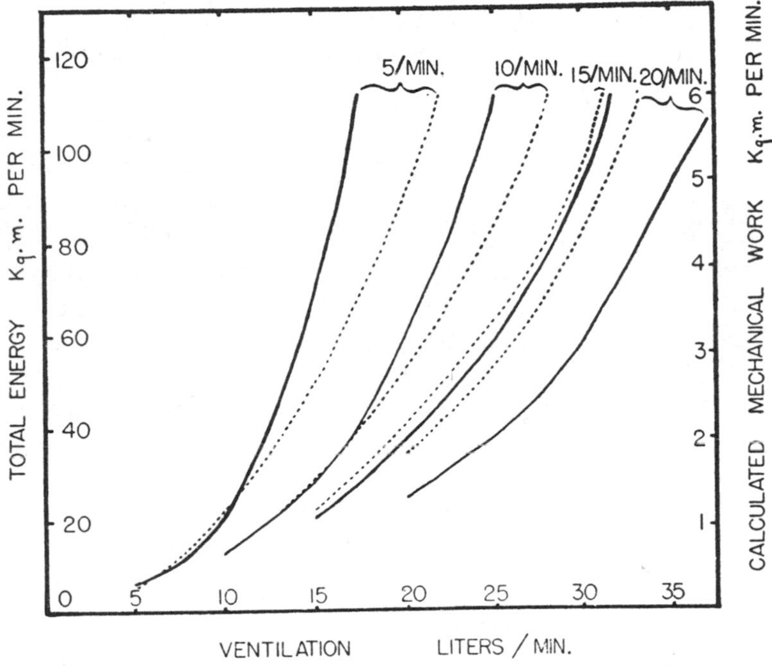

Fig. 9. WORK OF BREATHING at different ventilations and frequencies of breathing. *Left-hand scale of ordinates* refers to solid lines which represent total energy turnover as obtained by conversion of Liljestrand's (11) data for extra oxygen consumption. *Right-hand scale* refers to dotted lines which represent mechanical work calculated from *equation 11*.

conditions for minimal mechanical work are also those for maximal muscular efficiency.

At any rate it would seem that although 5 per cent is a representative efficiency for a considerable range of frequency-tidal combinations, the breathing under normal conditions of regulation may be usually carried out with a higher efficiency, in the order of 8 to 10 per cent.

It might be supposed that the relatively low mechanical efficiency of respiration could be attributed to insufficient opportunity for shortening of the intercostal muscles. Since they are arranged parallel to the circumference of the chest it might be supposed that they would have difficulty in shortening when the chest expands. Actually they are attached to the ribs in such a way that they can shorten an appreciable fraction of their length like any other muscles in the body. It is a general rule that muscles can shorten *in situ* only 50 per cent of the length of the individual fibers and the muscles of respiration are no exception in this respect. Isolated frog muscles, when stimulated, usually shorten, with no load, about one third of their resting length, and give maximal work and maximal efficiency when the load is such as to reduce this shortening to about one sixth. From this point of view, the muscles of respiration must operate under fairly efficient mechanical circumstances.

Maximal Work Obtainable from the Muscles of Breathing. The mechanical work done in the usual resting breathing may be estimated from figure 7 as being in the order of 0.4 to 0.5 kilogram meters per minute. Assuming an efficiency of 5 per cent this corresponds to a total energy requirement of about 0.0234 large calories per minute or 33.7 large calories per day. This amounts to only 1 or 2 per cent of the total resting metabolism; the fuel requirement for 24 hours of quiet breathing is only 10 grams of sugar, a fraction of a candy bar.

For comparison, it is interesting to estimate the maximal work output that can be obtained when the breathing system is operated at full capacity. This estimate may be made by three independent methods, which will now be described.

The maximal ventilation that an individual can perform is in the order of 150 liters per minute carried out at a frequency of 30 per minute. Under these conditions expiration can not be entirely passive, but if one assumes that the same amount of viscous and turbulent resistance must be overcome during expiration as during inspiration, and that the elastic energy stored during inspiration is available to aid expiration then inspiratory work rate can be calculated by *equation 11* and expiratory work rate by:

Rate of expiratory work =

$$\tfrac{1}{4}K'\pi^2(fV_T)^2 + \tfrac{2}{3}K''\pi^2(fV_T)^3 - \tfrac{1}{2}KfV_T^2 \qquad (15)$$

The total work per unit time is the sum of *equations 11* and *15*, or

Work rate =

$$\tfrac{1}{2}K'\pi^2(fV_T)^2 + \tfrac{4}{3}K''\pi^2(fV_T)^3 \qquad (16)$$

By *equation 16* it is calculated that the mechanical work required for maximal ventilation is 270 kilogram meters per minute or 9.0 kilogram meters per breath.

Another approach is to estimate the potential energy available for maximal inspiration and expiration from figure 1 of Rahn, Otis, Chadwick and Fenn (8) which shows the maximal inspiratory and expiratory forces available at various lung volumes. The total area bounded by the curves for these maximal forces gives the theoretical maximal work available during a single cycle consisting of a maximal inspiration and expiration. This method yields an estimate of 10.4 kilogram meters.

The maximal muscular forces available may also be estimated from anatomical data relating to the length, cross sectional area, and degree of shortening of the respiratory muscles. According to von Ebener (14) the lengths of the external and internal intercostals are 1.3 cm. and 1.6 cm. respectively, and in a full inflation or deflation of the chest the degree of shortening is about one eighth to one fourth of the muscle length for the former and one third to one half for the latter. The total cross sectional area of all the internal intercostals on one side of the chest is given by Weber, cited from Strasser (15, p. 143) as 97 $cm.^2$, and the corresponding figure for the external intercostals is 47 cm^2. Taking the force of contraction of these muscles as being similar to that for other human muscles (about 10 kg/cm^2 cross section) we have calculated the maximal work and entered the value in table 3, where the estimates by the other two methods are shown for comparison.

The value from the area of the *P-V* diagram is probably the most reliable

Table 3. Maximal work available for breathing

METHOD OF ESTIMATION	WORK/BREATH	WORK/MIN. AT 30 BREATHS/MIN.
	kg. m.	*kg. m.*
Equation 16	9.0	270
Area of P-V diagram	10.4	312
Anatomical data	8.0 – 13.5	240 – 405

since it is based on actual measurements on 15 individuals. The estimate by *equation 16* is of course a large extrapolation from rather scanty data and involves numerous assumptions. The calculation from the anatomical data must also be considered as only approximate. The work of the diaphragm is omitted from this calculation because we do not have the necessary data.

Considering the admittedly rough methods involved, the similarity of these values is quite gratifying and gives one confidence that the estimates are at least of the correct order of magnitude.

It is interesting to note that although the maximal ventilation is only about 15 to 20 times the resting ventilation, the rate of work required is about 500 times greater for the former. Of course, this maximal work output can be kept up for only short periods of time, but the margin of safety provided for emergencies is impressively large.

COMMENT

The above presentation should be regarded as only an approximate overall picture of the respiratory apparatus considered from the mechanical point of view along the lines sketched by Rohrer (3). Experimentally, the most inexactly estimated factor is probably the value for the non-elastic resistance of tissue since this determination was based on the assumption that the subjects were able voluntarily to relax completely and to permit the respirator to do all the work. Complete passivity is most likely not attained under these conditions, and the overlapping of the two sets of data shown in figures 3 and 5 is probably in part a manifestation of this inability to relax completely. Wirz (16) was able to describe the non-elastic resistance of the dog lung by an equation of the same form as our *equation 4* but he obtained negative values for the constant k_4. According to Bayliss and Robertson (6) and Dean and Visscher (7) at least a part of the non-elastic resistance of the lung is independent of velocity. For these various reasons we do not have confidence in the actual values obtained in our evaluation of non-elastic resistance of tissue. It seems likely, however, that we may have overestimated rather than underestimated the magnitude of this factor.

The approach employed in this analysis of the work of breathing, with emphasis on energy relationships and efficiency, is not to be justified so much by the importance of the magnitude of the work, which is generally relatively small, but rather as an aid in clarifying the interrelationship of some of the various factors involved.

In a more detailed analysis many factors would have to be included that are here omitted. For example, there is now good evidence that ventilation to various parts of the lungs is unequal (17, 18). It is also recognized that for optimal conditions of gas exchange a certain relationship should be maintained between blood flow and ventilation (19, 20). Since the breathing apparatus is a blood pump as well as an air pump, it may play an important part in the regulation of this ventilation/blood flow ratio. Certain patterns of breathing may be more efficient than others in this regard, and the selection by the body of particular tidal-frequency combinations may be related to this function.

Further study of respiratory mechanics should include investigation of the more detailed behavior of the respiratory muscles, their sequence of contraction and the behavior of the lungs in producing inequalities of ventilation. The work done by the breathing apparatus in moving blood as well as air should be evaluated, and the relationship between the pattern of air flow and that of blood flow should be considered.

SUMMARY

Relaxed human subjects were ventilated by a Drinker respirator while the velocity of respired gas flow and the pressure gradient between the mouth of the subject and the inside of the respirator were continuously and simultaneously recorded. From such experiments elastic resistance and total resistance to breathing were estimated. Resistance related to moving gas through the respiratory tract was measured on the same subjects by the method of interruptions. From the experimental data equations are derived that give an approximate description of the human breathing apparatus as a mechanical system. These equations permit the estimation of the work of breathing under various conditions, optimal frequencies of breathing, maximal mechanical work output of the respiratory muscles, and mechanical efficiency.

The authors wish to acknowledge the cooperation of Dr. Donald Proctor in some of the preliminary experiments and to thank Mr. William Doherty for technical assistance.

REFERENCES

1. Rohrer, F. *Arch. f. d. ges. Physiol.* 162: 225, 1915.
2. Rohrer, F. *Arch. f. d. ges. Physiol.* 165: 419, 1916.
3. Rohrer, F. *Handbuch der normalen und pathologischen Physiologie.* Berlin: Julius Springer, 1925, vol. 2, p. 70.
4. v. Neergaard, K. and K. Wirz. *Ztschr. f. klin. Med.* 105: 52, 1927.
5. Vuilleumier, P. *Ztschr. f. klin. Med.* 143: 698, 1944.
6. Bayliss, L. E. and G. W. Robertson. *Quart. J. Exper. Physiol.* 29: 27, 1939.
7. Dean, R. B. and M. B. Visscher. *Am. J. Physiol.* 134: 450, 1941.
8. Rahn, H., A. B. Otis, L. E. Chadwick and W. O. Fenn. *Am. J. Physiol.* 146: 161, 1946.
9. Otis, A. B. and D. F. Proctor. *Am. J. Physiol.* 152: 106, 1948.
10. Otis, A. B. and W. C. Bembower. *J. Applied Physiol.* 2: 300, 1949.
11. Liljestrand, G. *Skandinav. Arch. f. Physiol.* 35: 199, 1918.
12. Muller, E. A., H. Michaelis and A. Muller. *Arbeitsphysiol.* 12: 192, 1942.
13. Neilsen, M. *Skandinav. Arch. f. Physiol.* 74: 299, 1936.
14. von Ebner, V. *Arch. f. Anat. u. Physiol.* 4: 185, 1880.
15. Strasser, H. *Lehrbuch der Muskel und Gelenkmechanik.* Berlin: Julius Springer, 1908, vol. 2.
16. Wirz, K. *Arch. f. d. ges. Physiol.* 199: 1, 1923.
17. Fowler, W. S. *J. Applied Physiol.* 2: 283, 1949.
18. Rauwerda, P. E. *Unequal Ventilation of Different Parts of the Lung.* Thesis. Holland: Univ. Groningen, 1946.
19. Rahn, H. *Am. J. Physiol.* 158: 21, 1949.
20. Riley, R. L. and A. Cournand. *J. Applied Physiol.* 1: 12, 1949.
21. Barcroft, J. and R. Margaria. *J. Physiol.* 72: 175, 1931.
22. Lindhard, J. *Arch. f. d. ges. Physiol.* 161: 233, 1915.
23. Hansen, E. *Skandinav. Arch. f. Physiol.* 54: 50, 1928.

21

Physical Properties of Human Lungs Measured During Spontaneous Respiration[1]

JERE MEAD AND JAMES L. WHITTENBERGER. *From the Department of Physiology, Harvard School of Public Health, Boston, Massachusetts*

[*Editor's Note:* In the original, material precedes this excerpt.]

Methods of Analysis of the Measured Quantities

In this paper, elasticity-like properties are described in terms of volume change in liters per elasticity-like pressure difference change in centimeters of water. This ratio is the inverse of elastance, as defined by Bayliss and Robertson, and hence is compliance (C). This method of expressing the elasticity-like properties of the system has been chosen because the ordinary connotation of the term compliance has an implied polarity which elastance lacks. (The electrical analogue of compliance is capacitance.) In describing the nonelastic properties of the system, the nonelastic pressure differences are related to rates of volume change (gas flow rates). The ratio of nonelastic pressure difference (in centimeters of water) to the corresponding rate of flow (in liters/second) will be termed mechanical resistance (R). The terms viscous resistance and viscance are avoided since they imply that viscosity is the only property involved. The theoretical aspects of this analysis are essentially the same as those described by Rohrer and others.

Lung Compliance (C_L). At any instant during a respiratory cycle

$$\Delta P_L = \Delta P_{C_L} + \Delta P_{R_L} + \Delta P_{I_L} \qquad (1)$$

where ΔP_L is the instantaneous value for the total pressure difference from the airway opening to the surface of the lungs; ΔP_{C_L} = the pressure difference related to elastic forces, and hence is some function of volume (V); ΔP_{R_L} is the instantaneous pressure difference related to resistance forces, and hence is some function of the rate of volume change ($\dot{V}$); and ΔP_{I_L} is the instantaneous pressure difference related to inertial forces and hence is some function of the volume acceleration ($\ddot{V}$).

Equation 1 may be rewritten:

$$\Delta P_L = f(V) + f(\dot{V}) + f(\ddot{V}) \qquad (2)$$

The last term is dropped from the further analysis since under the conditions of the experiments it was considered to be of negligible magnitude. Experimental evidence supporting this simplification will be presented.

At instants during the respiratory cycle of zero volume change, that is at the volume extremes at end-inspiration and end-expiration, *equation 2* becomes

$$\Delta P_L = f(V) = \Delta P_{C_L} \qquad (3)$$

If the values of ΔP_L and the corresponding values of V are obtained for a range of tidal volumes taking end-expiration as 0 volume, a plot of $\Delta P = f(V)$ may be obtained. This is accomplished utilizing a cathode-ray oscilloscope as a co-ordinate plotting device with a voltage proportional to ΔP impressed on the X axis and that corresponding to V on the Y axis. In this case a single respiration takes the form of a closed loop (fig. 1*A*), the Y axis extremes representing the points of 0 flow. If with a series of respirations of differing depth the volume extremes can be shown to fall approximately along a straight line, this portion of the total plot of $\Delta P_L = f(V)$ can be expressed as

$$\Delta P_{C_L} = KV \qquad (4)$$

If compliance is volume/pressure difference, it may be seen that in that part of the curve defined by *equation 4*, the compliance is constant and is equal to $1/K$ (K representing the elastance).

Lung Mechanical Resistance (R). Considering the expression

$$\Delta P_L = \Delta P_{C_L} + \Delta P_{R_L} \qquad (5)$$

where $\Delta P_{C_L} = f(V)$ and $\Delta P_{R_L} = f(\dot{V})$, if $\Delta P_{C_L} = f(V)$ is known, ΔP_{R_L} may be solved for and the relationship $\Delta P_{R_L} = f(\dot{V})$ expressed. The solution is simplified if in the tidal range studied C_L can be shown to be about constant. In this case by substituting $\frac{1}{C_L} \cdot V$ for ΔP_{C_L} in 5 and transposing:

$$\Delta P_{R_L} = \Delta P_L - \frac{1}{C_L} \cdot V \qquad (6)$$

Since instantaneous values for ΔP_L, V, and $\dot{V}$ are available and C_L may be measured, a plot of $\Delta P_{R_L} = f(\dot{V})$ may be made.

In practice this is accomplished by utilizing the cathode-ray oscilloscope as a co-ordinate plotting device; $\dot{V}$ appears on the Y axis and ΔP_L on the X axis. A single respiration again takes the form of a closed loop. The points of intersection of the loop with the X axis correspond to the points of zero flow occurring between the phases of respiration. The distance along the X axis between the points of X axis intersection then must equal ΔP_{C_L}. If now a voltage proportional to V is impressed on the X axis plates so as to subtract from the ΔP_L voltage and the 'gain' of the V voltage is gradually increased from zero gain, the points of X axis intersection can be made to approach each other. When the 'gain' is adjusted so that the points of X axis intersection are superimposed, the subtracting voltage must equal $\Delta P_{C_L} = \frac{1}{C_L}.V$. The 'gain' setting is equivalent to the constant $\frac{1}{C_L}$. Thus an electrical solution of *equation 6* is obtained. At points of zero flow ΔP_{R_L} = 0. At all other points ΔP_{R_L} is represented by the abscissal distance from the zero flow point. Since $\dot{V}$ is expressed on the Y axis, a plot of $\Delta P_{R_L} = f(\dot{V})$ is obtained. As illustrated in figure 1*B*, the resulting plot consists of a curve which is essentially a single line for inspiration, and a similar curve opposite in sign for expiration. The mechanical resistance in $\Delta P/\dot{V}$ for any point on the curve is represented by the inverse slope of a straight line drawn from the origin through that point.

TABLE 1. LUNG COMPLIANCE IN 10 ADULT SUBJECTS

Subject	Sex	Age	Ht.	Wt.	V.C.	Compliance
		yr.	*cm.*	*kg*	*l*	*l/cm H_2O*
J. A.	M	33	162	61	4.86	0.20
M. B.	F	25	173	56	3.90	0.25
G. G.	M	34	183	81	5.25	0.26
S. K.	F	23	165	61	3.68	0.19
L. S.	F	25	158	50	3.48	0.18
D. T.	M	25	180	75	5.4	0.20
J. L. W.	M	38	187	86	6.85	0.30
E. B.	M	27	179	74	6.4	0.24
T. F.	F	24	161	58	3.28	0.14
J. M.	M	32	187	86	6.1	0.29
Mean						0.225

[*Editor's Note:* Material has been omitted at this point.]

DISCUSSION

In 10 healthy young adults, seated and with the esophageal balloon placed in the lowest fifth of the esophagus, the elastic component of intraesophageal pressure variation was found to be approximately linearly related to volume change over the midrange of lung volume change. Expressing this relationship in terms of compliance, the mean value for the 10 individuals was 0.225. Table 2 summarizes the results of previous workers, expressed in terms of compliance. This table is an extension of the table presented by Otis, Rahn and Fenn (15).

The low values reported by Christie and McIntosh (3) and Paine (5) are, at least in part, the result of their failure to obtain pressure measurement at instants of zero air flow. The inclusion of a resistance component of pressure difference would yield values for compliance lower than true static values.

It is difficult to find previous data on human lung resistance for comparison with our results. The calculations of Rohrer (16) concerned only the air-flow resistance of the respiratory tract. Furthermore, as has been pointed out by Gaensler (17), Rohrer made a dimensional error in his calculation of critical velocities which lead to the incorrect assumption that flow is laminar throughout the respiratory tract.

TABLE 2. COMPARISON OF HUMAN LUNG COMPLIANCE FROM OTHER WORKERS

Investigator	No. of Subjects	Lung Compliance *l/cm* H_2O
Rohrer (16)	Based on Donders' measurements on cadavers	0.22
v Neergaard and Wirz (2)	1 Tuberculous 1 Emphysematous	0.13 0.18
Christie and McIntosh (3)	5	0.08
Paine (5)	8	0.09
Otis, Rahn and Fenn (15)	8	0.21
Buytendijk (7)		0.22–0.33
Stead *et al.* (18)	10	0.23

Respiratory tract air-flow-resistance measurements in man have been reported by investigators (19, 13, 20) employing the technique of airway interruption for assessing alveolar pressure as developed by Neergaard and Wirz (19). In general, the resistances reported are somewhat greater than those reported here. We have compared resistance values obtained in the same individuals by the techniques of airway interruption and the method employed in the present investigation. These studies along with theoretical considerations lead us to conclude that the interrupter method does not afford a measure of respiratory tract air flow resistance, but rather approximates in normal subjects total lung resistance, i.e. air flow plus tissue resistance (21).

In the analysis of pulmonary compliance and resistance, the central assumption is made that the pressure recorded at the instant of zero air flow separating the phases of the respiratory cycle relates only to the elastic properties of the system. Corollaries of this assumption are that pressures relating to mass acceleration are negligible and that the system is truly 'static' at the instant of zero flow as measured by the pneumotachograph, i.e. that gas and tissue flow within the lungs has ceased. Furthermore, it is implied that the elastic forces are dependent only on the volume of the system and are independent of time.

The validity of these assumptions within the limits of function studied is best brought out by a consideration of the results obtained in the lung resistance measurements. Here the assumptions are implicit in the method used for subtracting the elastic component of pressure change, where a voltage equal to $(1/C) \cdot V$ is considered to define the elastic pressure. When this subtraction is accomplished during quiet respiration, the pressure points at zero flow become superimposed. The extent to which this superimposition is maintained under conditions of varied respiratory pattern, both in terms of rate and depth, is a measure of the validity of these assumptions. In general this superimposition was very closely maintained as long as the volume change remained within the range over which the measured compliance was constant. Figure 7 above is an illustration of this. In the 6 inspirations reproduced, the tidal volumes were between 0.5–1.0 liter produced from resting mid-position. The duration of the inspirations varied between 0.25 and 1.3 sec. with peak flow rates ranging from about 0.5–3 l/sec., and volume accelerations at the instants of zero flow ranging from +40 to +800 l/sec.^{2} at the beginning of the inspirations to −40 to −1000 l/sec.^{2} at the end of the inspiration.

Although the expression $\Delta P_{C_L} = (1/C)\Delta V$ seems to define the over-all elastic behavior of the lungs in the midrange of lung-volume change in the normal individuals studied, it should be emphasized that such an expression is by no means a complete expression of lung elastic behavior. Inasmuch as it is an incremental expression, it contains no information as to the absolute relationships of pressure and volume. For expression in absolute terms, information as to the percentage change of volume and pressure from the collapsed, i.e. unstressed, state would be necessary. Furthermore, the elastic behavior outside of the range of approximate linearity is undefined, and the time independence of compliance is established only over a short time span. An additional factor, namely the possible influence of the previous 'volume history' on elastic behavior, is unexplored in these measurements. In view of the importance of this factor in known elastomeric behavior of tissues, it is probable that failure to observe any such phenomena relates to the relatively limited range of stress encountered in these experiments as well as to the lack of precision of the measuring techniques.

Summary

A technique permitting analysis of the physical properties of the lungs simultaneously with respiration in spontaneously breathing human subjects is described in which variation in intraesophageal pressure is utilized as a measure of variation in intrapleural pressure. Lung compliance was found to have a mean value of 0.22/cm of water over the midrange of lung volume change in 9 healthy young adults. Lung resistance expressed in terms of centimeters of water/liter/second was found to have a mean value of 2 in 7 subjects at a flow of 1 l/sec. The curvilinear relationship of flow to the resistance component of pressure variation was found to be closely approximated by the expression $\Delta P_R = K_1\dot{V} + K_2\dot{V}^2$ up to flow of 2 l/sec., mean values for K_1 and K_2 being 1.74 and 0.28 in 7 subjects. Lung resistance was found to be inversely related to lung volume over the vital capacity range in 3 normal subjects, the order of magnitude of change being approximately twofold. Lung resistance was found to be approximately the same for the inspiratory and expiratory phases except during rapid respiration where inspiratory resistance continued to fit the parabolic expression as defined during less rapid respiration, while expiratory resistance transiently showed as much as twentyfold increase from these levels.

The authors have been aided by the contributions of a number of individuals. Robert A. Waters suggested the use of linear differential transformers in the construction of the pressure transducers. W. J. Mead designed and constructed the transducer units. Arthur Miller designed much of the electronic equipment. The excised tracheal resistance plots were obtained with the assistance of E. P. Radford, Jr. The authors are also grateful for a very cooperative group of test subjects.

REFERENCES

1. Rohrer, F. *Nomalen und path. Physiol.* 2: 70, 1925.
2. von Neergaard, K. and K. Wirz. *Ztschr. klin. Med.* 105: 35, 1927.
3. Christie, R. V. and C. A. McIntosh. *J. Clin. Investigation* 13: 279, 1934.
4. Bayliss, L. E. and G. W. Robertson. *Quart. J. Exper. Physiol.* 29: 27, 1939.
5. Paine, J. R. *J. Thoracic Surg.* 9: 550, 1940.
6. Dean, R. B. and M. B. Visscher. *Am. J. Physiol.* 134: 450, 1941.
7. Buytendijk, H. J. Electrische Drukkerij. Groningen: Oppenheim, N. V., 1949, vol. I.
8. Otis, A. B., W. O. Fenn, and H. Rahn. *J. Applied Physiol.* 2: 592, 1950.
9. Dayman, H. *J. Clin. Investigation* 30: 1175, 1951.
10. Lawton, R. W. and D. Joslin. *Am. J. Physiol.* 167: 111, 1951.
11. Fry, D. L., W. W. Stead, R. V. Ebert, R. I. Zubin and H. S. Wells. *J. Lab. & Clin. Med.* 40: 664, 1952.
12. Silverman, L. and J. L. Whittenberger. *Methods in Medical Research.* J. H. Comroe, Jr., (editor in chief). Chicago: Yr. Bk. Pub., 1950, vol. 2, p. 104.
13. Otis, A. B. and D. F. Proctor. *Am. J. Physiol.* 152: 106, 1948.
14. di Rienzo, S. *Radiology* 53: 168, 1949.
15. Otis, A. B., H. Rahn and W. O. Fenn. *Am. J. Physiol.* 146: 307, 1946.
16. Rohrer, F. *Arch. ges. Physiol. (Pflügers)* 162: 225, 1915.
17. Gaensler, E. A. and J. V. Maloney, Jr. *J. Lab. & Clin. Med.* 39: 935, 1952.
18. Stead, W. W., D. L. Fry, and R. V. Ebert. *J. Lab. & Clin. Med.* 40: 674, 1952.
19. von Neergaard, K. and K. Wirz. *Ztschr. klin. Med.* 105: 51, 1927.
20. Vuilleumier, P. *Ztschr. klin. Med.* 143: 698, 1944.
21. Mead, J. and J. L. Whittenberger. In preparation.

22

Reprinted by permission of the American Physiological Society from *J. Appl. Physiol.*, **8**(4), 427–443 (1956)

Mechanical Factors in Distribution of Pulmonary Ventilation[1, 2]

ARTHUR B. OTIS, COLIN B. McKERROW, RICHARD A. BARTLETT, JERE MEAD, M. B. McILROY, N. J. SELVERSTONE[3] AND E. P. RADFORD, JR. *From the Department of Surgery, The Johns Hopkins University School of Medicine, Baltimore, Maryland and the Department of Physiology, Harvard School of Public Health, Boston, Massachusetts*

THIS paper is presented jointly from two laboratories since it involves identical theoretical concepts arising simultaneously and independently, albeit from different approaches by the two teams of investigators. The Boston group had made the observation that the compliance of the lungs of patients with pulmonary emphysema appeared to change with the frequency of breathing (1), and the possibility occurred to them that this phenomenon and the uneven ventilation associated with this disease might have a common mechanical basis. The Baltimore group was likewise searching for a possible mechanical basis for the phenomenon of uneven alveolar ventilation which had been well demonstrated in other laboratories (2, 3) by experiments showing nonuniform distribution of various relatively insoluble reference gases.

With regard to the latter problem, our thinking has proceeded from the hypothesis that uneven ventilation involves temporal as well as spatial differences in the distribution of gas flow in the various units of the lung (cf. 'sequential ventilation' of Fowler (2)). Temporal and spatial differences in the volume change in various parts of the lungs might conceivably arise from either of two situations. In the first place, one might postulate that all pulmonary pathways are mechanically similar, but that the driving force (intrapleural pressure surrounding them) is not the same for all. Evidence for local variations in intrapleural pressure has appeared in the literature (4). A second possibility, and one which forms the basis of this report, is that the lungs are composed of a population of elements or pathways which are not all similar mechanically and that because of these mechanical differences they operate asynchronously even when subjected to the same driving force. The existence of local variations in driving force is not precluded, but it is not necessary to postulate it.

Similarly, in considering a possible explanation for the observations that the compliance of the lungs as a whole may alter with frequency of breathing, one might postulate that the compliance of the individual pathways varies with frequency. One might then be led to search for some reflex or other physiological mechanism responsible for the change. On the other hand, if one postulates a population of pathways the mechanical properties of which are dissimilar but invariant with frequency, it can be shown that the behavior of the overall system would be expected to vary with frequency of breathing even though the fundamental properties of each component remain unchanged.

In the pages that follow we shall first develop the latter concept theoretically, and then indicate graphically some of its possible implications by presenting results of experiments with a mechanical model. Next some experiments on human subjects will be described, and the results interpreted in light of the theory. Finally, the possible importance of this concept in connection with the intrapulmonary distribution of inspired gas will be discussed.

THEORY

Rohrer (5) was the first to show that the volume-elastic and flow-resistive properties

Received for publication July 5, 1955.

[1] The study at the Johns Hopkins University School of Medicine was supported by funds provided under Contract AF 18(600)-342 with the U.S.A.F. School of Aviation Medicine, Randolph Field, Texas.

[2] The study at the Harvard School of Public Health was aided by a grant from the National Foundation for Infantile Paralysis, Incorporated.

[3] Work performed during the tenure of a Fellowship in the Medical Sciences administered by the National Research Council for the Rockefeller Foundation.

of the lungs could be analyzed by separating the pressure to which the lungs are subjected into its static and dynamic components. The relationship between pressure, volume and flow may be expressed algebraically. One such expression, similar to that used by Otis, Fenn and Rahn (6) is as follows:

$$\Delta P = KelV + K_1\dot{V} + K_2\dot{V}^2 \qquad (1)$$

where ΔP is the pressure difference across the lung, Kel is the ratio of pressure change to the volume change (V) measured at instants of no air flow, and the remainder of the expression represents the pressure-flow characteristics of the airway and tissue resistance in the range of lung volume, V, ($\dot{V}$ expressing the rate of flow).

It is possible to construct a model with a single volume-elastic unit and a single flow-resistance unit (e.g. a rubber bellows connected to a glass tube) which conforms mechanically to expression 1, and indeed, for purposes of simplicity, it is sometimes useful to think of the lungs as a whole in terms of such a system. As we shall attempt to show, however, this simple description is, under some circumstances, inadequate when applied to the lungs as a whole, although we shall assume that it is generally valid for any single pulmonary pathway of which the lungs are composed.

In this theoretical analysis the following assumptions have been made: *a*) the lungs are made up of many separate pathways, each with its own flow-resistive and volume-elastic properties; *b*) inertial factors are negligible up to a frequency of 2 cps (7); *c*) the resistive and elastic characteristics of each pathway are linear (i.e. K_2 of *equation 1* is zero); *d*) the pressure changes to which the lungs are subjected may be approximated by sine waves; *e*) the pressure changes to which the individual pathways are subjected are the same as, or directly proportional to, the overall pressure changes for the lungs. Having made these assumptions, it is possible to make certain predictions about the mechanical behavior of the lungs using techniques developed to account for the behavior of electrical circuits.

Behavior of a Single Pathway. Subject to the above approximations a single pulmonary pathway may be regarded mechanically as consisting of a volume-elastic part having a *compliance*, C, and a part having a *resistance*, R, in series (see fig. 1*A*). By definition

$$C = \frac{V}{P_1} \qquad (2)$$

$$R = \frac{P_2}{\dot{V}} \qquad (3)$$

where V is the volume at a given pressure difference P_1 across the compliance, and $\dot{V}$ is the flow produced by a given pressure difference P_2 across the resistance. These equations are analogous to equations which define electrical capacitance and electrical resistance, respectively. If the total pressure across the system at any moment is ΔP, then

$$\Delta P = \frac{1}{C} V + R\dot{V} \qquad (4)$$

This expression is *equation 1* expressed in terms of compliance and a linear resistance (Kel = 1/C; K_1 = R and K_2 = 0). Since the compliance and resistance of a single pathway are constants, the total pressure will be determined at any instant by the volume of the unit and the rate and direction of flow at that instant. If the volume is undergoing cyclic variation in a particular pattern, it is possible to describe the associated pattern of applied pressure by solving *equation 4* at successive points during the cycle. On the other hand, if the pattern of applied pressure is known, it is not possible in general to construct the associated pattern of volume change from *equation 4* in any simple fashion. In this analysis the latter solution was desired. This was accomplished by limiting the form of the pressure pattern to a sine wave and applying equations which have been developed by electrical engi-

TABLE 1. ANALOGOUS QUANTITIES IN MECHANICAL AND ELECTRICAL SYSTEMS

Mechanical			Electrical		
Quantity	Symbol	Units	Quantity	Symbol	Units
Volume	V	liter	Charge	Q	coulomb
Flow	$\dot{V}$	l/sec	Current	I	ampere
Pressure	P	cm H_2O	Voltage	E	volt
Resistance	R	cm H_2O/l/sec	Resistance	R	ohm
Compliance	C	l/cm H_2O	Capacitance	C	farad

neers to describe the behavior of analogous electrical circuits.

Our hypothetical pulmonary pathway is analogous to an electrical circuit consisting of a capacitor and a resistor connected in series (shown at right in fig. 1*A*)[4]. If such a system is subjected to a sinusoidally varying driving pressure, then

$$\Delta P = \Delta Pm \sin 2\pi ft \qquad (5)$$

where $\Delta Pm = \frac{1}{2}$ the amplitude of the driving pressure, f = the frequency, and t = time. (ΔP can be considered as varying around a mean pressure which in a volume-elastic system must be greater than zero if complete collapse is to be avoided. This mean pressure, along with the compliance of the unit, determines the mean volume or 'mid-position' of the system, but does not enter into the present analysis, since it does not influence the relationship between the imposed pressure variation and the resulting volume variation.)

The flow, $\dot{V}$, will vary as follows:

$$\dot{V} = \dot{V}m \sin (2\pi ft + \theta) \qquad (6)$$

where

$$\dot{V}m = \frac{\Delta Pm}{\sqrt{R^2 + \left(\frac{1}{2\pi fC}\right)^2}} \qquad (6A)$$

and

$$\theta = \tan^{-1} \frac{1}{2\pi fRC} \qquad (6B)$$

That is to say the flow pattern will also be a sine wave but will lead the pressure curve in time by an amount indicated by the magnitude of the *phase angle* θ. As the equation shows, θ depends on the frequency, the compliance, and the resistance. Increasing either f, C or R diminishes the phase angle between the driving pressure and the resulting flow. If the system were a purely elastic one with no resistance, the phase angle would be 90°, i.e. the flow would lead the pressure by $\frac{1}{4}$ cycle. If the system had no elasticity (infinite compliance), which would be equivalent electrically to a short across the capacitor, then the phase angle would be 0° and flow and pressure would be exactly in phase. At very high frequencies θ approaches 0° and pressure and flow are nearly in phase. At very low frequencies θ approaches 90°, and flow leads pressure by nearly $\frac{1}{4}$ cycle.

[4] The reader is referred to text books of electrical engineering for the derivation of many of the equations used in this analysis. The analogous quantities are listed for convenience in table 1.

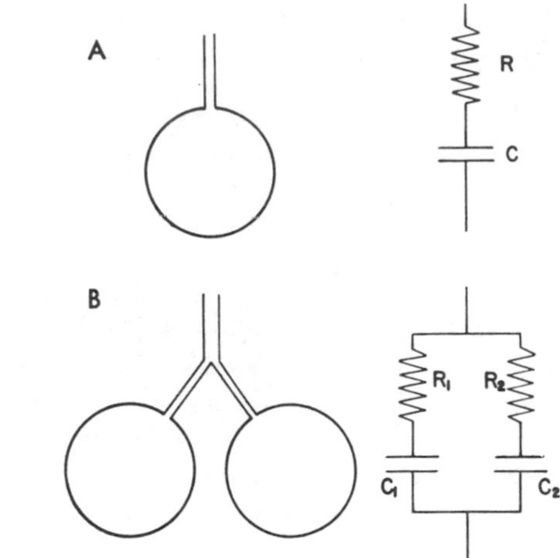

FIG. 1. *A*, Analogy between a single pulmonary pathway and an electrical circuit consisting of a resistor and condenser connected in series. *B*, mechanical and electrical analogies of two pulmonary pathways connected in parallel.

The tidal volume is given by the integral of *equation 6* between the limits $\frac{2\pi - \theta}{2\pi f}$ and $\frac{\pi - \theta}{2\pi f}$.

$$V_T = \frac{\Delta Pm}{\pi f \sqrt{R^2 + \left(\frac{1}{2\pi fC}\right)^2}} \qquad (7)$$

For a given pressure amplitude, tidal volume will decrease with an increase in R and increase with an increase in C. Increasing the frequency with Pm constant will diminish tidal volume.

The product, RC, which appears in *equation 6B*, has the dimension of time, and is called the *time constant* of the system. The larger the time constant, the smaller will be the phase angle between pressure and flow. The temporal behavior of a single pulmonary element in response to a given sinusoidal driving pressure is therefore a function of its time constant.

Rearrangement of *equation 6A* shows that the quantity

$$\sqrt{R^2 + \left(\frac{1}{2\pi fC}\right)^2}$$

expresses the amplitude ratio of pressure and flow. In a purely resistive system this ratio defines the resistance of the system. In a system which includes volume-elasticity as well as resistance, this ratio is called the *impedance* of the system, Z. By inspection it may be seen that at high frequencies the impedance approaches the flow resistance, while at low frequencies the impedance depends increasingly on the compliance of the system.

For a given pressure amplitude the peak flow rate depends on Z. Increasing R will diminish peak flow; increasing C will increase it. Increasing f, with Pm constant, will increase the peak flow.

It is important to note that if the expression

$$\dot{V} = \frac{P}{Z} \qquad (8)$$

is used to calculate flow from a known pressure curve, only the magnitude of flow curve is obtained. To specify flow completely in its correct temporal relationship to pressure, the amount by which it leads the pressure curve must also be stated in terms of its phase angle, θ.

For this purpose use is often made of the *vector impedance*

$$\bar{Z} = Z \underline{|\theta} \qquad (9)$$

where Z indicates the relative magnitudes of the flow and pressure amplitude (*equation 8*), and θ indicates the phase of flow with respect to pressure.

If impedance is expressed in this fashion then

$$\dot{V} = \frac{P}{\bar{Z}} \qquad (9A)$$

In this equation the relationship between flow and pressure is expressed with regard to phase relationship as well as magnitude.

An alternative method of expressing the vector impedance, and one which is especially useful for certain numerical calculations as will be shown later, is in terms of the complex number:

$$\bar{Z} = R - j\frac{1}{2\pi fC} \qquad (10)$$

where $j = \sqrt{-1}$

In such calculations use will be made of the reciprocal relationships $1/Z$ or $1/\bar{Z}$ which are known as the *admittance* and *vector admittance*, respectively.

Behavior of Pulmonary Elements in Parallel. The mechanical and electrical analogues of two pulmonary pathways connected in parallel are shown schematically in figure 1*B*. If such a system is subjected to a sinusoidal driving pressure each pathway behaves in accordance with the equations given in the previous section.

In such a network, consisting of two or more separate pathways in parallel, the distribution of the overall flow in the separate pathways and the timing of the flow events depends on the distribution of the impedance of the separate pathways.

If the separate impedances are identical they will all operate exactly in phase with each other and the magnitude of the total admittance will be the simple arithmetic sum of the separate admittances.

$$\frac{1}{Z} = \frac{1}{Z_1} + \frac{1}{Z_2} \qquad (11)$$

From this it follows that the volume flowing during a complete cycle in the pathway common to the whole system will be the sum of the volume flowing in the component pathways.

With a change in frequency the separate impedances will show identical changes, the proportional distribution of flow will remain unaltered, and the timing of events for any single pathway will always be the same as the timing for the entire network.

This will also be true if the impedance of the separate pathways are not the same, but change proportionately with frequency. In this case the distribution of impedance will also remain unchanged with frequency, and the timing of pressure and flow events will be the same for all pathways at a given frequency.

It can be shown (APPENDIX I) that the proportionate change of impedance with frequency is the same in different pathways if the time constants of the separate pathways are equal. If the separate pathways have different timc constants, the phase angles between flow and pressure will be different and the flows will be out of phase with each other. The instants of zero flow in the separate pathways will not correspond, and there will be gas flowing between the separate pathways at the instants of zero flow in the common path. In this case *equation 11* does not apply and the total admittance of the system must be expressed in the vector form:

$$\frac{1}{\bar{Z}} = \frac{1}{\bar{Z}_1} + \frac{1}{\bar{Z}_2} \qquad (12)$$

With a change in frequency, the impedance of the separate pathways will not change proportionately, and hence the distribution of flow and of volume change will be altered.

These points are illustrated in figure 2 which is a schematic representation of a two-pathway system. The two compliances are equal. The flow resistance of one pathway is greater than the other, and hence the time constant of the higher resistance pathway is greater. During very slow pressure cycling the impedances of the pathways are nearly equal, and hence the tidal volumes are about the same. The overall compliance is the sum of the individual compliances. At higher rates of cycling the impedance of the pathways depends increasingly on the pathway resistances, and the low resistive pathway receives more than one-half of the total volume moved. The over-all compliance in this case is less than at slow rates. At rapid rates the phase difference between the pathways becomes accentuated. At the end of inspiration, when flow has dropped to zero in the common path, the low time constant path is already expiring while the high time constant path is still inspiring At the end of expiration gas is passing from the high to the low time constant pathway. As a result, the sum of the individual tidal volumes is greater than the overall tidal volume, the difference representing the volume of gas that passes back and forth between the two pathways ('pendelluft').

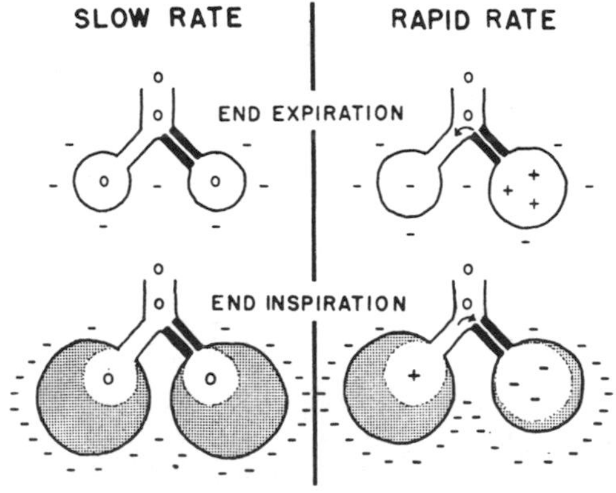

FIG. 2. Two-pathway system illustrating behavior at slow and rapid rates. +, — and o indicate pressure relative to atmospheric. Shading indicates volume change.

In the further development of the theory, we have considered chiefly the influence of the distribution of pathway impedances on the overall dynamic pressure-volume relationships of the lungs, since the latter are measurements that can be made experimentally. In any network of separate parallel pathways, each with resistance and compliance elements in series, the behavior of the network at a given frequency may be duplicated by a single resistance element and a single compliance element in series. This follows from a basic theorem in alternating current network theory (8). If the time constants of the separate pathways are equal, the equivalent or effective resistance and compliance of the network will be the same at all frequencies. If this were the case for the lungs, a simple model, such as the one shown in figure 1*A*, would have the same mechanical behavior as the lungs. On the other hand, if the time constants of the separate pathways are not equal, the effective compliance and resistance will change with frequency. In this case no simple model would be adequate, except at a fixed frequency.

Expressions for calculating the effective compliance and resistance for a two-pathway network will now be given. The steps leading to these expressions are shown in APPENDIX II.

In a two-pathway network, made up of known resistance and compliance elements, R_1, C_1, R_2 and C_2, the effective compliance,

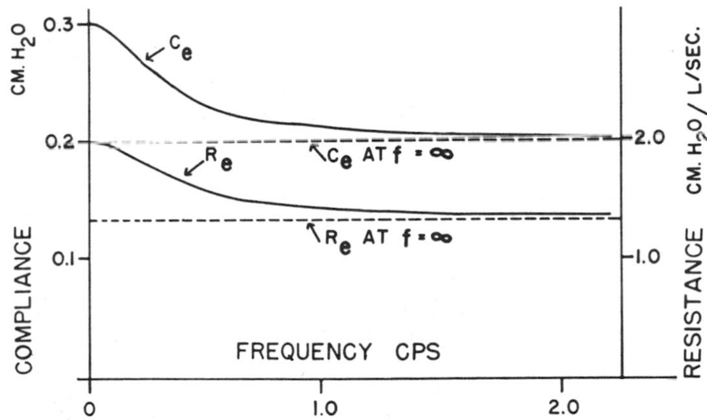

FIG. 3. Effective compliance, Ce, and effective resistance, Re, of a two-pathway system as functions of frequency. ($R_1 = 2$, $C_1 = 0.1$, $T_1 = 0.2$, $R_2 = 4$, $C_2 = 0.2$, $T_2 = 0.8$.)

Ce, and effective resistance, Re, may be expressed as follows:

$$Ce = \frac{\omega^2(T_2 C_1 + T_1 C_2)^2 + (C_1 + C_2)^2}{\omega^2(T_1^2 C_2 + T_2^2 C_2) + (C_1 + C_2)} \quad (13)$$

$$Re = \frac{\omega^2 T_1 T_2(T_2 C_1 + T_1 C_2) + (T_1 C_1 + T_2 C_2)}{\omega^2(T_2 C_1 + T_1 C_2)^2 + (C_1 + C_2)^2} \quad (14)$$

where

$$\omega = 2\pi f,\ T_1 = R_1 C_1 \quad \text{and} \quad T_2 = R_2 C_2$$

When the time constants of the pathways are equal, i.e. $T_1 = T_2$, these expressions are simplified and become independent of frequency:

$$Ce = C_1 + C_2 \quad (15)$$

$$Re = \frac{T}{C_1 + C_2} = \frac{1}{\frac{1}{R_1} + \frac{1}{R_2}} = \frac{R_1 R_2}{R_1 + R_2} \quad (16)$$

These equal time constant expressions may be generalized to fit a network of n-pathways, thus:

if

$$T_1 = T_2 = T_3 \cdots = Tn = T$$

then

$$Ce = C_1 + C_2 \cdots + Cn \quad (17)$$

and

$$Re = \frac{T}{C_1 + C_2 \cdots + Cn} = \frac{1}{\frac{1}{R_1} + \frac{1}{R_2} \cdots + \frac{1}{Rn}} \quad (18)$$

When the time constants are unequal, both Ce and Re change with frequency. Figure 3 is a graph of Ce and Re as a function of frequency for the two elements case (*equations 13, 14*). It may be seen that both decrease as frequency is increased. Furthermore, both approach specific limits at the extremes of frequency. These limits may be predicted by solving *equations 13* and *14* as ω approaches 0 and ∞. As generalized to a system of n-pathways:

$$\lim_{\omega \to 0} Ce = C_1 + C_2 \cdots + Cn \quad (19)$$

$$\lim_{\omega \to \infty} Ce = \frac{\left(\frac{1}{R_1} + \frac{1}{R_2} \cdots + \frac{1}{Rn}\right)^2}{\left(\frac{1}{R_1 T_1} + \frac{1}{R_2 R_2} \cdots + \frac{1}{Rn\,Tn}\right)} \quad (20)$$

$$\lim_{\omega \to 0} Re = \frac{C_1 T_1 + C_2 T_2 \cdots + Cn\,Tn}{(C_1 + C_2 \cdots Cn)^2} \quad (21)$$

$$\lim_{\omega \to \infty} Re = \frac{1}{\frac{1}{R_1} + \frac{1}{R_2} \cdots + \frac{1}{Rn}} \quad (22)$$

At very low frequencies Ce approaches the equal time constant case, while Re approaches a value determined by the separate pathway compliances and time constants. At very high frequencies Re approaches the equal time constant case, while Ce approaches a value determined by the time constants and resistances of the separate pathways.

Having solved for Ce and Re as a function of frequency, it is possible to solve for the tidal volume of the network at a given fre-

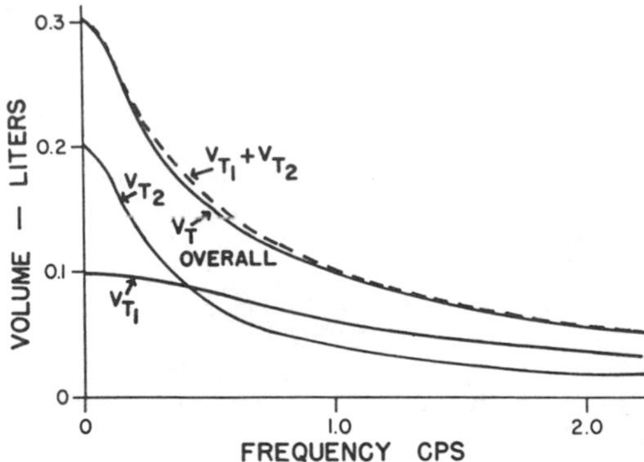

FIG. 4. Tidal volumes of the system VT and of the individual pathways, V_{T1} and V_{T2} for the example shown in fig. 2 as functions of frequency. Difference between the dotted line ($V_{T1} + V_{T2}$) and VT indicates the volume passing back and forth between the pathways (pendelluft).

quency and pressure amplitude. If the tidal volumes of the separate pathways at a given frequency are also known, it is possible to calculate the volume of gas passing back and forth between the pathways as a function of frequency, for, if the sum of the individual tidal volumes exceeds the overall network tidal volume, this additional volume change must take place between the pathways.

The tidal volumes of the network and of the individual pathways at a given frequency may be expressed as follows:

$$Vt = C(\Delta Pc) \qquad (23)$$

where ΔPc is the change in pressure occurring between the instants of no flow at the extremes of VT. For a sinusoidal pressure variation with an amplitude ΔP, $\Delta Pc = \Delta P \sin \theta$, where tan $\theta = \frac{1}{2\pi fRC.}$ Thus:

$$V_T = C(\Delta P \sin \theta) \qquad (24)$$

This expression is equivalent to *equation 7*.

Figure 4 is a graph of the overall tidal volume, and the individual tidal volumes as a function of frequency, for the network illustrated in figure 2 at a pressure amplitude of 1 cm H_2O. The upper dotted line is the sum of the individual tidal volumes. The volume difference between the dotted line and the overall tidal volume represents the volume passing back and forth between the pathways. This volume has a maximum value of 5.5% of the overall tidal volume in the example shown.

The proportion of gas transferred between pathways is dependent on the relative impedances of the overall system. An expression for calculating this 'pendelluft' as a proportion of overall tidal volume is

$$\frac{V_P}{V_T} = \frac{Z(Z_1 + Z_2)}{Z_1 Z_2} - 1 \qquad (25)$$

where VP is the volume of 'pendelluft', VT the effective tidal volume of the overall system and Z_1, Z_2 and Z are the impedances of the separate branches and of the overall system, respectively. Since the values for the impedances vary with frequency the proportion of 'pendelluft' will also do so, and for any system composed of a pair of elements having differing time constants there will be a frequency at which the proportion of pendelluft is maximal. The greatest possible pendelluft occurs in a system consisting of a pure resistance R_1 (time constant = ∞) and a pure compliance C_2 (time constant = 0) connected in parallel and driven at a frequency such that $R_1 = \frac{1}{2\pi fC_2}$. In such a case the proportion of pendelluft is 41.1%. As pairs of elements having less discrepant time constants are chosen the proportion of pendelluft decreases and of

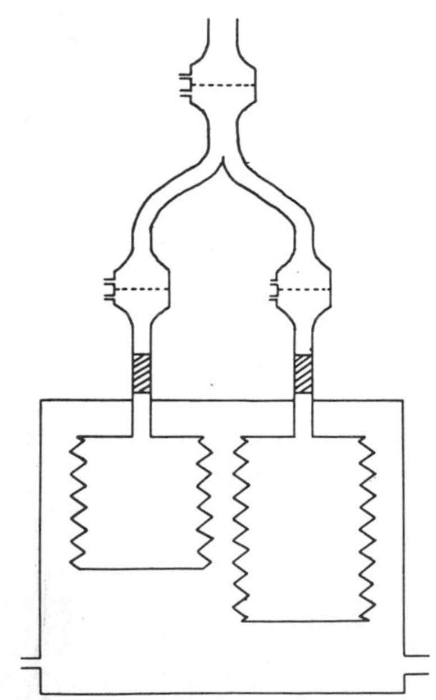

FIG. 5. Schematic diagram of a mechanical model of two pulmonary pathways connected in parallel. For description see text.

course reaches zero in the equal time constant case.

RESULTS

Model Experiments. The model used is shown schematically in figure 5. It consists of two 'pulmonary pathways' enclosed in an 'intrapleural space' and connected in parallel as indicated. The compliant component was constructed by sealing a Lucite disc over each end of a rubber bellows of the type used in the Kreiselmann resuscitator. A hole was drilled in the center of one of the discs to accommodate a length of 1-inch o.d. Lucite tubing which was sealed in place. A component having a higher compliance was constructed by cementing two bellows together, the result being a bellows twice as long as each original bellows.

The flow resistive components indicated on the diagram were made by mounting discs of sintered bronze or of wire gauze in the lumen of $\frac{15}{16}$ inch i.d. brass tube. The latter could be easily connected by rubber tubing to the Lucite tubes leading from the bellows.

The intrapleural space consisted of a box 15 x 15 x 11 inches made of wood except for the removable front which was a sheet of Lucite, held in place with screws and sealed with a rubber gasket.

Two openings fitted with glands and rubber gaskets allowed the emergence of the Lucite tubes leading from the bellows, and held them

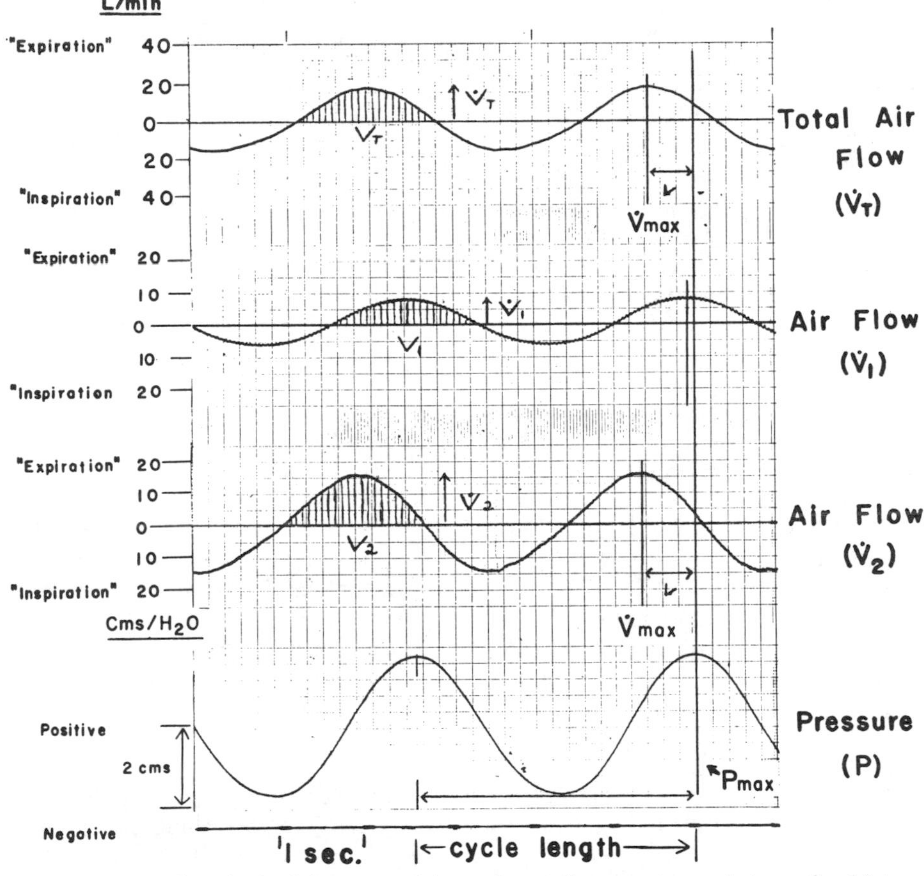

FIG. 6. Typical recording obtained from a model experiment. Lowermost record shows the driving pressure (relative to atmospheric) within the box. The two central records show the flows in each separate pathway and the topmost record the flow in the common pathway. Sensitivity of the top channel was set to equal $\frac{1}{2}$ that of the central channels. A vertical line has been drawn through a point of maximal pressure. Points of maximal air flow have also been indicated on the flow curves by vertical lines. Difference in time by which the flow curves lead pressure curves is indicated by the horizontal distance between the point of maximal flow and that of maximal pressure. Phase angles are these differences divided by the time for a complete cycle and multiplied by 360°. Shaded areas are proportional to the tidal volumes.

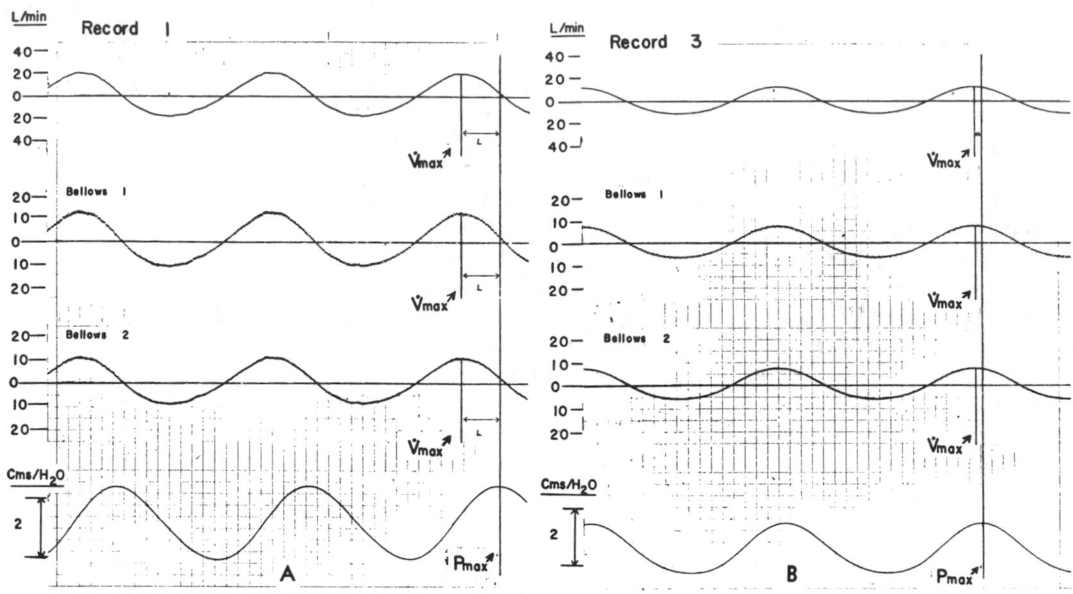

FIG. 7. *A*, recording in which the separate pathways have equal time constants $C_1 = C_2 = 0.08$ l/cm H_2O; $R_1 = 2.0$ cm. H_2O/l/sec. *B*, recording in which the separate pathways have equal time constants, the resistances being relatively high, $C_1 = C_2 = .08$ l/cm H_2O; $R_1 = R_2 = 16$ cm. H_2O/l/sec.

firmly in place. An opening on the side of the box was connected to a pump and another opening served for measuring the pressure within the box. The pump produced an approximately sinusoidal variation of the pressure within the box and both its frequency and displacement could be varied.

Pneumotachograph screens were arranged as indicated to record the flow from each element and the combined flow from the two elements.

The pressure fluctuations in the box and the rates of air flow were measured using electrical pressure transducers and recorded with a direct writing oscillograph.

Experiments were performed in which compliance, resistance and rate of cycling were varied. Figure 6 and its accompanying legend is presented for the orientation of the reader. Each of the following records is presented to illustrate the effects of altering some particular variable as explained below, and may be interpreted in the light of the previous theoretical section.

In figure 7*A* the resistances of the separate pathways are equal and relatively small (2.0 cm H_2O/ l/sec.). The compliances are also equal (0.08 l/cm H_2O). Hence, the time constants of the two are equal, and the separate flows are exactly in phase with each other and with the combined flow. Because of the low resistance, the time constants are relatively short and the flow curves lead the pressure by a substantial amount ($\theta = 73°$). Since the two pathways have the same impedance, the separate flows and volumes changes are identical.

In figure 7*B* the two pathways are also identical, but the resistances have each been increased approximately eight times. The flows are all exactly in phase with each other; but since the time constants are relatively large, the flows lead the pressure by a relatively small amount as compared with the case in figure 7*A*. Also the flows and tidal volumes are markedly reduced owing to the greater impedance.

Figures 8*A* and 8*B* illustrate the effects of an alteration in frequency of 'breathing' when the separate pathways have identical compliances (.08 l/cm H_2O) but differing resistance R = 17 cm H_2O/l/sec. for pathway 1 and 2 cm H_2O/l/sec. for pathway 2. In figure 8*A* the frequency of breathing is .217/sec. (13/min.). The pathway with the high resistance has a markedly smaller ventilation than the other element and since it has a longer time constant, it leads the pressure curve considerably less. Figure 8*B* shows that increasing the frequency to .73/sec. (44/min.) has produced an even greater disparity in the magnitudes of ventilation of the two pathways. This

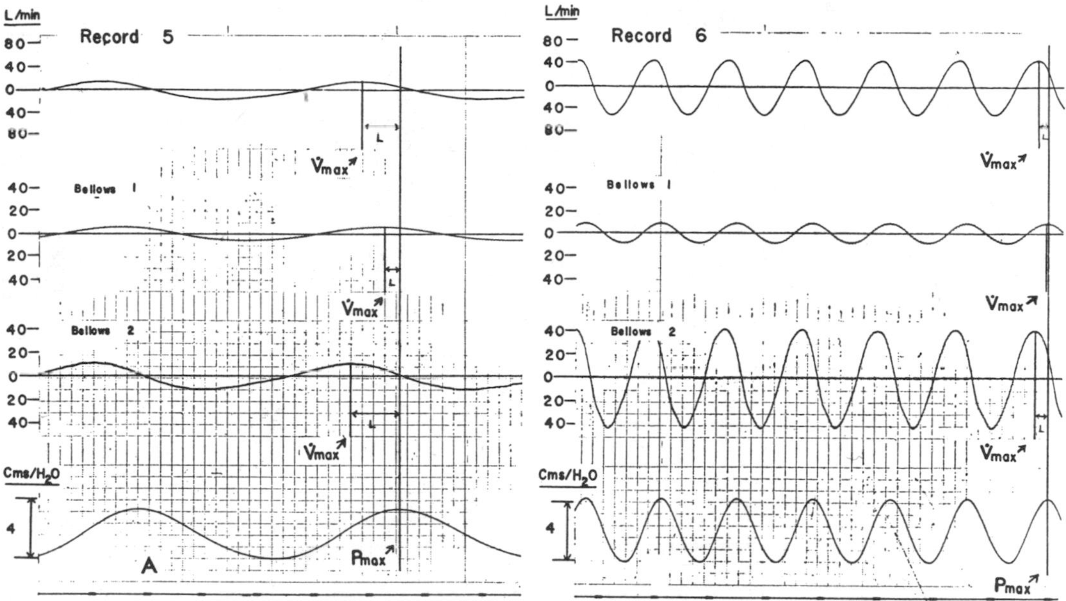

FIG. 8, *A* and *B*. Effect of alteration in frequency, $C_1 = C_2 = .08$; $R_1 = 17$, $R_2 = 2$. In *A* the frequency is 13/min. and in *B* 44/min.

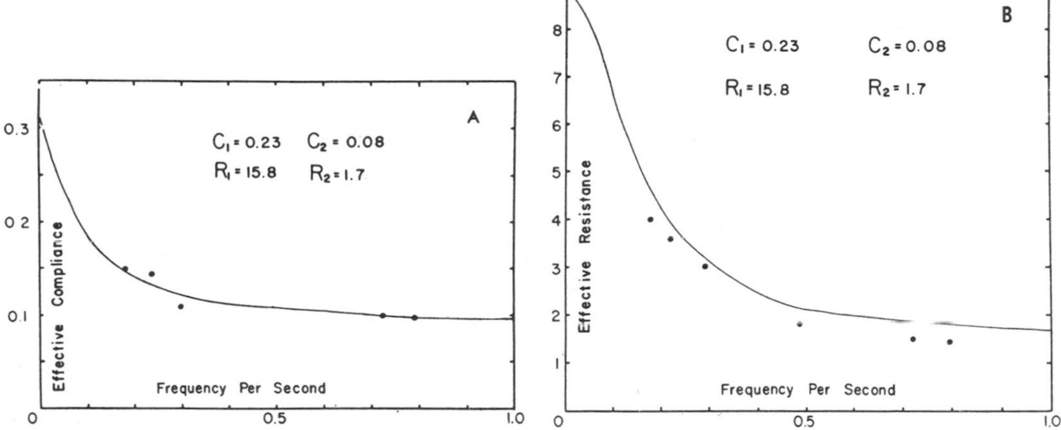

FIG. 9, *A* and *B*, change in effective compliance and resistance with frequency when $C_1 = 0.25$, $C_2 = 0.08$, $R_1 = 15.8$, $R_2 = 1.7$. Curves are drawn from theoretical calculations. Points were obtained from measurements on the model.

occurs because the impedance of a pathway with a relatively low resistance is altered much more by a change in frequency than is that of one with a relatively high resistance. The increased frequency has also reduced the phase angle of both pathways.

Figures 8*A* and 8*B* also illustrate the 'pendelluft' that occurs when phase differences between the pathways exist. During part of each cycle flows are in opposite directions in the two pathways i.e., one is inspiring while the other is expiring and vice versa. This means that gas is transferred between the two pathways as well as between each pathway and the outside and that the sum of the separate tidal volumes is greater than the total tidal volume.

The records shown can be further analyzed by integrating the flow curves and plotting pressure-volume diagrams. From these diagrams the compliance of each pathway and the effective compliance of the combination

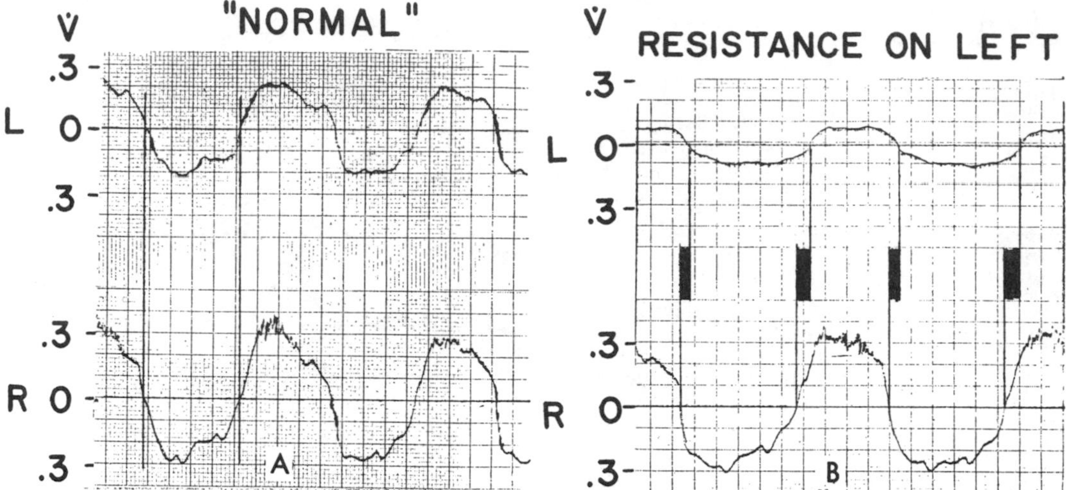

FIG. 10. *A*, flows from each branch of a Carlens catheter in the bronchi of a human subject. *B*, the same but with a resistance inserted in the branch leading to the left bronchus.

can be measured, and by reference back to the flow curves the corresponding resistances can also be determined. This procedure has been applied to several records obtained at various frequencies with the separate elements having values for compliance and resistance as follows:

$C_1 = 0.23$; $R_1 = 15.8$; $T_1 = 3.63$;
$C_2 = 0.08$; $R_2 = 1.7$; $T_2 = 0.136$

Values obtained for the effective compliance and resistance of the system as a whole are shown in figures 9*A* and 9*B*, together with theoretical curves. It is evident that the effective compliance and resistance both diminish with frequency and that the former is always less than the sum of the separate compliances while the latter is always greater than would be predicted by simple addition of the reciprocal resistances.

Test of Theory on a Human Subject.[5] In an attempt to demonstrate qualitatively that the sort of behavior shown by the mechanical model could occur in human lungs the following experiment was performed. A Carlens differential bronchial catheter was inserted in a human subject and a pneumotachograph was attached to each branch of the catheter. The recording shown in figure 10*A* was obtained, which shows that flows in the two bronchi were roughly equal and exactly in phase with each other. A resistance was then inserted in the branch of the catheter leading to the left bronchus, the pneumotachographs were reconnected and another record was taken. Figure 10*B* shows that the addition of the resistance not only reduced the flow in the left bronchus, but also produced a phase difference between the two flows, the side with the added resistance lagging the 'normal' side, as would be expected theoretically and from the behavior of the mechanical model.

Further Experiments on Human Subjects. The mouth-to-esophagus pressure difference was used as a measure of the changes in transpulmonary pressure. A thin-walled latex balloon, 10–15 cm long and of 5–6 ml capacity, sealed around a thin polyethylene tube with multiple side openings was passed into the esophagus through the nose. The balloon was placed so that its tip was a few centimeters above the cardiac sphincter, and was adjusted to 1 ml air volume. The balloon catheter was connected to a differential manometer (9). The other side of the manometer was connected by tubing to the mouthpiece assembly through a multiple side-hole manifold in the mouthpiece at a point where the mouthpiece cross-section was 25 sq. cm. Volumes were recorded by means of a 7-liter Krogh spirometer. Voltage changes proportional to volume were obtained from a rotational transducer[6] mounted at the

[5] We wish to thank Dr. Bruce Armstrong of the Veterans Administration Hospital, Baltimore, Md., for his cooperation in carrying out this experiment.

[6] Microsyn Type 1C-D18-L; Doelcam Corporation, Boston, Mass.

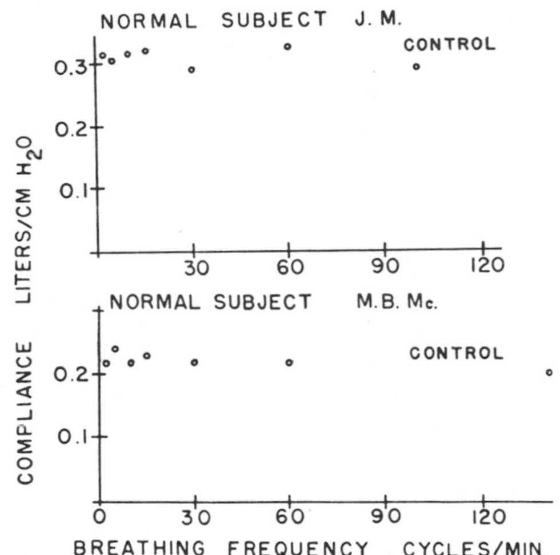

FIG. 11. Pulmonary compliance as a function of frequency in two normal subjects.

TABLE 2. PULMONARY COMPLIANCE IN FOUR NORMAL SUBJECTS AT SLOW AND RAPID RATES OF BREATHING

Subj.	Resp. Rate/min.	Compliance l/cm H_2O	Resp. Rate/min.	Compliance l/cm H_2O
E.B.	13	0.21	56	0.21
M.McL.	10	0.12	120	0.11
N.S.	10	0.25	60	0.24
E.P.R.	10	0.14	60	0.14

fulcrum of the spirometer. During the experiments subjects rebreathed from the spirometer, the duration of the runs being short enough to permit this.

Subjects breathed with tidal volumes of approximately 1 liter at various rates. Changes in mid-position were minimized by having the subject expire to the same volume level with each breath. Tracings were obtained of pressure, volume and flow on a Sanborn Polyviso at a paper speed of 50 mm/sec. The compliance of the lungs was measured as the ratio of volume change to the difference in pressure at the instants of maximum and minimum volume and expressed in liters per centimeter H_2O. Measurements were made for 10 or more breaths at each breathing frequency to eliminate errors due to the variation in pressure associated with the heart beat.

Figure 11 shows a graph of the compliance of the lungs plotted against the rate of breathing in two normal subjects. The compliance was not altered significantly over a range of from 2 to more than 100 breaths/min. Table 2 shows the results obtained in four additional normal subjects studied at two widely separated frequencies.

Figure 12 shows results obtained in two normal subjects studied immediately following inhalation of an aerosol of 3% histamine. The dose was sufficient to produce a two- to threefold increase in respiratory resistance as measured during quiet breathing. No respiratory distress was apparent and no significant change in vital capacity or mid-position was observed. In both cases a definite and progressive fall in pulmonary compliance was observed as the rate of breathing increased.

Similar graphs obtained in a patient with bronchial asthma experiencing a mild attack (pulmonary resistance measured during quiet breathing = 5.5 cm H_2O at 1 l/sec.) and a patient with advanced pulmonary emphysema are shown in figures 13 and 14. In both instances pulmonary compliance fell as breathing frequency increased. It was not possible for the patient with emphysema to maintain a fixed mid-position as he increased his rate of breathing, but the fall in compliance was much greater than could be accounted for on the basis of mid-position shift alone.

Figure 15 shows a similar graph in a patient with asthma before and after inhalation of a broncho-dilator agent (1:100 adrenaline aerosol). It can be seen that the fall in compliance

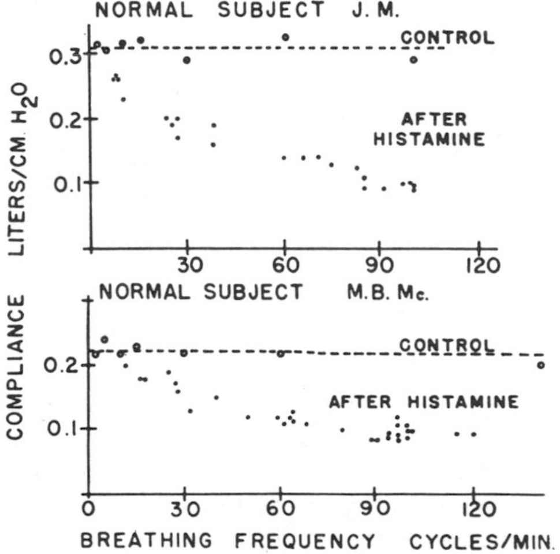

FIG. 12. Pulmonary compliance as a function of frequency in two normal subjects before and after inhalation of histamine aerosol.

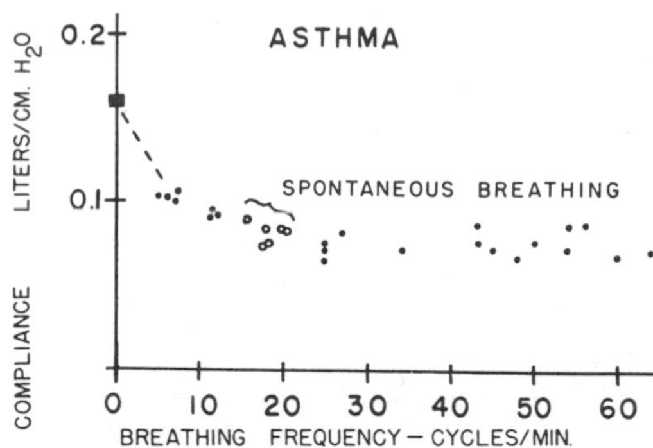

FIG. 13. Pulmonary compliance as a function of frequency in a patient with asthma.

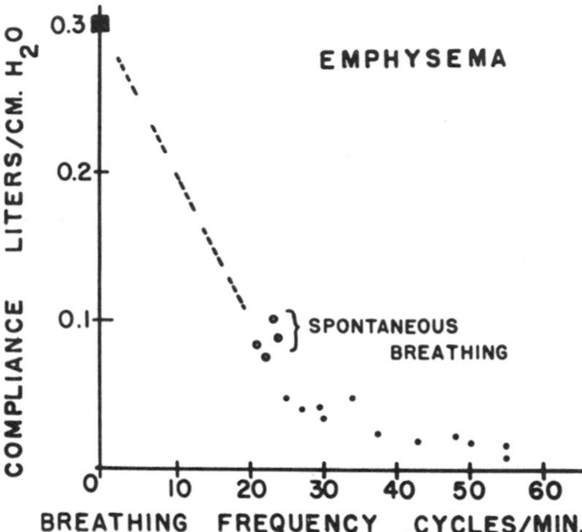

FIG. 14. Pulmonary compliance as a function of frequency in a patient with emphysema.

with increasing frequency is less after the inhalation of adrenaline.

DISCUSSION

The results of the human experiments may be interpreted in the light of the theoretical analysis and its confirmation with models. The theoretical analysis presented has been based on simple networks with known linear resistances and compliances subjected to sine waves of pressure change. The lungs in reality have multiple pathways with nonlinear resistances and compliances and are subjected to a wide variety of pressure waves. The step from theory to experimental results is a large one; nevertheless, certain conclusions may be drawn.

From theoretical considerations it was predicted that the overall mechanical behavior of systems comprising separate pathways in parallel should be influenced in a particular way by the distribution of mechanical properties amongst the separate pathways. These predictions may be summarized at this point: the overall volume-elastic and flow-resistive properties of such systems remain unchanged as the frequency of pressure cycling is changed only if the impedance of the separate pathways changes proportionately with frequency. This condition is common to all systems in which the time-constants of the separate pathways are the same. In contrast to this, systems with time-constant discrepancies undergo disproportionate changes in the impedances of the separate pathways as the frequency of pressure cycling is changed. In this case the overall volume-elastic and flow-resistive properties are different at different frequencies: the effective compliance and effective resistance both decrease as the frequency of pressure cycling increases.

It should be pointed out that these predictions are not restricted to linear systems or to sine waves of applied pressure. The qualitative implications of proportionate, in contrast to disproportionate changes in pathway impedance with frequency, would be the same for nonlinear systems subjected to pressure wave forms other than sine waves. Effective compliance and effective resistance would remain insensitive to frequency in the first case and decrease with increasing frequencies in the second case. Quantitative predictions from theoretical grounds, however, would be extremely complex.

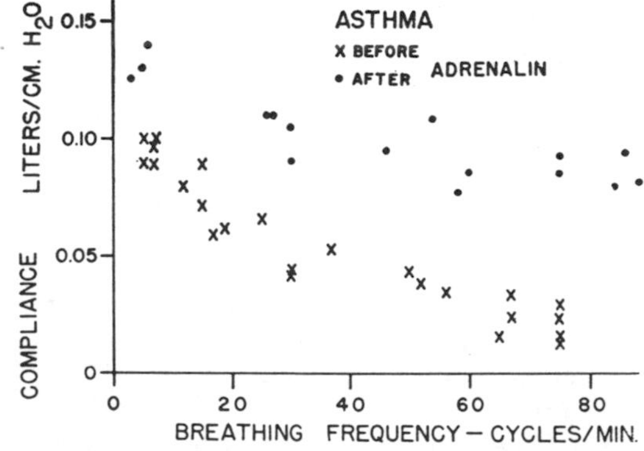

FIG. 15. Pulmonary compliance as a function of frequency in a patient with asthma before and after adrenaline inhalation.

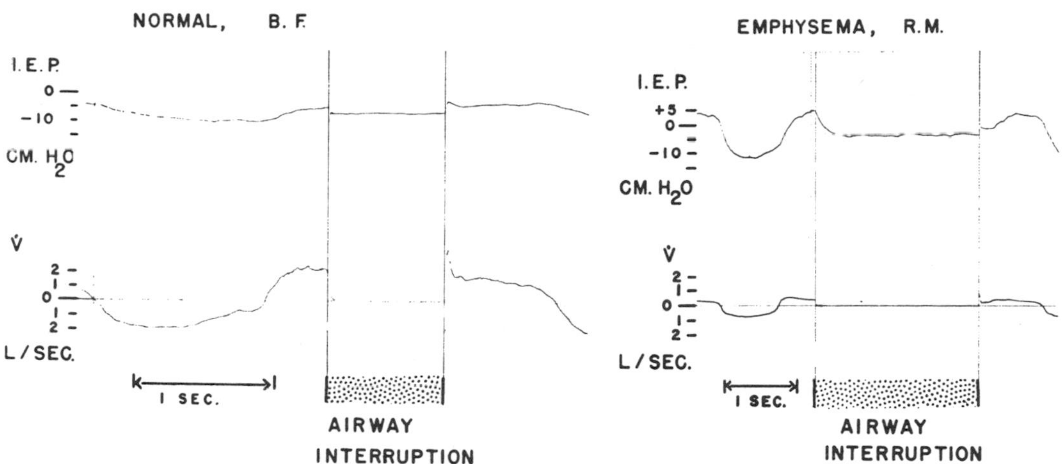

FIG. 16. Tracings of pressure and flow during airway interruption in a normal subject and a patient with emphysema.

The finding that the compliance of the lungs did not change appreciably with the frequency of respiration in normal subjects suggests that the impedances of the separate component pathways change proportionately with frequency. In a linear system this is equivalent to saying that the time-constants of the separate elements must be the same.

Marked reductions in pulmonary compliance with increased rates of breathing were found in normal subjects following the inhalation of histamine aerosols, and in two disease states. These results suggest that substantial time-constant inequalities of the separate pathways may exist in abnormal lungs.

The possible pertinence of these findings to the problem of the distribution of ventilation within the lungs will now be considered. There are two general methods in current use for the detection of uneven alveolar ventilation (10, 11). One consists essentially in the measurement of the washout rate of N_2 during the breathing of oxygen over a period of several breaths. The finding of an abnormally slow washout is taken as evidence of uneven ventilation. Such a criterion is consistent with the concept that the lungs consist of pathways which are ventilated synchronously but unevenly as regards volume.

In the second method the instantaneous nitrogen concentration is measured continuously during a single expiration following the inspiration of a single breath of oxygen. A rising 'alveolar plateau' is taken as evidence of uneven ventilation. This criterion requires, as has been suggested by Fowler (12), that the diluting gas (oxygen) be distributed unevenly not only spatially but also temporally. For example, suppose that the diluting gas were unevenly distributed spatially during inspiration. This would lead to inequalities in the concentration of nitrogen in the various pulmonary pathways. If during the succeeding expiration all the pathways emptied synchronously the *mixed* alveolar gas which is under observation would have a uniform nitrogen composition. Nonuniformity of the expired alveolar gas requires, therefore, that the emptying occur asynchronously from the different pathways. In other words there must be a temporal difference in the operation of the pulmonary pathways, at least during expiration, and such a difference is not precluded during inspiration.

In the case of the mathematical and mechanical models described above it has been shown that such temporal and spatial differences in ventilation will occur when the time-constants of the component pathways are different. The results of the experiments on human subjects suggest that time-constant inequalities exist in abnormal lungs. We would conclude from this that the concepts developed in this report may have practical significance in the production of uneven alveolar ventilation.

In normal lungs the time-constants of the separate pathways appear to be nearly equal. Since there is an infinite variety of distributions of compliance and flow-resistive properties within the lungs that could satisfy the equal time-constant case, nothing can be concluded from the observations made as to the particular distribution of volume change within normal lungs. It may be concluded, however, that whatever the volume distribution within normal lungs may be, it apparently does not change appreciably with the breathing frequency.

Some additional experiments were performed which test a corollary of these considerations. If a decrease in compliance with increased breathing frequency reflects an altered distribution of ventilation, it would be expected that sudden interruption of the air stream at the mouth during rapid breathing should be followed by a period of continuing gas flow within the lungs as the dynamically distributed volume is redistributed to conform with the static, or 'zero frequency' distribution. The transpulmonary pressure difference, as measured between the mouth and the esophagus would change as this redistribution took place and should reflect the time course of the redistribution. Figure 16 shows tracings of pressure and flow in a normal subject and in a patient with emphysema during airway interruption, produced by means of a solenoid-driven shutter valve in the mouthpiece assembly. In the normal subject it took about 0.02 seconds for the pressure to reach a constant level, while in the patient with emphysema equilibration took 0.5 seconds. Equilibration times in five additional subjects with emphysema were from three to twenty times as long as in normal subjects, where equilibration invariably took place in 0.03 seconds or less.

The rapid equilibration observed in normal subjects is consistent with the previous conclusion that the distribution of ventilation in normal lungs is little influenced by dynamic factors. The prolonged equilibration observed in patients with pulmonary emphysema is independent evidence supporting the conclusion that dynamic factors may play a role in the production of uneven ventilation.

It is of interest to consider some further implications of the theory and the results which pertain to the overall mechanical behavior of the lungs. In the past, two methods have been used to measure the elastic characteristics of the lungs during life. One relates the tidal volume observed during continuous breathing to the change in transpulmonary pressure between the instants of zero air flow at the extremes of the tidal volume (9, 13–15). In the framework of this report this method measures the effective compliance of the lungs. The other relates stepwise volume change of the lungs to corresponding steps in transpulmonary pressure (16, 17). At each step the volume is maintained constant for a brief interval either voluntarily (16) or by momentarily closing off the airway by means of a valve in the mouthpiece assembly (17). The volume-step method is essentially a static determination and thus in the framework of this report should indicate the zero frequency compliance of the lungs.

The finding that lung compliance of normal subjects as measured by the two methods give similar values at comparable mid-positions (9, 17) is to be expected since the compliance of normal lungs apparently does not alter with breathing frequency. In instances where the effective compliance decreases with increased frequencies of breathing the volume step method gives higher values than the continuous volume-cycle method. This is illustrated in figures 13 and 14 where the 'zero-frequency' values were obtained by the volume-step method. Depending on the method used, strikingly different conclusions might be drawn as to lung elasticity in these instances. The static compliance for the patient with emphysema is if anything higher than would be found in a normal subject of similar size. On the other hand, the values obtained during spontaneous breathing are considerably below normal.

Actually both values are significant in determining the volume behavior of the lungs during spontaneous breathing. Their separate significance becomes apparent when transpulmonary pressure and lung gas volume are considered on an absolute rather than an incremental scale. The forces applied by the thorax to the lungs may be considered to be made up of a steady component which influences the average volume of the lungs (the mid-position), and a changing component which influences the volume increment (the tidal volume) of each breath. The steady component of this force along with the static compliance of the lungs determines the average volume or mid-position of the lungs. The changing component, along with the effective resistance and effective compliance of the lungs for the particular frequency and shape of the pressure pattern, determines the tidal volume.

SUMMARY

A theoretical analysis of the effects of local differences in mechanical properties on the distribution of ventilation within the lungs and on the overall mechanical behavior of the lungs has been presented. The theory has been tested with a model system and has been applied to measurements made on human subjects.

For the purpose of the analysis the lungs have been considered to be made up of a number of parallel pathways each consisting of a compliance (C) and a resistance (R) in series. By using methods which apply to analogous electrical circuits it has been concluded that the distribution of ventilation would be uninfluenced by changes in breathing frequency only if the time-constants (the products of R and C) of the separate pathways are the same. On the other hand, if the time constants differ, the distribution of ventilation would alter with changes in breathing frequency. Furthermore, these changes would be accompanied by changes in the overall mechanical behavior of the lungs: both the compliance and resistance of the lungs would decrease as the breathing frequency increased.

The theoretical analysis has been tested with a model consisting of two parallel pathways and the results were consistent with the theory. In normal young adults pulmonary compliance did not change over a wide range of breathing frequencies. It is inferred from this result that the time constants are substantially the same for the separate pathways in normal lungs and that the distribution of ventilation is independent of the breathing frequency. In contrast, pulmonary compliance dropped with increased breathing frequencies in normal subjects with induced bronchospasm and in patients with asthma and emphysema. These observations suggest that considerable time-constant inequalities of the separate pathways existed in these instances, and that the distribution of ventilation altered with changes in breathing frequency.

APPENDIX I

To prove that the proportionate change in impedance with frequency is the same in different pathways in parallel (each consisting of single flow-resistive and volume-elastic elements in series) if the products of the resistance and compliance of the separate pathways are equal:

For each pathway the magnitude of the impedance, Z, may be expressed:

$$Z = \sqrt{R^2 + \frac{1}{(\omega C)^2}} = \frac{1}{C}\sqrt{T^2 + \frac{1}{\omega^2}}$$

where $T = RC$, and $\omega = 2\pi f$.

The proportional change of Z with change in frequency from ω_1 to ω_2 may be expressed:

$$\frac{Z_1}{Z_2} = \frac{\frac{1}{C}\sqrt{T^2 + \frac{1}{(\omega_1)^2}}}{\frac{1}{C}\sqrt{T^2 + \frac{1}{(\omega_2)^2}}} = \sqrt{\frac{T^2 + \frac{1}{(\omega_1)^2}}{T^2 + \frac{1}{(\omega_2)^2}}}$$

Thus, for each pathway the proportional change in Z depends only on frequency and the product of the pathway compliance and resistance, T. If all pathways have equal values of T, then their impedances must change proportionately with ω.

APPENDIX II

Development of the expressions for *equivalent compliance* and *equivalent resistance* for two-pathway systems, each pathway consisting of single flow resistance and volume-elastic elements in series.

The admittance of a pathway, Y, is the inverse of the pathway impedance, Z.

$$\bar{Y} = \frac{1}{\bar{Z}}$$

The admittance of parallel system is equal to the sum of the individual pathway admittances. Let $\bar{Y}_0$ equal the total admittance, and $\bar{Y}_1$ and $\bar{Y}_2$ equal the separate pathway admittances. Then

$$\bar{Y}_0 = \bar{Y}_1 + \bar{Y}_2$$

To solve for $\bar{Y}_0$ in terms of the impedance, it is convenient to use the complex form which permits an algebraic solution. In complex form $\bar{Z} = R - j\frac{1}{\omega C}$, where j is equal to $\sqrt{-1}$, and $\omega = 2\pi f$; all terms with the coefficient $-j$ lag the remaining term by 90°.

Expressed in complex form:

$$\bar{Y}_1 = \frac{1}{\bar{Z}} \quad \frac{1}{R_1 - j\frac{1}{\omega C_1}} = \frac{\omega C_1}{\omega R_1 C_1 - j}$$

and

$$\bar{Y}_2 = \frac{1}{\bar{Z}_2} = \frac{1}{R_2 - j\frac{1}{\omega C_2}} = \frac{\omega C_2}{\omega R_2 C_2 - j}$$

$$\bar{Y}_0 = \bar{Y}_1 + \bar{Y}_2 = \frac{\omega C_1}{\omega R_1 C_1 - j} + \frac{\omega C_2}{\omega R_2 C_2 - j}$$

$$= \frac{\omega^2 C_1 C_2(R_1 + R_2) - j\omega(C_1 + C_2)}{(\omega^2 R_1 C_1 R_2 C_2 - 1) - j\omega(R_1 C_1 + R_2 C_2)}$$

$$\bar{Z}_0 = \frac{1}{\bar{Y}_0} = \frac{(\omega^2 R_1 C_1 R_2 C_2 - 1) - j\omega(R_1 C_1 + R_2 C_2)}{\omega^2 C_2 C_1(R_1 + R_2) - j\omega(C_1 + C_2)}$$

Let $A = \omega^2 R_1 C_1 R_2 C_2 - 1$

$B = \omega(R_1 C_1 + R_2 C_2)$

$K = \omega^2 C_2 C_1 (R_2 + R_1)$

$M = \omega(C_1 + C_2)$

$$\text{Then } \bar{Z}_0 = \frac{A - jB}{K - jM}$$

Multiplying numerator and denominator by $K + jM$:

$$\bar{Z}_0 = \frac{AK + BM}{K^2 + M^2} - j\frac{BK - AM}{K^2 + M^2}$$

$$Z_0 = Re - j\frac{1}{\omega Ce}$$

where Re is the *effective resistance* and Ce is the *effective compliance*. Thus:

$$Re = \frac{AK + BM}{K^2 + M^2} \text{ and } Ce = \frac{K^2 + M^2}{\omega(BK - AM}$$

The values for Re and Ce in *equations 14* and *13* in the text were obtained by substituting in these expressions the values for A, B, K and M and letting $R_1C_1 = T_1$ and $R_2C_2 = T_2$.

REFERENCES

1. Mead, J., I. Lindgren and E. A. Gaensler. *J. Clin. Investigation* 34: 1005, 1955.
2. Fowler, W. E. *Physiol. Rev.* 32: 1, 1952.
3. Rauwerda, P. E. *Unequal Ventilation of Different Parts of the Lung and the Determination of Cardiac Output.* Groningen: Groningen Univ. 1946.
4. Wiggers, C. J., M. M. Levy and G. Graham. *Am. J. Physiol.* 151: 1, 1947.
5. Rohrer, F. *Arch. ges. Physiol.* 162: 225, 1915.
6. Otis, A. B., W. O. Fenn and H. Rahn. *J. Appl. Physiol.* 2: 592, 1950.
7. DuBois, A. B. *Federation Proc.* 12: 35, 1953.
8. Cruft Electronics Staff. *Electronic Circuits and Tubes.* New York: McGraw-Hill, 1947, p. 110.
9. Mead, J. and J. L. Whittenberger. *J. Appl. Physiol.* 5: 779, 1953.
10. Fowler, W. E., E. R. Cornish, Jr. and S. S. Kety. *J. Clin. Investigation* 31: 40, 1952.
11. Comroe, J. and W. Fowler. *Am. J. Med.* 10: 408, 1951.
12. Fowler, W. S. *J. Appl. Physiol.* 2: 283, 1949.
13. von Neergaard, K. and K. Wirz. *Ztschr. klin. Med.* 105: 35, 1927.
14. Christie, R. V. and C. A. McIntosh. *J. Clin. Investigation* 13: 279, 1934.
15. Bayliss, L. E. and G. W. Robertson. *Quart. J. Exper. Physiol.* 29: 27, 1939.
16. Buytendijk, H. J. *Electrische Drukkerij.* Groningen: Openheim, N. V., 1949, vol. 1.
17. Stead, W. W., D. L. Fry and R. V. Ebert. *J. Lab. & Clin. Med.* 40: 674, 1952.

23

EXPERIMENTAL STUDIES ON THE MOVEMENT OF FLUIDS THROUGH TUBES OF VERY SMALL DIAMETER

J. L. M. Poiseuille

This excerpt was translated expressly for this Benchmark volume by Karen Lewis, Editorial Assistant, Cardiovascular Research Institute, University of California, San Francisco, from "Recherches expérimentales sur le mouvement des liquides dans les tubes de très petits diamètres," C.R. Acad. Sci., ***11,*** *961–967 and 1041–1048 (1840)*

M. de Prony, drawing on the research of Bossut, Couplet, and Dubuat done on conduction tubes whose diameters varied from 27 to 490 mm and whose lengths varied from 9 to 2280 m, established a flow formula that satisfied hydrodynamic requirements. If the hydrodynamicists can neglect an examination of fluid movement in tubes with much smaller diameters, such is not the case for physiologists, who must consider the passage of fluids through tubes with diameters of about 0.01 mm. However, several authors, Dubuat, Gerstner, and Girard, were concerned with the movement of fluids in tubes of a much smaller caliber than that of those corresponding to M. de Prony's formula; but the tubes they used, although much smaller, were still larger than 1 mm. It was thus necessary to study liquid flow in tubes approaching the capacity of capillary vessels in seeking to discover properties pertaining exclusively to them. This is the goal we intend to accomplish in the *Memoires* we have the honor of submitting for the judgment of the Academy.

Actually, M. Navier, starting with hypotheses formed a priori on the reciprocal actions of fluid molecules in movement, arrived analytically at an equation for liquid movement in pipes with very small diameters; but this formula, which coincides with one that M. Girard had already considered, although his own experiments did not confirm it, must, to be valid, agree with results obtained experimentally.

To clarify the question we are working on, we have been led to examine the influence of the following on the amount of liquid that passes through these small-diameter tubes: (1) pressure, (2) length of the tube, (3) diameter, and (4) temperature.

I. INFLUENCE OF PRESSURE ON THE AMOUNT OF LIQUID PASSING THROUGH TUBES OF VERY SMALL DIAMETER

We measured the pressure, not by the height of a column of fluid, but with a manometer open to the air, using either mercury or distilled water; in addition, we assured ourselves directly that it made no difference whether we used one or the other pressure at the very slow flow we studied. This condition allowed us to obtain the pressure at will and, so to speak, instantaneously, with the help of a force pump. We worked from a pressure of a few millimeters of mercury up to 8 atm.

The tubes were glass, with a 4- to 5-mm external diameter, an internal diameter varying from 0.013 to 0.65 mm, and a length from approximately 2 to 800 mm.

We used distilled water for liquid.

Since the mean value of the quantity of liquid flowing, called product, was 1 cc in several hours, we could not collect the liquid in a graduated test tube. One can imagine that, for such a slow flow, this manner of gauging the products would have caused large errors in the time determinations. Besides, it was absolutely necessary to always operate at the same temperature; to operate as we have just outlined, with the tube exposed to room air, the flow would have been at ambient rather than constant temperature.

The amount of liquid flowing is actually determined by the capacity of an ordinary spherical glass bulb, whose volume varied with the tube used in the experiment. To each end of the bulb, we joined supplementary tubes of approximately 0.75 mm diameter. On each of these tubes, one above and one below the bulb, we placed, with the help of a file, lines or marks at equal distance from the bulb and perpendicular to the axis of the tubes; we joined the tube of small diameter used in the experiment to the lower tube.

After having loaded the bulb and the tube with distilled water, we determined with a chronometer the time it took for the liquid to flow from the upper mark to the lower mark; this time represented the duration of the experiment.

We determined the beginning and end of an experiment by the use of a microscope positioned at the coincidence of a horizontal thread placed at the ocular with the marks on the tube.

The volume of air that presses on the moving liquid changes from the beginning to the end of the experiment by the total capacity of the bulb; to prevent a variation in pressure that would occur from this change, we used a large, very thick copper cylinder air tank, with a capacity of approximately 60 liters.

One advantage of the bulb is the ability to work with a constant temperature determined in advance; in fact, it is necessary only to immerse the bulb and tube in a beaker of distilled water maintained at the same level throughout the experiment, with a thermometer whose bulb is placed at the level of the experimental tube. With this arrangement, the liquid movement takes place in a tube connecting two beakers. Briefly, this is the apparatus we adopted; without mentioning here the research needed to measure the exact pressure, we shall report succinctly the experiments that are the object of this first *Memoire*.

The constant temperature at which we generally worked was 10°C; the mercury and distilled water manometers were all brought to this reference temperature from the laboratory temperature, which was variable.

Tube A, 100.5 mm long, had the following diameters at its ends*:

$$\text{Open end}\begin{cases} d = 0.1390 \\ D = 0.1410 \end{cases}\ \text{mm} \qquad \text{Opposite end near the bulb}\begin{cases} d = 0.1405 \\ D = 0.1430 \end{cases}\ \text{mm}$$

At pressures of 385.870, 739.114, and 773.443 mm Hg, the vial emptied in 3505.75, 1803.75, and 1750 s, respectively.

In comparing the time intervals to the corresponding pressures, we easily see that they are inversely related.

We cut approximately 25 mm from this tube, which, now reduced to 75.8 mm, gave the following results:

At pressures of 97.764, 147.832, 193.632, 387.675, 738.715, and 774.676 mm Hg, the bulb emptied in 10,361, 6851, 5233, 2612.5, 1372.5, and 1308 s, respectively. We see, as before, that the time intervals are inversely related to the pressures.

When 51.1 mm long, the tube showed the same inverse relation between time and pressures.

But if tube length was reduced to 25.55, 15.75, 9.55, and 6.75 mm, this relation no longer held; the higher the pressure, the longer is the time interval than that predicted by the relation described.

For example, we take tube B, of smaller diameter than tube A:

$$\text{Open end}\begin{cases} d = 0.1117 \\ D = 0.1135 \end{cases}\ \text{mm} \qquad \text{Opposite end}\begin{cases} d = 0.115 \\ D = 0.1145 \end{cases}\ \text{mm}$$

For tube lengths of 100.05, 75.05, and 49.375 mm, the time intervals were inversely related to the pressures. When the length of the tube was reduced to 23.575 mm, this relation, which no longer held for tube A at this reduced length, still held for this narrower tube B; however, the relation did not exist for the shorter lengths of 9 and 3.9 mm; as for tube A, the time intervals corresponding to higher and higher pressures were proportionately longer.

Tube C had smaller diameters than tube B:

$$\text{Circular open end}\quad D = 0.084\ \text{mm} \qquad \text{Opposite end}\begin{cases} d = 0.085 \\ D = 0.086 \end{cases}\ \text{mm}$$

The preceding relation held for tube lengths of 100.325, 74.95, 49.7, and 24.4 mm, as well as for 10.15 mm, whereas this was not true with this latter length for tube B, and even less for tube A.

* In this and the succeeding paper, Poiseuille gives two measurements for diameter, *d* and *D*; although not so stated in either paper, these refer to the two diameters of the tube when it is not perfectly circular.

Analogous findings have been made for tube D, of even smaller diameter than tube C. The diameters were as follows:

$$\text{Open end}\begin{cases} d = 0.0460 \text{ mm} \\ D = 0.0470 \text{ mm}\end{cases} \qquad \text{Opposite end}\begin{cases} d = 0.0425 \text{ mm} \\ D = 0.0445 \text{ mm}\end{cases}$$

The same was true for tube E, with the following diameters:

$$\text{Open end}\begin{cases} d = 0.0286 \text{ mm} \\ D = 0.0296 \text{ mm}\end{cases} \qquad \text{Opposite end}\begin{cases} d = 0.02933 \text{ mm} \\ D = 0.03000 \text{ mm}\end{cases}$$

This diameter is only three times larger than that of mammalian capillaries; in this case, the correlation established for pressures is valid for any length, even as short as 2 mm.

It was important to determine if this law would still hold for tubes with much larger diameters than those previously described; we chose one with a diameter of 0.65 mm, that is, 500 times larger than the former tube studied. With a tube length of 800 mm, we found an inverse relation between time intervals and pressures, as with 400 and 383 mm; but the law did not hold for 200 mm and shorter lengths, whereas for that just demonstrated, this relation was true for much shorter lengths, providing the diameter of the tube was smaller.

In the experiments reported here, the pressure was never higher than 1 atm; we wanted to make sure that the law was still valid for much higher pressures; in fact, we determined that for diameters varying between 0.013 and 0.1316 mm the law applied up to 6136 mm Hg, that is, for a pressure of more than 8 atm. The explosion of one of the machines at 10 atm prevented us from investigating higher pressures.

From the experiments we report on here, experiments performed on nearly 300 tubes with quite different lengths, and with a caliber varying from 1 to 2500, it appears that, when the same amount of liquid flows through a tube, the transit times are inversely related to the pressures.

This relation, which appears moreover to be independent of temperature, since it was not modified when working at 8, 11, and 19°C, will let us establish easily the relation between products and pressures during the same interval of time.

If a is the amount of fluid flowing at pressure P during the time interval t, then at pressure mP, the same amount of fluid a will flow in a time interval of t/m; thus with mP pressure, ma fluid will flow during time interval t. The products of outflow and units of pressure are proportional to the pressure exerted. Call Q the products corresponding to the pressures P; then for the movement of fluids in tubes under consideration, $Q = kP$, k being a constant for a given tube. We shall soon see that this coefficient is a function of the length of the tube, of its diameter, and of the temperature during the experiment.

This relation between products and pressures does not depend on limits to the velocity of flow, since for any tube shortened to a certain length this relation is abolished, even though the fluid velocity is in between those of two tubes for which the law holds.

Results from these observations indicate that for a given diameter the tubes have to be longer than a determined limit of length—otherwise the law is not valid. As we have just seen, this limit decreases with a decrease in the diameter of the tube. Thus, the law of pressures is still valid for a length as small as 2 mm, when the diameter of the tube is 0.03 mm. We are led to believe that the direct relation between products and pressures would still exist for a 0.01-mm tube, with a length of 0.5 or 0.3 mm, which is the size of mammalian capillary vessels in the network that they form between arteries and veins.

In an upcoming lecture, we shall be honored to expound to the Academy the laws relating to the length of tubes, their diameters, and the temperature.

II. INFLUENCE OF LENGTH ON THE AMOUNT OF LIQUID PASSING THROUGH TUBES OF VERY SMALL DIAMETER

To determine the possible influence of the length of the tube, we investigated the time interval of flow for the same amount of liquid at the same pressure and the same temperature, using tubes of different lengths.

This project required the use of perfectly cylindrical glass tubes which do not exist; they are all conical; however, in choosing among many hundreds of tubes, we found a certain number that, although not perfectly cylindrical, could be considered as such, with only slight differences of 0.001 to 0.002 mm at the two ends, for widths of 100 to 150 mm. We took the precaution of noting these small differences in diameter of each tube and took this into account in the results obtained.

The diameters were measured in two ways. In the first, we used a *camera lucida* adapted to the Amici horizontal microscope, after having determined the magnification power for the lenses, using a micrometer. In the other, we passed a certain amount of mercury many times through the tube whose diameter we were measuring, each time measuring the length of the corresponding mercury column; we collected all these small amounts of mercury and determined the weight with a Fortin scale, and then the volume; we divided the total volume by the sum of the mercury columns, and we then obtained, at the constant temperature we worked at, the surface area of a section of the tube perpendicular to its axis, and consequently the diameter of the tube, or the mean diameter if it is oval. Either method gave the same results, but the latter required a lot of time: we preferred the former, which in addition, had the advantage of giving the small differences existing between the measurements of the diameter of the tube, when it is oval, which is more often the case.

The lengths of the tubes were determined with a Gambey compass; a sliding vernier was adapted to it, giving 20ths and, when necessary, 40ths of a millimeter.

According to what we know about the law of pressures, it did not matter if we used a particular pressure for the flow; we adopted a pressure of 775 mm mercury and a temperature of 10°C.

We will now report on the results obtained. The length of the tube is 100.325 mm, the diameters are

$$\text{Circular open end} \quad D = \overset{mm}{0.0845} \qquad \text{Opposite end} \begin{cases} d = \overset{mm}{0.085} \\ D = 0.086 \end{cases}$$

We cut off various portions successively, to lengths of 100.325, 74.95, 49.7, 24.4, 10.15, and 6.025 mm.

We notice that the original tube had a detectably smaller cross section at the open end than at the opposite end, and therefore each shorter tube had a progressively larger diameter than the preceding one.

The time intervals for the liquid flow in the bulb for these lengths are 2090.8, 1560, 1028.4, 497, 203.14, and 131.2 seconds (s), respectively.

Let us suppose for one moment that the time intervals are directly related to the tube lengths, and we are seeking, according to this hypothesis, the time interval of an experiment, comparing it to the one immediately preceding it; we will get:

for the second experiment,	1562 s instead of 1560 s;
for the third,	1034 s instead of 1028.4 s;
for the fourth,	504 s instead of 497 s;
for the fifth,	206 s instead of 203.14 s.

We see that the time intervals obtained experimentally were always smaller than the calculated time intervals but only by a few seconds; we are already led to believe that the hypothesis of time intervals being directly related to lengths is valid; if this is so, the time intervals obtained experimentally must be perceptibly smaller than the hypothetical ones, because the shorter tubes had a perceptibly larger cross section than the one directly preceding it, to which we are comparing it, and the corresponding time interval of flow of the same amount of liquid must necessarily be perceptibly smaller.

But if the tube, instead of having the open end of smaller diameter than the end near the bulb, as previously, has the opposite arrangement; if we have

$$\text{Open end} \begin{cases} d = \overset{mm}{0.0460} \\ D = 0.0470 \end{cases} \qquad \text{Opposite end near bulb} \begin{cases} d = \overset{mm}{0.0425} \\ D = 0.0445 \end{cases}$$

and if we proceed with respect to this tube as we just did previously, we then had experimental time intervals several seconds longer than those obtained by calculation, because each smaller length of tube would have a slightly smaller cross section than the preceding one. From this we would like to conclude that time intervals are directly related to lengths.

The first tube, reduced to 6.025 mm, which at this length did not obey the law of pressures, also did not maintain the relation that we just obtained for 100.325, 74.95, 49.7, 24.4, and 10.15 mm. But, just as we observed concerning the law of pressures, when the tube is 6.025 mm long, the time interval is proportionally longer than that which would be expected from the direct relation of time to length. As such, the sixth experiment, by comparison to the fifth, would yield, according to the preceding relation, 120.5 s, while we obtained 131.2 s experimentally.

Analogous findings are supplied by tubes with diameters of 0.1416 and 0.1134 mm. For a tube of smaller diameters

$$\text{Open end}\ \begin{cases} d = 0.0286 \\ D = 0.0296 \end{cases}\ \text{mm} \qquad \text{Opposite end}\ \begin{cases} d = 0.02933 \\ D = 0.03000 \end{cases}\ \text{mm}$$

and lengths of 23.1, 8.5, and 2.1 mm, the time intervals are 2003.4, 734.9, and 178.1 s, respectively; seeking, as before, the time intervals of an experiment by comparison with the previous one, we find 737.18 s instead of 734.9 s and 181.3 s instead of 178.1 s.

Finally, a tube with a diameter of 0.01394 mm, and consequently quite similar to capillary vessels in mammals, yields, for lengths of 18.50 and 1.25 mm, time intervals of 1240 and 84.5 s, respectively; the time intervals of the second experiment by comparison to the first would be 83.5 s instead of 84.5 s, using the law of lengths.

From the preceding data we can conclude that the time interval of flow for the same amount of liquid at the same pressure and the same temperature, for the tubes of very small diameter that we worked with, is directly related to the lengths.

The tube with a diameter of 0.65 mm that we studied in the preceding paragraph also confirms this law, for lengths of 800 and 400 mm.

Let a be the amount of liquid flowing through a tube of length L during the time interval t. If the length of the tube becomes L/m, the time interval required for the same amount of liquid to flow will be, according to the preceding law, t/m; then the amount of liquid flowing through the L/m tube will be ma; the products are inversely related to the lengths of tubes.

We can now introduce length L of the tube in the preceding formula $Q = kP$. If $k = k'/L$, then $Q = k'(P/L)$, the coefficient k' being a function only of the diameter of the tube and the temperature, as we will soon see.

With the law of lengths existing at the same time as the law of pressures, we can say that the relation just established occurs for tubes 0.01 mm in diameter, where the lengths are 0.3 to 0.5 mm. From this we can conclude, all things being equal, that any capillary network whose vessels would be 2, 3, or 4 times shorter than the capillary vessels of another network would be perfused by a two-, three-, or fourfold amount of liquid than the former one.

III. INFLUENCE OF DIAMETER ON THE AMOUNT OF LIQUID PASSING THROUGH TUBES OF VERY SMALL DIAMETER

In the interest of answering this question, we determined the amount of liquid that flowed through tubes of different diameter, at the same pressure, at the same temperature, during the same time interval using tubes of the same length.

It is rare to find cylindrical tubes and equally so for circular tubes; we chose among a large number of tubes and selected those that could be considered cylindrical, approaching a circular shape, with a somewhat oval opening; but considering it elliptical, we were able to obtain the average diameter of the tubes, without detectable error.

Without entering into the details of our calculations, which are easy to conceive of according to the preceding, we are going to report the results of our experiments, performed on seven tubes of the same length with diameters varying from 0.013 to 0.652 mm.

The pressure is 775 m Hg, the temperature 10°C, and the time interval 500 s. Rounding the figures in the table, the ratio of the diameters of the seven tubes (M to F) were related as 1 : 2 : 3 : 6 : 8 : 10 : 50; it was easy to see that the products were in direct relation to the fourth power of the diameters.

Tubes	*Diameters (fractions of millimeters)*	*Products (cubic millimeters)*
M	0.01394	1.4648
E	0.02938	28.8260
D	0.04373	141.5002
C	0.08549	2067.3912
B	0.11340	6398.2933
A	0.14160	15532.8451
F	0.65217	6995870.2463

In fact, according to this relation, in looking for the product of tube M, compared to tube E, the calculated value is 1.4650 mm³ instead of the 1.4648 mm³ that we obtain from the experiment. Proceeding in this manner to tubes E and D, the product of E is 28.808 mm³ instead of the 28.826 mm³ obtained from the experiment.

	*mm*³		*mm*³
The product of tube D compared to C is	141.63	instead of	141.500
The product of tube C compared to B is	2066.93	instead of	2067.39
The product of tube B compared to A is	6389.24	instead of	6398.29
The product of tube A compared to F is	15547.10	instead of	15532.84

If we are seeking the product of a tube by comparing it to another with a much larger cross section, M to D, for example, for the product of M, we get 1.46415 mm^3 instead of 1.4648.

The diameter of tube F is about 50 times greater than that of M, and consequently has a cross section 2500 times larger; the product of tube M compared to F is 1.46448 instead of 1.4648 mm^3.

The product of C compared to F is 2065.92 mm^3 instead of 2067.39 mm^3.

All other combinations of two tubes giving equally satisfying results, we are allowed to conclude that the products, all other factors being equal, vary as the fourth power of diameters.

In including this result with those previously obtained, the equation of movement for liquids in our small tube will be, if D is the diameter, $Q = k''(PD^4/L)$, k'' being a constant coefficient for a given temperature and for the same force of gravity.

We determined the value of k'' for each of these tubes, replacing Q, P, D, and L with their corresponding numbers; and, by supposing that the time interval for flow is 1 s, we obtained:

For tube M	$k'' = 2495.50$
For tube E	$k'' = 2496.00$
For tube D	$k'' = 2494.42$
For tube C	$k'' = 2497.77$
For tube B	$k'' = 2496.20$
For tube A	$k'' = 2492.67$
For tube F	$k'' = 2495.00$

These values of k'' differ very little, as we can see, the mean being 2495.224. The previous equation becomes $Q = 2495.224\ (PD^4/L)$ at a temperature of 10°C.

If the pressure, instead of being determined by the weight of mercury, as we have just been doing, was measured by the weight of distilled water, the formula would be, at 10°C, $Q = 183.783(PD^4/L)$. The equation for velocity, coming from equation $Q = k''(PD^4/L)$, is $V = (4k''/\pi)\cdot(PD^2/L)$ (π representing the ratio of circumference to the diameter). Then, the flow, in tubes of very small diameter, is inversely related to their length, and proportional to pressure and to the square of their diameter.

M. Navier's formula, deduced by analysis from a priori hypothesis on the steady state of fluid molecules in movement, is $V = H(PD/L)$ (H

being a constant coefficient); this formula differs from the former one by having the first power of the diameter of the tube instead of the second power.

The dimensions of capillary vessels of animals are such that the laws of fluid flow established here apply perfectly; so that, if one considers the capillary system of two organs, if the diameter of capillaries of one of them is twice that of the second, the amount of fluid flowing through the former one will be, all other things being equal, 16 times greater than in the latter.

It would be important to consider if the equation $Q = k''(PD^4/L)$ would exist even for tubes having a larger diameter than those studied here. Dubuat, Gerstner, and Girard's experiments, performed on tubes whose diameters were 1 to 4 mm, do not satisfy our formula; but the results obtained on the tube with 0.65 mm diameter, much wider than all our tubes, coinciding with the former ones when the latter is long enough, led us to think that the tubes used by these authors were not long enough with respect to their diameter to fit the formula $Q = k''(PD^4/L)$ for the flow described. We then decided to work on tubes of greater diameter, with an increased length; but our apparatus, which was already inconvenient for the 0.65-mm-diameter tube, cannot be used for long tubes. It would have been necessary to build another one, quite different from the one we used, requiring some conditions that were impossible to achieve in our laboratory. But with the help of M. Savant, who put at our disposal part of his hydraulic observatory in the Collège de France, we hope to be able to extend this research to much longer tubes, to determine the upper limit to which the law of movement of fluids in very small diameter tubes is valid.

Now we would like to express the k'' value, which is 183.78 at 10°C, as a function of temperature. We worked from 0 to 45°C, increasing by 5° steps; we observed that for the small-diameter tubes, the amount of liquid flowing at 45°C was about 3 times greater than at 0°C. But as we fear to abuse the Academy's time, we will report this expression of k'' value at a future lecture.

24

THE RESISTANCE TO FLOW IN THE HUMAN AIR PASSAGES AND THE INFLUENCE OF THE IRREGULAR BRANCHING OF THE BRONCHIAL SYSTEM ON THE COURSE OF RESPIRATION IN DIFFERENT REGIONS OF THE LUNGS

Fritz Rohrer

These excerpts were translated by Renward Mangold, Bern, Switzerland, from "Der Strömungswiderstand in den menschlichen Atemwegen und der Einfluss der unregelmässigen Verzweigung des Bronchialsystems auf den Atmungsverlauf in verschiedenen Lungenbezirken," Pfluegers Arch. ***162,*** *225–227, 252–256, 292–299 (1915)*

There is a series of experimental investigations (Gad, Ewald, Block) on the flow in the upper respiratory tract that furnishes data on the essential factors (respiratory volume, lateral pressure, temperature and humidity of the respiratory air, etc.). On the other hand, due to the inaccessibility of this part of the airways, little is known so far on the flow of air in the bronchial system and its cause, that is, the difference in pressure between the alveoli and the tracheal bifurcation.

In general, the experimental investigation of a certain problem in research has to precede theoretical considerations. If, however, the possibilities of conducting an experimental investigation are very small, as they are in this case, it may be permissible to begin with a theoretical reconstruction of the event.

The flow of air in the respiratory tract is a purely physical event and the laws governing it are fairly well known. If these laws are applied to this special case with consideration of all the possible factors, we may assume with a high degree of probability that we approach the real conditions very closely.

H. v. Recklinghausen[1] tried in this way to determine alveolar pressure by replacing the bronchial system by a system of tubes, with regular dichotomous branching. He found (in adults) with quiet respiration a difference of pressure between the alveoli and atmospheric air of 0.129 cm H_2O at the peak of expiration. This is a value that is so low in comparison with the lateral pressure in the trachea as measured by other investigators that it seemed desirable to go through the calculations once more on a broader basis, especially since there has been much progress in physical research of events during flow, and methods have been developed that permit the calculation of flow in irregularly branching systems of tubes (bronchial system).[2] The mathematical procedure of Blaess has been derived for turbulent flow. A similar method of calculating streamlined flow in systems of branching tubes has not yet been published. I shall devote a considerable part of the present study to this question, which is of some importance considering the role of flow in branching tubes in physiology in general.

As a basis for our calculations of flow of air in the lungs, we have taken the bronchial system of the right lung, which has been measured down to the lobular bronchi of 1-mm diameter.

Based on this material we shall try to solve two further problems of respiratory physiology that have not yet been given due consideration: (1) the influence of the irregular anatomy of the bronchial system on the respiration in different sections of the lung, and (2) the dimensions of the dead space.

[*Editor's Note:* Material has been omitted at this point.]

BRONCHIAL SYSTEM

Morphology of the Bronchial Tree

Because there are no data in the literature on complete measurements of the bronchial system, it was first necessary to obtain this basis for the calculations of flow.

The method of casts, which has given excellent results in the study of the form of branching of the bronchial tree (Aeby, Narath, Birch-Hirschfeld), is less suitable for the exact determination of cross sections, which are above all important in our study. By the hydrostatic pressure of the casting mass of high specific gravity, the trachea and main bronchi (Braune and Stahel)[3] are dilated and, naturally, the medium and fine bronchi even more so.

I therefore proceeded to the measurement of the bronchi in the dead lung directly by means of calibrated bougies, a method that in other fields of medicine (urology) also serves to determine the caliber of canals. The diameter of the bougies used fell between 1 and 10 mm, with steps of 0.5 mm each. The bougies had a longitudinal scale with graduations of 0.5 cm for a length of 5 cm from their slightly rounded distal tip on.

Measurements were made successively, beginning at the main bronchus and continuing down to bronchi of a diameter of 1 mm.

Control was partly visual but mainly tactile. Because a psychophysiologic factor, that is, the tactile threshold for differences in resistance, is of some importance here, it was no use to increase the number of steps in the diameter of the bougies. In the big, noncollapsed bronchi, it is relatively easy to find out which size of bougie just fills the lumen, and it is also not difficult to feel what size just unfolds the smaller, collapsed bronchi. A bifurcation of the bronchus can be felt as a slight resistance to the bougie, which is introduced with a light touch, and then the length of the bronchus is read on the 0.5-cm scale, the millimeters being estimated. Once the diameter and length of the bronchus are determined, it is split open lengthwise and the length is verified directly whenever possible with a rule, especially if two bronchi of the same caliber follow each other and the bougie has passed the first bifurcation. At the main bronchi and the connecting bronchi between upper and middle lobe, where the cross section is not circular, two diameters are measured with the rule, one perpendicular to the other. Because the collapsed medium and small bronchi are opened up during this method of measurement, the values correspond to a state of the lung that immediately precedes the collapsed state. The measured values for the collapsed lung (see Rohrer, p. 250) also correspond to this state, since with the folding of the bronchial walls a further outflow of air is prevented. For the sake of simplicity, we can therefore assume that this state of the lung can still be described as a collapsed lung.

After this method had been tried on another lung, the whole bronchial system of the right lung of a 48-year-old patient of 166-cm height, who died of a carcinoma of the colon, was measured down to the bronchi of 1-mm diameter.

The measurement was done on a fresh preparation during three successive days; in the intervals the lung was kept in the cold room of the pathology–anatomy institute. The excellent reproductions in the paper by Birch-Hirschfeld[4] served as a continuous orientation in the morphologic features of the bronchial system. The results of the measurements were successively plotted on a scale of 2 : 1 and the values for length and diameter added. At eight places the bougie penetrated into the pulmonary tissue during the measurement of bronchi of a diameter of 1.5 mm. In these cases the average value for the length of bronchi of the same caliber was taken.

That we can consider the 467 bronchi of 1-mm diameter found in the right lung as being lobular bronchi can be proved by the value for the size of the lobule obtained from this number, the weight of the lung (355 g), and its volume (675 cc).

If we take the weight of the bronchi and blood vessels as about $\frac{1}{3} = 120$ g $= 120$ cc, the volume of a single lobule would be $\frac{555}{467} = 1.19$ cc. A sphere of the same volume has a diameter of approximately 1.3 cm. For the polyhedric lobules, the diameters have to be taken slightly greater, at about 1.5 cm, a value that falls very well into the measured range of 0.6–2.8 cm.[5]

As it would take up too much space to reproduce the tables of measured values, I present two statistical tables to orient one on the structure of the bronchial system of the right lung. The first table shows the part the bronchi of different caliber take in the total structure of the bronchial system, and the second indicates the distribution of the sums as well as the average values for the length of the bronchi for the individual lobules and for the whole lung.

mm	*Number of bronchi*	*Total length of bronchi (cm)*	*Average length of bronchi (cm)*	*Total contents of bronchi (cc)*
17	1	3.0	—	6.8
12	1	2.9	—	3.3
9	2	2.3	—	1.5
8	1	0.4	—	0.2
7.5	1	1.4	—	0.6
6	2	2.0	—	0.6
5.5	6	5.1	0.85	1.2
5	5	6.5	1.30	1.3
4.5	8	8.1	1.01	1.3
4	22	23.5	1.07	2.9
3.5	24	22.3	0.93	2.1
3	36	31.0	0.86	2.2
2.5	67	59.6	0.89	2.9
2	86	73.5	0.85	2.3
1.5	204	160.4	0.79	2.8

For the main bronchi and the connecting bronchi between upper and middle lobes where the lumen is not circular, the cross section was calculated from the two diameters 18 : 16 mm and 13 : 11 mm, respectively, according to the formula for an ellipse. In the table, the average value for the diameters of 17 and 12 mm, respectively, has been used.

	No. of lobules	*No. of bronchi*	*Total length of bronchi (cm)*	*Average length of bronchi (cm)*	*Total contents of bronchi (cc)*
Right lung	467	466	402	0.86	32
Upper lobe	163	162	128.9	0.80	7.2
Middle lobe	104	103	89.4	0.87	4.4
Lower lobe	200	199	177.8	0.89	10.4

It is interesting that for the individual lobules as well as for the whole lung the number of bronchi is smaller by one than the corresponding number of lobules. This is a general relationship that is valuable wherever there is a branching system with regular or irregular dichotomy; the number of afferent* branches is equal to the number of terminal branches minus one.

The total length of all bronchi (402 cm) is small if we consider that the distance of the lobules from the bifurcation reaches up to 20 cm in the

* Rohrer uses the words *zuführenden* and *ausführenden*, translated here as *afferent* and *efferent*, repectively.

collapsed lung, whereas the increase in length of the afferent tubular network for each lobule amounts to 0.86 only. The average length of the bronchi increases slightly if we go down from the upper lobe to the lower lobe, corresponding to an increasing distance from the bifurcation.

To complete this review, a small table on the bronchioles of the 467 lobules of this right lung is provided. Together with the values for the bronchial system, we obtain the sums for the entire right lung:

Diam (mm)	*Number of bronchi*	*Total length of bronchi (m)*	*Average length of bronchi (mm)*	*Total contents of bronchi (cc)*
1	467	1.87	4	1.5
0.82	934	3.03	3.27	1.6
0.67	1,868	4.99	2.67	1.8
0.55	3,736	8.18	2.19	1.9
0.45	7,472	13.38	1.79	2.1
0.37	14,944	21.98	1.47	2.3
0.3	29,888	35.9	1.2	
0.24	59,776	58.6	0.98	
0.2	119,552	95.6	0.8	320
Alveolar ducts	358,656	466.2	1.3	

Total number of all bronchi and bronchioles	239,103
Total number of bronchi, bronchioles, and alveolar ducts	597,759
Total length of all bronchi, bronchioles, and alveolar ducts	713.75 m
Total contents of efferent systems	43.2 cc

It is interesting to note the great number (about 600,000) and length (about 700 m) of all tubular elements (bronchi, bronchioles, and alveolar ducts) of this lung. A total volume of 43.2 cc for the contents of the whole efferent system (bifurcation to intralobular bronchioles of the fifth order) is important; 32 cc of the 43.2 belong to the interlobular bronchi and 11.2 cc to the intralobular bronchioles.

The volume ratio between right and left lung according to measurement is 675 : 450 cc = : 0.67 ($\frac{2}{3}$). The ratio is here somewhat smaller than usual.

According to the measurements made by Braune and Stahel,[6] the left lung is 74.9 percent ($\frac{3}{4}$) of the right on an average basis. Since we have intentionally chosen a special case and considered all its characteristics, we shall base our calculations on this measured ratio of 1 : $\frac{2}{3}$.

The left lung has to be equal to a certain fraction of the right lung. Therefore, all the values determined for the right lung, such as numbers, lengths, and volumes, have all to be reduced in the ratio 1 : $\frac{2}{3}$. Consequently, we have to assume about 311 lobules for the left lung and, correspondingly, 310 interlobular bronchi.

A few values concerning sums of both lungs together are remarkable: the number of lobules of about 778, the number of all bronchi, bronchioles, and alveolar ducts of about 1 million, the tremendous length of all air passages of about 1200 m, the total content of all air spaces of about 0.6 liters, and above all the air content of the efferent system of 72 cc. Of the latter, 53.3 cc are attributed to the interlobular bronchi, and 18.7 cc to the intralobular bronchioles.

[*Editor's Note:* Material has been omitted at this point.]

SIZE OF THE DEAD SPACE

The dead space is, anatomically defined, equal to the total volume of the inflow and outflow system. In the collapsed lung we found this to be 162 cc.

The change in dimension of the bronchi on expansion of the lungs takes place, as we have seen, according to type 3 (pp. 247 and 278). If a is a coefficient of volume change of the lung, the volume (J) of the bronchial system will be $J' = \sqrt{a} \times J$ (p. 248). The change in dimension of the main stem bronchus and the immediately following branches is probably less than in the other bronchi. We shall therefore add the volumes of the bronchi with a diameter above 7.5 mm, which is 20.6 cc, to the invariable volume of the upper respiratory passages of 90 cc: 20.6 + 90 = 110.6 cc. The total volume of the bronchi of less than 7.5-mm diameter is 51.4 cc. We thus have the value of the dead space: $(110.6 + 51.4) \times \sqrt{a}$. For the principal states of respiration we obtain the following values:

	Volume of air in lungs (liters)	a	*Dead space*
State of collapse	0.6	1	160
Maximal expiration	1.2	2	180
Ordinary expiration	2.8	4.67	220
Ordinary inspiration	3.3	5.5	230
Maximal inspiration	4.9	8.17	260

On the passage from maximal expiration to maximal inspiration, the volume of the dead space of the lungs increases by about 80 cc. For the average state of expansion of about 3 liters, we can calculate a volume of about 225 cc for the dead space.

The value is considerably greater than the generally accepted one of 140 cc found by Loewy.[7] Loewy obtained this value in three different ways:

1. By injection of the air passages of the collapsed lung: 144 cc. This value corresponds to the one of 143.3 cc found by us in the collapsed lung (p. 260) and corresponds to the upper passages plus interlobular bronchi.
2. By analysis of samples of expiratory air at the beginning of expiration

for their carbon dioxide content. At the start of expiration, the dead space is filled with atmospheric air. The first portion of expiratory air containing little carbon dioxide seems to correspond to the volume of the dead space. It was shown in the course of the investigation that a high degree of mixing of expiratory air takes place. Only about 75 cc contains a small amount of carbon dioxide.[8] Loewy did not draw any further conclusions from these experiments.[9]

The mixing found by Loewy has two causes:

a. As the air in the center of a tube reaches twice the average velocity of flow (p. 231), alveolar air rich in carbon dioxide will already have passed through the central part of the tubes when the volume flow corresponds to only half the dead space.

b. As about one third of the dead space is more peripheral than the openings of the most central lobules into the bronchial system, alveolar air from these lobules has already arrived when the dead space has emptied to only two thirds.

Since both factors are important to an equal degree, it follows that the volume flow poor in carbon dioxide, found experimentally by Loewy to be 75 cc, corresponds to only $\frac{1}{2} \times \frac{2}{3} = \frac{1}{3}$ of the volume of the dead space. We therefore obtain a value for the dead space of 3×75 cc = 225 cc, which corresponds with the value that we determined.

This mixing of the respiratory air found by Loewy makes it possible to distinguish between anatomical and physiological dead space during small breaths.

Breaths with a tidal volume a little above 75 cc already carry alveolar air from the most central lobules on expiration and bring atmospheric air into these same lobules on inspiration; even the most peripheral lobules are reached by atmospheric air on inspiration if the tidal volume exceeds about 110 cc, that is, half the dead space. The physiological value for the dead space may go down to one third of the anatomical value with small tidal volumes.

On the other hand, it is important to find at what volume of respiration both values coincide. The tidal volume must reach about twice the volume of the dead space, that is, about 450 cc, to make the physiological dead space equal to the anatomical dead space. In this case all the air rich in carbon dioxide contained in the in- and outflow system reaches the alveoli on inspiration and is replaced by atmospheric air, which is then expired without any change.

For breaths between about 80 and 450 cc, we may assume that the physiological dead space increases progressively from the lower value of 75 cc to the upper limit of 225 cc. For a tidal volume of 250 cc, for instance, which is somewhat below the average of this range, we would have a value of about 140 to 150 cc for the physiological dead space. This value corresponds to the one observed by Loewy and explains his third observation[10]:

3. Loewy did experiments on respiration below atmospheric pressure

with a tidal volume of about 250 cc and, taking the conditions for partial pressure of oxygen of the alveolar air as a basis, found 140 cc to be the most likely value of the dead space. This number obtained by Loewy is of very limited value and can be explained by the difference between physiological and anatomical dead space on shallow breathing. For respiration with a tidal volume above 450 cc, especially for ordinary breathing, we always have to assume an average value of the dead space of about 225 cc.

For the exchange of oxygen, the size of the dead space at the end of an inspiration is the determining factor; for the exchange of carbon dioxide, it is the size at the end of expiration. On ordinary breathing this factor may be neglected; on maximal depth of breathing it favors the exchange of carbon dioxide by a volume of about 80 cc.

The composition of the alveolar air depends on the size of the dead space. In the following table the values are presented that have been derived from our and from Loewy's determinations[11] of the dead space for an ordinary tidal volume of 500 cc:

	Dead space = 140 cc	*Dead space = 225 cc*
Quotient of ventilation	$\frac{1}{9}$	$\frac{1}{12}$
CO_2 content of alveolar/air	5.6%	7.4%
Partial pressure	40 mm Hg	53 mm Hg
O_2 content of alveolar air	14.6%	12.6%
Partial pressure	104 mm Hg	90 mm Hg

The resulting composition of the alveolar air again points to an active secretory activity of the respiratory epithelium.

The importance of the dead space for the working economy of respiration will be the subject for another investigation.

SUMMARY

1. The viscosity of respiratory air is for all physiological conditions, with slight variations, $\eta = 0.0001873$ (dyne).

2. The flow of air in the respiratory passages is streamlined during respiration (capillary flow according to Poiseuille's law). On maximal breathing the critical velocity is never exceeded in any section of the air passages, during quiet respiration the lower limiting velocity is not reached anywhere.

Changes in cross section and direction can be taken separately into consideration as local extra resistances.

These conditions are not influenced by the nonstationary character of respiration nor by phonation.

3. Simple laws of summation can be derived for the calculation of the

resistance to streamlined flow in branching systems of tubes as well as for the calculation of the additional resistances.

4. Considering all morphological details as exactly as possible, the following relationship between volume flow in the trachea, in liters per second, and difference of pressure between atmospheric and alveolar air can be found for the almost collapsed lungs:

$$P_{alv} = 0.8(V + V^2) \text{ cm } H_20$$

(The most important data on the structure of the bronchial system of the collapsed lungs can be found on pp. 254–256.)

This equation seems to be valid for all states of expansion of the lungs. This conclusion is reached primarily by analogy with the small changes of resistance in the pulmonary vascular system during expansion of the lungs, as determined experimentally by Cloetta.[12]

The alveolar pressure gradient at the height of an ordinary inspiration is 0.36–0.6 cm H_2O.

For volume flows above 5 liters/s, for instance during coughing, the formula $p = V^2$ cm H_2O (V in liters) can be used as an approximation.

5. The resistance to flow in the bronchi beyond the bifurcation shows a rise and fall repeated 2 to 3 times. In bronchi of 4- to 6-mm diameter, the velocity of flow may exceed by 1.7 times the velocity in the trachea, in the lobular it is only $\frac{1}{3}$ to $\frac{7}{10}$ of the velocity in the trachea, and in the respiratory bronchioles of the third order it is only $\frac{1}{30}$ to $\frac{7}{100}$ of the tracheal velocity.

6. The nasal passages and the narrow bronchi (intralobular and interlobular bronchi of a diameter below 3 mm) account for most of the resistance to flow. About one tenth of the total resistance is due to pharynx, trachea, and major bronchi. Nine tenths of the extra resistance is caused by changes in cross section and direction in the upper air passages. The glottis alone produces two thirds of the sum of extra resistances. Only about one tenth of the extra resistance is due to the bronchiolobular system.

7. During quiet respiration, the extra resistances contribute very little to the fall in pressure between bifurcation and alveoli (one twelfth); the distribution of the volumes depends almost entirely on the resistances to tubular flow. Since more than 90 percent of these resistances arise in the most peripheral parts of the bronchiolobular system, the conditions for flow are the same as if each lobule had an isolated direct connection with the trachea.

The calculations for the distribution of volumes and pressures in the lungs in two extreme cases show that the alveolar pressure is constant within the physiological limits of volume distribution. They also show that for the individual lobules the quotient of volume flow (of the lobular bronchus per second) and pressure gradient between trachea and alveoli (*Vp* quotient) is a systemic constant, independent of the form of distribution. Compared to the average value, the *Vp* quotient is about

1.3 for the most central, and about 0.65 for the most peripheral lobules. With the same bronchiolobular pressure gradient, the volume flow of the central lobules is therefore about twice as high as for the peripheral ones, and, on the other hand, with the same volume flow the pressure gradient to the most peripheral lobules is about twice as high as that to the most central ones.

8. These particular conditions for the individual lobules are determined by the interaction of three systems of forces: (a) the pressure gradient between alveolar and atmospheric air, (b) the elastic force of retraction of the lung tissue, and (c) the forces of traction acting from outside on the lung. The sum of the first two forces is in equilibrium with the third force in any section of the lung at any given time. The force of traction acts uniformly throughout the entire lung.

The relationship between the force of traction *p,* the average force of elastic retraction *P,* and the difference of pressure P_{alv} can be expressed for the entire lung in a simple equation:

$$p = P_{el_0} \pm (4.5 \times Q) \pm 0.8\ (V + V^2)$$

P_{el_0} is the force of elastic retraction in cm H_2O at the beginning of a breath (for the usual state of expiration it is 10 cm H_2O), Q is the change in volume in liters in a given interval of time, V is the momentary volume flow in the trachea in liters/unit time, + is for inspiration, and − for expiration.

For the individual lobules the equation assumes the following form:

$$p = P_{el_0} \pm (3.5 \times q) \pm (P_{bif}) \pm (c \times V)\ \text{cm } H_2O$$

B_{bif} is the momentary pressure gradient in the upper air passages to the bifurcation in cm H_2O, q is the change in volume in cubic centimeters that has taken place in the lobule, and V is the volume flow in the lobular bronchus. The constant c is 0.283 for the average lobule, 0.218 for a central lobule, and 0.436 for a peripheral lobule.

The irregular structure of the bronchial system causes an irregular distribution of air at the beginning of a breath and an irregular distribution of pressure during the further course of a breath. At the beginning of each breath, the same difference in pressure exists for all alveoli, and correspondingly the volume flow is twice as high for the central lobules as for the peripheral ones according to the *Vp* quotient.

After this initial phase during a breath, the final stage is approached asymptotically, where the volume flow is the same in all lobular bronchi. This process takes place so rapidly for uniform and for accelerated volume flow that 0.5 s is after the start of a breath the final stage is practically reached, almost independent of the spirometrical curve.

The increase and decrease in lobular volume on inspiration and expiration show a similar change as the volume flow, but here the curves approach each other more slowly. Uniformity is practically reached here, too, 0.5 to 1 s after the beginning of a breath.

After the first half-second and for the rest of a phase of breathing, the pressure gradient between the bifurcation and the alveoli of the central lobules is only half as great as between the bifurcation and the alveoli of the peripheral lobules. The ratio for the total difference in pressure between alveolar and atmospheric air is $\frac{3}{4}$: 1 for central and peripheral lobules. At the height of an ordinary inspiration the alveolar pressure gradient is as follows:

Average	*cm H_2O*
Entire lung	0.36–0.6
Most central lobules	0.32–0.54
Most peripheral lobules	0.46–0.77

We may assume that similar conditions exist for the bronchi as for the most central lobules, that is, a rapid change in dimensions at the beginning of a breath. As the circular elastic force of the bronchi is higher than the average force of elastic retraction of the lung tissue, this change will appear only when high pressure gradients exist, such as during coughing, as has been shown by bronchoscopic observations.

During coughing the conditions are similar to the beginning of a breath, but the difference between peripheral and central sections of the lung is accentuated by the importance of the additional resistance at the high rates of volume flow. In the bronchi of the central lobules, the volume flow at the beginning of a cough is about three times as high as in the bronchi to the peripheral lobules.

During deep breathing the situation for the most central sections and for the sections situated medially above the hilus is exceptional. Their volume change is less than in the rest of the lung.

9. The volume of the dead space can be calculated to be 225 cc for an average state of lung expansion; it changes by 80 cc between maximal expiration (about 180 cc) and maximal inspiration (about 260 cc).

The value accepted generally until now of 140 cc (Loewy) can be found under particular conditions, for instance in shallow breathing, where only part of the dead space is physiologically important. The physiological dead space can be as low as one third of the anatomical dead space on shallow breathing.

REFERENCES

1. Recklinghausen, H. v., *Pfluegers Arch.,* **62:**451–493, 1895.
2. Blaess, *Die Strömung in Röhren und die Berechnung weitverzweigter Leitungen.* Verlag Oldenbourg, München, 1911.
3. Braune and Stahel, *Arch. Anat. Entwicklungsgesch.,* p. 13, 1886.
4. Birch-Hirschfeld, *Dtsch. Arch. klin. Med.,* **64:**58–128, 1899.

5. Kölliker's *Handbook of Histology,* p. 38.
6. Braune and Stahel, *op. cit.,* pp. 5–44.
7. Loewy, *Pfluegers Arch.,* **58**:416–427, 1894.
8. *Ibid.,* p. 422.
9. *Ibid.,* p. 423.
10. *Ibid.,* pp. 424–427.
11. Bohr, in Nagel's *Handbuch d. Physiologie d. Menschen,* **1**:139, 1905.
12. Cloetta, *Pfluegers Arch.,* **152**:358, 1913.

25

THE PNEUMOTACHOGRAPH; AN APPARATUS FOR DETERMINING THE VELOCITY OF RESPIRED AIR

Alfred Fleisch

This excerpt was prepared expressly for this Benchmark volume by Hans Hahn, North Senior Fellow, Cardiovascular Research Institute, University of California, San Francisco, from "Der Pneumotachograph: ein Apparat zur Geschwindigkeitsregistrierung der Atemluft," Pfluegers Arch., ***209,*** *715–716 (1925)*

[*Editor's Note:* In the original, material precedes this excerpt.]

DESIGN OF THE PNEUMOTACHOGRAPH

Ninety tubes, each 20 cm long, 2 mm wide, with both ends conically widening, are put together in a bundle in such a way as to prevent any passage of air in between the tubes (Figure 1). All 90 tubes merge into a common collecting tube which tapers off so that its smallest diameter is 2.5 cm. The mouthpiece is attached to this tapered end. Two branching tubes are soldered on to one of the 90 tubes at right angles (i.e., two T-junctions are created), which are 5.5 cm from either end and 9 cm from each other. Similar branching connections are attached to another tube but the distance between these is 18 cm. For a third and fourth tube the distances are 4 and 1.5 cm, respectively. These four pairs of branching tubes are used for measuring pressure differences. Since

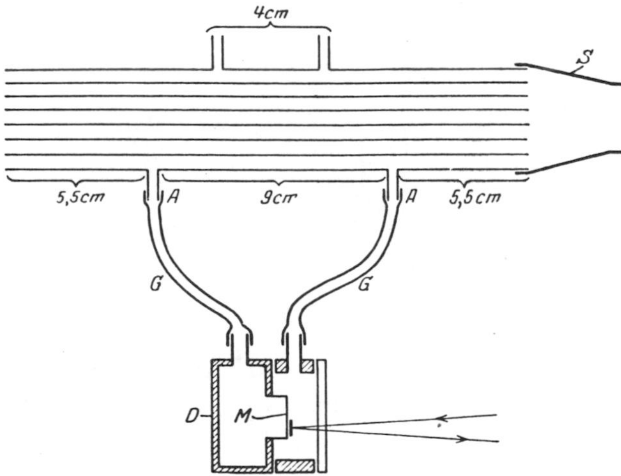

Figure 1 (Reproduced from *Pfleugers Arch.,* **209** (1925);

these are bigger the farther the tubes are apart, the four pairs give a choice of four different deflections, the ratios of which are 18 : 9 : 4 :1.5. The six openings not in use in any one experiment are, of course, plugged.

From the two openings that are used, two identical pieces of rubber tubing lead to the differential manometer *D,* the membrane of which is a piece of condom rubber 14 mm in diameter. During air flow, the pressure difference between the two openings causes a deflection of the rubber membrane *M,* which is transmitted by a light beam reflected from a small mirror glued to the rubber surface.

Care must be taken to prewarm the air inspired through the pneumotachograph; otherwise water will condense from expired air inside the tubular system.

26

Reprinted from *J. Clin. Invest.*, **35**, 327–335 (1956)

A NEW METHOD FOR MEASURING AIRWAY RESISTANCE IN MAN USING A BODY PLETHYSMOGRAPH: VALUES IN NORMAL SUBJECTS AND IN PATIENTS WITH RESPIRATORY DISEASE [1]

By ARTHUR B. DuBOIS, STELLA Y. BOTELHO, and JULIUS H. COMROE, Jr.

(From the Department of Physiology and Pharmacology, Graduate School of Medicine, University of Pennsylvania, Philadelphia, Pa.)

(Submitted for publication October 17, 1955; accepted December 5, 1955)

Satisfactory methods, utilizing measurements of transthoracic or transpulmonary pressure and airflow, are now available for determining "non-elastic" pulmonary resistance. However, the non-elastic pulmonary resistance has two components, tissue resistance and airway resistance, and no valid direct method is available for measuring either of these components separately in man. Since airway resistance is the ratio of alveolar pressure during flow to airflow, airway resistance alone could be measured if there were a method for determining alveolar pressure during flow. This report presents a new method for accomplishing this measurement, and gives data for airway resistance obtained in normal subjects and in patients with respiratory disease.

Of previous attempts to measure airway resistance, one of the earliest was the painstaking study by Rohrer (1) who made anatomical measurements on the tracheobronchial tree of a human lung post mortem and calculated the cumulative resistance to airflow of the entire system using Poiseuille's law and turbulence theory. The first important experimental study of pulmonary resistance in the living animal was made by von Neergaard and Wirz who, in 1927 (2), analyzed intrapleural pressure into two major components, "dynamic" (which is essentially resistive) and "static" (which is predominantly elastic in nature). This approach made it possible to obtain values for total pulmonary resistance, though not for airway resistance alone. Bayliss and Robertson (3), reasoning that airway resistance, but not tissue resistance, would vary with the viscosity of the gases breathed, ventilated isolated animal lungs with gases of different density and viscosity; from the changes in pressure and volume during artificial ventilation with different gases, they calculated the fraction of non-elastic pulmonary resistance attributable to airway resistance. Studies based upon the revised principle of utilizing several different gas mixtures of different density and viscosity have been carried out more recently in man by Fry, Ebert, Stead, and Brown (4) and McIlroy, Mead, Selverstone, and Radford (5) who made the point that gas combinations which have equal kinematic viscosities should be selected. The results using this technique have been at variance to date, possibly owing to other factors affecting airway resistance (5).

A number of investigators have measured mouth pressure immediately after interruption of airflow with the belief that in such a static system, mouth pressure equals alveolar pressure. Von Neergaard and Wirz (6), Vuilleumier (7), Otis, Fenn and Rahn (8), and Mead and Whittenberger (9), using such a technique, found that brief interruption of the airstream gave a pressure at the mouth of about the same magnitude as the "dynamic" component of ventilatory pressure; however theoretically the alveolar pressure, after airflow has stopped, is not necessarily the same as before the airflow stopped, because there is adequate time for a major change in alveolar pressure to occur during the transition from flow to no flow (9). There are no measurements which compare alveolar pressure during interruption and during airflow because until now it has not been possible to measure alveolar pressure during airflow.

METHOD

Airway resistance (R) is the ratio of alveolar pressure (P_A) to airflow ($\dot{V}$) at a particular time. Since airflow can be measured readily with a pneumotachograph, the method of measuring airway resistance presented in this

[1] These studies were aided (in part) by a contract between the Office of Naval Research, Department of the Navy, and the University of Pennsylvania, NR 112-323.

paper centers on the determination of alveolar pressure as it exists during airflow. The general principle of the method is as follows: The subject sits and breathes inside an airtight box (body plethysmograph) similar to those which have been used to estimate the volume of gas in the lungs (10) or abdomen (11) by application of Boyle's law relating gas volumes and pressures. If there were no airway resistance, the alveolar pressure would be equal to the ambient pressure in the plethysmograph throughout the respiratory cycle and neither pressure would fluctuate, provided the R. Q. were 1 and there were no change in temperature or saturation of the gas in the plethysmograph-lung system. However, to make gas flow through the airway during expiration, alveolar pressure must exceed box pressure and to make gas flow during inspiration, alveolar pressure must be less than box pressure. Since the total amount of gas in the plethysmograph-lung system is constant, an increase in gas pressure inside the lungs of the subject, as during expiratory effort, must cause a decrease in pressure in the remainder of the gas in the plethysmograph. Therefore, at any instant, the resulting pressure change in the box must be opposite in sign to the pressure change in the lungs. By means of a very sensitive capacitance

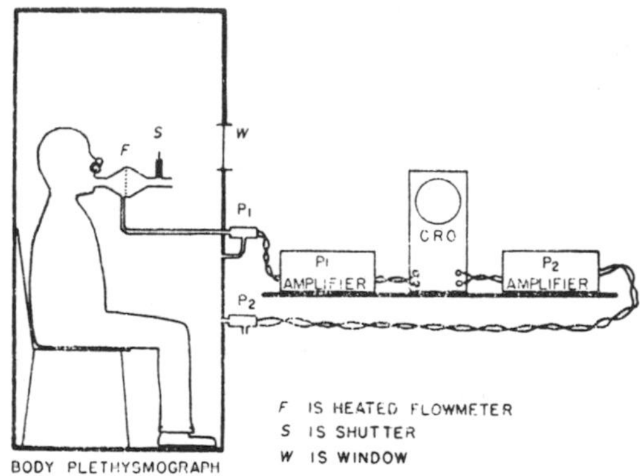

FIG. 1. APPARATUS FOR MEASUREMENT OF AIRWAY RESISTANCE

A. With shutter, S, open, air from plethysmograph is breathed through heated flowmeter, F. Flow is recorded on the Y-axis of the cathode ray oscillograph, CRO, by means of pressure transducer, P_1. Simultaneous change in body volume is recorded on the X-axis of the cathode ray oscillograph by means of pressure transducer, P_2. Alveolar gas is compressed during expiration and expanded during inspiration.

B. With shutter closed, there is no airflow. Mouth pressure (in equilibrium with pressure in the tracheobronchial tree) is recorded on the Y-axis of CRO by means of pressure transducer, P_1. Change in body volume is recorded on the X-axis of CRO by means of P_2. Lung volume is computed by means of Boyle's law for gases.

Airway resistance is computed by combining the results of A (shutter open) and B (shutter closed).

manometer, the pressure changes in the plethysmograph can be measured continuously during the respiratory cycle.

The measured value, change in plethysmographic pressure, can be used to calculate change in alveolar pressure if one also knows the initial alveolar gas volume and the initial alveolar pressure (which is assumed to be equal to atmospheric pressure at end expiration when there is no gas flow). However, this calculation is time-consuming and airway resistance can be determined much more quickly by the following procedures: 1) Changes in airflow are plotted simultaneously against plethysmographic pressure changes (which are proportional to changes in alveolar pressure) on the two axes of a cathode ray oscillograph (CRO). 2) Immediately thereafter, changes in plethysmograph pressure are plotted against mouth pressure on the cathode ray oscillograph under *static* conditions, as the subject makes inspiratory-expiratory efforts against a closed airway; since mouth pressure equals alveolar pressure in a static system, this second step serves to relate changes in plethysmograph pressure to changes in alveolar pressure in each subject. Thus, alveolar pressure is effectively measured during flow since the alveolar pressure for a given plethysmograph pressure is the same whether or not flow is interrupted provided the ratio of lung to plethysmograph gas volume is constant. The difference between this method and previous interrupter methods is that the interruption of flow in the present method is merely the means of calibrating the changes in plethysmograph pressure in terms of alveolar pressure; the values for resistance are always obtained during uninterrupted airflow. The details of the method will now be described:

1. *Measurement of changes in pressure in the body plethysmograph simultaneously with flow:* The plethysmograph is a metal chamber with the proportions of a telephone booth but having an air tight door; its internal volume is approximately 600 liters. Attached to this box is a sensitive Lilly capacitance manometer [2] which responds to a pressure of 0.05 cm. H_2O by one inch horizontal deflection on a cathode ray oscillograph; [3] it measures pressure changes in the box with reference to atmospheric pressure (Figure 1).

The subject sits inside and breathes the air in this closed chamber. The box can be vented to the atmosphere by a valve.[4] At the end of the two-minute warm up time, the subject, who wears a noseclip, places his mouth on a flowmeter-shutter apparatus (which is suspended from the box ceiling by means of curtain rods with spring sockets) and pants to and fro for 5 to 15 sec. through the flowmeter [5] (volume 0.3 liter and sensi-

[2] Lilly capacitance manometer, Technitrol Engineering Co., Philadelphia, Pa.

[3] Cathode Ray Oscillograph, Type 304 A, Allen B. Dumont Co., Clifton, N. J.

[4] Solenoid valve, Automatic Switch Co., Orange, New Jersey.

[5] Flowmeter, Technitrol Engineering Co., Philadelphia, Pa.

tivity 1.34 liters per sec. per in. deflection) which is warmed by an electric current passing through a loop of nichrome wire.

When the subject breathes, airflow is recorded on the Y-axis of the cathode ray oscillograph and plethysmograph pressure (which is proportional to alveolar pressure) is recorded on the X-axis; the slope of the line generated on the cathode ray oscillograph is $\dot{V}/P_P$ where $\dot{V}$ is airflow and P_P is plethysmograph pressure (Figure 2).

Breaths of normal tidal volume produce an artefact caused by the instantaneous warming and wetting of inspired air and the cooling and condensation of expired air; because the rate of the latter is less than of the former, this produces a net effect in the direction of increased pressure in the box with each breath. Shallow breathing through the heated flowmeter reduces the size of the artefact. As long as the front between plethysmograph air and pulmonary air remains inside the metallic heated flowmeter, this artefact is eliminated. This artefact is also eliminated when the subject rebreathes in a rubber bag containing hot water, which serves to keep the respired air at constant conditions of temperature and saturation throughout the respiratory cycle.

Although most previous investigators using other methods have measured resistance to breathing at a normal breathing frequency and tidal volume, rapid, shallow breathing such as panting has certain theoretical and practical advantages: It minimizes the temperature, saturation and R. Q. effects to the extent that they can be neglected. It improves the signal to drift ratio because it allows completion of each respiratory cycle in a fraction of a second. Gradual thermal changes and very small leaks in the box become insignificant compared to

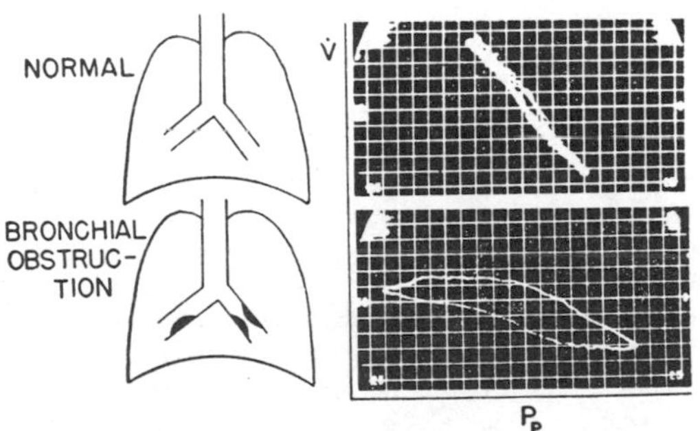

FIG. 2. PHOTOGRAPH OF CATHODE RAY SCREEN (SHUTTER OPEN)

Airflow on the Y-axis has calibration of 1.3 L. per sec. per inch deflection. Change in body volume on the X-axis has calibration of 14 cc. per inch deflection (normal subject), and 27 cc. per inch, case No. 20, bronchial obstruction. Zero flow is in center of screen. Although a simple 'S' shaped resistance line was characteristic of normal subjects, patients who had predominantly expiratory obstruction generally showed the looping of resistance, which was increased in association with expiratory flow, or volume, as in this case, or both.

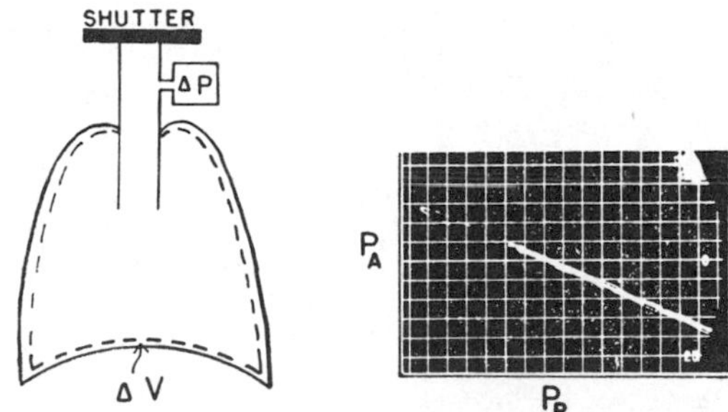

FIG. 3. PHOTOGRAPH OF CATHODE RAY SCREEN (SHUTTER CLOSED)

Mouth pressure on Y-axis has calibration of 7.1 cm. H_2O per inch deflection. Change in body volume on the X-axis has calibration of 14 cc. per inch deflection. Atmospheric pressure in center of screen. Grid lines in Figure 2 and Figure 3 are 0.2 inch.

the volume changes attributable to compression and decompression of alveolar gas.

Certain objections may be raised to the use of panting: a) The volume of gas in the lungs during panting is often different from the volume during quiet breathing because the subject chooses a lung volume which offers the least sensation of obstruction to breathing, b) the subject may tend to open maximally his upper airway (mouth and glottis), c) the subject breathes so shallowly that gas distribution is not limited by stiff regions of the lung, but the gas follows only the pathways of least resistance and d) panting at very low tidal volumes leads to a rise in P_{CO_2} and a decrease in P_{O_2} in the airways during the period of the test. On the other hand it has been shown that the over-all resistance to breathing can be measured by a pump at 6 cycles per second (12), that the frequency response of the chest wall is satisfactory in this frequency range (13) and that respiratory resistance measured in cats is not different when measured at high and low frequencies (14). However, further studies are needed to determine the exact magnitude of changes in airway resistance produced by the panting procedure *per se*. The present measurements of airway resistance were made at panting frequencies which were approximately 2 cycles per second. This frequency is well within the limit of both capacitance manometers since their frequency responses were flat to at least 35 cycles per second.

2. *Method of relating plethysmographic pressure changes to alveolar pressure changes:* To relate changes in plethysmograph pressure to changes in alveolar pressure, the following procedure is performed: The operator activates a rotary solenoid (9) which occludes the distal end of the flowmeter. The subject continues to pant and records are made continuously of mouth pressure (Y axis) and plethysmograph pressure (X axis) (Figure 3). (The pressure gauge[6] formerly used to record differential

[6] Venous pressure head, Technitrol Engineering Co., Philadelphia, Pa.

pressure across the flowmeter now measures mouth pressure with respect to box pressure. Ideally, it should now measure mouth pressure with respect to atmospheric. The 1 per cent error was insufficient to warrant the technical difficulty of changing over the back side of the gauge. However it is necessary to reduce the sensitivity of this gauge by a factor of ten at the same time that the rotary solenoid is activated; its sensitivity is now 7 cm. H_2O per inch deflection.) Since there is no airflow during the period of occlusion, mouth pressure equals alveolar pressure and the slope of the line generated on the cathode ray oscillograph is now P_A/P_P where P_A is alveolar pressure and P_P is plethysmograph pressure. Since the same manometer is used to record P_P both with the shutter open and closed, P_P of both slopes is the same.

The lines produced on the oscilloscope are traced[7] or photographed (f 5.6, bulb exposure, Plus-X film, with plus 2 diopter supplementary lens) or both. The total time in the box is approximately 5 minutes. The flowmeter is then calibrated with a recording spirometer to measure airflow and the mouth pressure gauge is calibrated with a water manometer.

3. *Calculation of airway resistance:* To determine the airway resistance, it is necessary to know the ratio of alveolar pressure to airflow at the mouth, $P_A/\dot{V}$. The experiments yielded two slopes. First, with the shutter open, the slope $\dot{V}/P_P$ was measured on the S shaped line from the point of 1 liter per second of inspiratory flow to the point of 1 liter per second of expiratory flow.[8] Second, the slope P_A/P_P is generated with the shutter closed. The total airway resistance is calculated by taking the ratio of slopes:

$$R = \frac{P_A/P_P}{\dot{V}/P_P}$$

where P_A is alveolar pressure, $\dot{V}$ is airflow, P_P is plethysmograph pressure (the same with shutter open and closed), and R is resistance.

A correction is made on the total airway resistance for the volume of the dead space by assuming that the average resistance to airflow is halfway down the tracheobronchial tree: The slope P_A/P_P is multiplied by the ratio of total gas volume occluded by the shutter to gas volume proximal to the point of mean resistance to gas flow. The total volume is measured immediately at the end of the test by the plethysmographic method (15). The volume proximal to the resistance is the total volume minus the volume of the flowmeter (0.3 liter) and half the volume of the tracheobronchial tree (0.1 liter). Resistance of the flowmeter-shutter breathing apparatus is measured (0.5 to 0.7 cm. H_2O per liter per sec.) and subtracted from the total airway resistance to obtain airway resistance of the subject. The values for airway resistance are expressed in cm. H_2O per liter per sec.

4. *Experimental accuracy:* The method of tracing and reading the image from the cathode ray oscillograph permits a 5 per cent error of slope. Since two different slopes are used in the calculation of resistance, the sum of the errors may be 10 per cent. There is a slight reading error in calibration of the flowmeter and mouth pressure gauge; however errors in calibration of the box pressure gauge are automatically cancelled in the calculation of resistance. Since these reading errors are of a random nature, the over-all accuracy is improved by repeating the measurement of airway resistance several times and averaging the results.

The advantage of tracing is that it permits calculation of the airway resistance without delay; however the slopes can be read more accurately from a photograph than from a pencil tracing.

5. *Validity:* The validity of the plethysmograph method for airway resistance was tested by determining the total resistance before and after various degrees of resistance were interposed between the flowmeter and the subject's mouth. The added resistances were 2.7, 5.9, and 10.9 cm. H_2O per liter per sec.; these caused an increase in airway resistance as measured by the plethysmograph method of 2.2, 5.9, and 9.3 cm. H_2O per liter per second, respectively. The discrepancies were within the combined reading errors of the methods for measuring the values of the added resistances and the airway resistance.

6. *Other possible sources of error:* Since the total gas volume, which is used to correct for the volume of the dead space in calculating resistance is determined by a plethysmograph method (15), a gross check of this method was done as follows: The total gas volume was determined before and after the subject inspired measured volumes from a recording spirometer. The inspired volumes were 1.1 liters, 2.4 liters, and 3.7 liters and the compressible gas was found to increase by 1.0 liters, 2.2 liters, and 3.5 liters, respectively. The presence of abdominal gas might conceivably produce an error in the calculated volume of compressible gas in the lungs. If the abdominal gas were compressed during expiration and expanded during inspiration, the total apparent compressible volume would be greater than the lung volume, whereas if the abdominal gas were expanded during expiration and compressed during inspiration, the calculated volume would be less than the lung volume. However, if the calculated gas volume during voluntary efforts against the closed shutter were equal to the calculated volume during voluntary panting through the flowmeter, there would be no error in the calculation of airway resistance, because the plethysmograph pressure terms which would be affected cancel during the calculation. Errors in box calibration are eliminated for the same reason. Abdominal pressure changes measured by a gastric balloon and box pressure were recorded on two normal subjects and four patients during panting through

[7] "Oscillotracer," R. A. Waters, Inc., Waltham, Mass.

[8] Some subjects showed increased end expiratory resistance, forming a loop in the appropriate portion of the pressure-flow curve. This loop was probably caused by partial or complete collapse of some of the air passages as the subject expired toward residual volume. In these subjects the mean slope was measured after drawing a line along the imaginary center, or long axis of the loop.

the flowmeter and against the closed shutter and the relationship between abdominal and box pressure showed no significant difference with the shutter open or closed. The calculated volume, shutter-open, would therefore be the same as with the shutter closed. The conclusion is that abdominal gas cancels out in the calculation of airway resistance. More detailed accounts of the accuracy of the plethysmographic method of determining thoracic gas volume and abdominal gas volumes will be the subject of separate reports (15, 16).

The R. Q. might conceivably produce an error in the determination of airway resistance by the plethysmographic method since there is a gradual absorption of gas when the mean R. Q. is less than 1.0. For example, if oxygen consumption is 300 cc. per minute and the CO_2 output is 240 cc. per minute the mean R. Q. is 0.8 and the net gas absorption is 60 cc. per minute ("respiratory exchange difference") or 1 cc. per sec. During inspiration, the respiratory exchange difference is slightly greater, and during expiration, it is slightly less than the mean. Upon rebreathing the dead space gas, the respiratory fluctuations disappear, but the trend of the respiratory exchange differences changes, as in breath holding, causing a slight increase in the net rate of gas absorption. Neither the mean trend nor the respiratory fluctuations are large enough to interfere with the measurement of airway resistance or lung volume because, during panting, pressure changes are sufficiently rapid and the volume changes due to compression of lung air are large enough that the R. Q. effect is small by comparison, even in subjects with normal airway resistance.

7. *Other tests:* Those performed on the patients included vital capacity, maximal expiratory flow rate over the range 200 to 1,200 cc., maximal breathing capacity using a Tissot spirometer and lung compliance using an esophageal balloon, capacitance manometer, spirometer with potentiometer, and cathode ray oscillograph.

RESULTS AND DISCUSSION

1. *Normal subjects*

Twenty-one subjects who had no signs, symptoms, or history of respiratory disease were studied; ten of these were tested on two different days, and eleven were tested on only one day. The mean airway resistance of the 21 normal subjects was 1.5 cm. H_2O per liter per sec., at a flow of one liter per second, panting. The standard deviation was $\pm$ 0.49 and the range 0.6 to 2.4 (Table I). In those subjects tested on two different days, the standard deviation of the mean of the differences between determinations was $\pm$ 0.37. Because this small series contains men and women in all age groups, breathing at different lung volumes, these data are presented only to give an approximate range of normal values; larger groups in all decades are now being studied in order to define normal values more precisely.

In this series, the sensitivity of the manometers was adjusted so that the most accurate readings

TABLE I

Airway resistance in normal subjects (panting) *

Subject	Age (*yrs.*)	Sex	Height (*ft., in.*)	Weight (*pounds*)	Plethysmographic thoracic gas volume (*liters, BTPS*) No. 1	No. 2	Airway resistance (*cm. $H_2O/L./sec.$*) No. 1	No. 2
1. F. K.	33	M	5′10″	165	3.9	3.9	1.6	1.3
2. J. M.	32	M	5′5″	133	2.4	2.8	1.6	1.3
3. L. C.	28	M	5′9½″	180	5.3	1.8	1.4	1.7
4. E. H.	30	F	5′4¾″	137	2.0	2.3	2.1	1.7
5. L. D.	28	M	5′7″	160	3.0	2.7	1.6	1.8
6. P. C.	23	F	5′3″	101	2.4	2.8	1.8	1.1
7. M. E.	22	F	5′10″	145	3.5	4.0	1.4	1.3
8. A. V.	40	M	6′½″	190	3.4	5.2	1.1	0.7
9. C. C.	29	M	5′9″	145	3.6	3.5	2.0	1.7
10. A. D.	30	M	6′3″	200	2.9	3.7	1.3	1.8
11. B. L.	29	M	5′11″	175	5.2	—	1.4	—
12. J. T.	29	F	5′5″	110	1.9	—	1.9	—
13. D. T.	28	F	4′10″	93	2.4	—	2.4	—
14. E. B.	37	M	5′10½″	160	4.5	—	0.6	—
15. M. J.	51	M	5′11″	185	4.2	—	0.9	—
16. S. D.	57	M	5′3″	150	3.0	—	2.3	—
17. R. N.	37	M	5′11″	150	3.7	—	1.7	—
18. M. M.	33	M	6′3″	185	3.9	—	1.0	—
19. R. C.	51	M	5′10½″	168	5.4	—	0.9	—
20. C. M.	35	M	6′1″	150	4.8	—	1.9	—
21. R. D.	27	F	5′8½″	117	3.5	—	1.3	—

* Subjects 1–21, mean airway resistance = 1.50 cm. H_2O per L. per sec., S.D. $\pm$0.49. Subjects 1–10, mean of the differences between No. 1 and No. 2 measurements of airway resistance = 0.15 cm. H_2O per L. per sec., S.D. $\pm$0.37.

of the S-shaped curve on the cathode ray oscillograph were made at flow rates of 1 liter per sec. Mean values of airway resistance measured at flow rates of 0.75 liter per sec. are approximately 0.1 cm. H_2O per liter per sec. less and those measured at 0.5 liter per sec. are approximately 0.2 cm. H_2O per liter per sec. less than values obtained at flow rates of 1.0 liter per sec. The values obtained represent those for a specific pattern of mouth breathing; the resistance to airflow through the nasal passages may be appreciable as indicated by measurements of pressure differential between nasopharynx and one nostril, which we have found to range from 1 to 4 cm. H_2O per liter per sec. at

TABLE II

Airway resistance in thirty patients

Subject	Age (*yrs.*) and sex	Disease	Duration of disease (*yrs.*)	Chief symptom*	Vital capacity (*L.*)	Max. expir. flow rate (*L./min.*)	Max. breathing capacity (*L./min.*)	Lung compliance (*L./cm. H_2O*)	Plethysmographic thoracic gas volume (*L.*)	Airway resist. (*cm. H_2O/ L./sec.*)	Measured at flow rate of (*L./sec.*)
1. W. M.	42 M	? Silicosis	2	DOE, slight	4.6	530	168	0.22	3.9	1.9	1.0
2. E. M.	48 F	Scleroderma	3	Cough	2.1	170	114		3.0	1.6	1.0
3. R. D.	44 M	Scleroderma† (biopsy)	3	Dyspnea, occasional	1.5		145	0.04	1.6	0.6	0.9
4. M. C.	44 F	Chr. bronchitis‡		DOE	2.4			0.15	3.5	5.5	0.8
5. J. L.	65 F	Asthma‡	31	DOE, 1 flt.	2.5	72		0.08	4.1	9.8, 7.0§	0.7
6. J. C.	55 M	Asthma and stenosis of the glottis‡	25	Parox. dyspnea	4.5	124	43		3.5	7.2	1.0
7. N. P.	56 M	Chr. bronchitis‡	18	DOE and cough	3.4	93	44		7.3	3.4	1.0
8. W. H.	54 M	Asthma‡	21	DOE	3.3	29		0.26	6.7	5.2	0.9
9. I. B.	67 M	Asthma	12	Dyspnea at rest	1.8	22	22	0.06	6.5	6.8 1.9‖	0.58
10. J. J.	56 M	Asthma	37	DOE, 1 flt.	2.4	17			3.7	6.8	0.68
11. A. A.	64 F	Asthma	15	DOE, occasional	2.0	115			2.8	3.1	0.5
12. C. C.	54 M	Pulm. fibrosis†‡	1	"Chest cold"	1.2	260	50	0.011	2.6	2.8	0.7
13. S. T.	21 M	Asthma		Asympt.	5.5	270		0.21	2.9	3.2	0.8
14. C. K.	63 F	Asthma	12	Dyspnea at rest	1.5	58		0.05	2.6 2.3	6.8§ 6.8	0.7
15. B. J.	38 M	Asthma	30	Dyspnea at rest	1.9	13		0.06	5.6 5.5	7.5§ 6.9	0.5
16. R. H.	51 M	Asthma		Dyspnea, slight	2.1	44		0.13	6.1	5.9	0.8
17. L. B.	53 M	Asthma	47	Dyspnea, occasional	2.6	35		0.27	5.1	4.5	0.9
18. E. N.	42 F	Asthma		Asympt.	2.2	77	43	0.20	3.5	3.9	0.7
19. G. D.	53 M	Emphysema	3	DOE, slight	2.6	66		0.11	5.6	7.7	0.5
20. W. L.	51 M	Silicosis	11	DOE, 1 flt.	2.1	19	26	0.14	5.1	10.8	0.5
21. S. S.	63 F	Asthma		Asympt.	2.2	49		0.08	3.9	8.3	0.7
22. B. J.	28 M	Asthma	10	Dyspnea	2.3	19			6.0	4.7	0.9
23. M. H.	9 F	Pulm. fibrosis	1	Dyspnea, ½ flt. Resp. rate 72/min.	0.2				1.0	5.2	0.6
24. J. H.	61 M	Pneumoconiosis	9	DOE, 1 block	2.4	26	60		4.6	6.4	0.5
25. M. C.	62 M	Pneumoconiosis	2	DOE, 1 flt.	3.1	99	46		4.8	2.3	0.5
26. H. P.	44 M	Asthma	16	Asympt.	2.6	132			3.2	2.2	0.9
27. E. C.	47 F	Hay fever	30	Asympt.	2.8	140			3.2	2.2	0.5
28. G. L.	58 M	"Alveolar cell" Ca†	1	DOE, severe	0.9		72	0.013	2.1	2.2	0.7
29. L. F.	55 M	Asthma ?	17	Asympt.	1.9	57?		0.12	4.1	1.7	0.7
30. E. W.	26 F	Normal preg.	0.7	Asympt.					3.7	2.6	1.0

* DOE = Dyspnea on exertion; flt. = flight.

† Biopsy of lung showed: No. 3, interstitial fibrosis; No. 12, pulmonary fibrosis; autopsy showed: No. 28, no tracheobronchial obstruction.

‡ Bronchoscopy showed: No. 4, chronic tracheobronchitis; No. 5, bronchiectasis and purulent tracheobronchitis; No. 6, stenosis of glottis (laryngoscopy); No. 7, bilateral tracheobronchitis; No. 8, allergic tracheobronchitis; No. 12, no abnormalities.

§ Patients 5, 14 and 15, airway resistance measurement was repeated on a subsequent day.

‖ After subcutaneous injection of epinephrine.

flow rates of 0.25 liter per sec. in normal subjects with no subjective complaints of nasal obstruction. Therefore the resistance of the total airway in subjects breathing through the nose would be greater than the values obtained in this study. The resistance predicted by Rohrer from anatomical measurements of the tracheobronchial tree in a cadaver was 1.6 cm. H_2O per liter per sec. It is not possible to make a comparison of these data with data obtained by other investigators using different methods for several reasons: a) Some of the methods purporting to measure airway resistance alone actually include other factors as well and are not specific tests of airway resistance, b) the specific breathing pattern used in this test differs from that used by other investigators. However, a comparison with the esophageal pressure method for pulmonary resistance, reported in detail in reference 17, yielded mean normal pulmonary tissue resistance of approximately 0.2 cm. H_2O per liter per second at 0.5 liter per second.

2. Patients with respiratory disease

No attempt will be made here to present a complete analysis of the mechanical factors in breathing in patients with respiratory disease. However this test for airway resistance has been applied to a sufficient number of patients to evaluate its practicality, limitations and usefulness in diagnosis and treatment.

The method cannot of course be used in patients who are too sick or too weak to sit in the plethysmograph. Patients with bilateral paralysis of the lower extremities would have to be lifted in and out of the box. No patients refused to enter the box but one "normal" subject refused to enter the box because of claustrophobia. Several patients were unable to breathe at flow rates as great as 1.0 liter per sec.; in these the resistance was calculated at flow rates of 0.5 to 1.0 liter per sec. Many of the patients with high resistance showed loops similar to that in Figure 2, bottom, compatible with expiratory obstruction. The 30 patients, including one child aged nine years, studied in this series were all able to follow directions and complete the test satisfactorily. Data obtained upon these 30 patients are presented in Table II and Figure 4. Since there is no other method available for direct measurement of airway

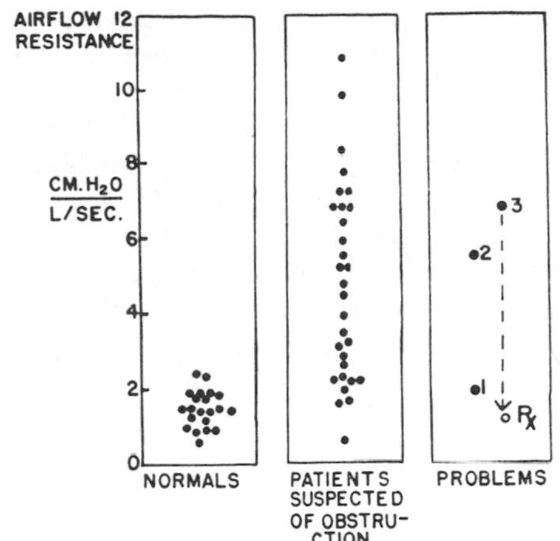

FIG. 4. SUMMARY OF AIRWAY RESISTANCE VALUES IN NORMAL SUBJECTS, PATIENTS WITH SUSPECTED OBSTRUCTION AND IN THREE PROBLEM CASES

The three problem cases are as follows:

1. W. M. Case No. 1 (Table II), was referred for evaluation of possible pulmonary disability due to suspected pneumoconiosis: Objective pulmonary function tests were of value in ruling out impairment of function.
2. M. C. Case No. 4 (Table II), was tested to distinguish between dyspnea accompanying anxiety versus organic disease. This method revealed evidence of organic tracheobronchial obstruction.
3. I. B. Case No. 9 (Table II), was evaluated for effect of bronchodilator drugs on respiratory obstruction. It was found that his obstruction was not of the 'fixed' type, but reversible by administration of epinephrine subcutaneously.

resistance, the reliability of this method cannot be checked experimentally except for evidence of false positive or false negative indication of tracheobronchial obstruction. For example, since patients 1 to 3 had a maximal breathing capacity in the normal range, it is unlikely that they had any significant increase in airway resistance; their values (0.6 to 1.9 cm. H_2O per liter per sec.) fell in the normal range. Patients 4 to 8 had known partial obstruction in their large airways by bronchoscopic examination and all had increased airway resistance by the present test.

The values for airway resistance in patients 9 to 24 were increased and in all of these there were clinical reasons for expecting either increased airway or tissue resistance. Patients 25 to 28 were borderline cases with high normal values for airway resistance and clinical findings suggestive of partial obstruction. Patient 29 had airway resistance within one standard deviation of the normal mean, but his maximal expiratory flow rate was less than normal. This means that the low value for maximal expiratory flow rate was caused by factors other than increased airway resistance; some of these might be partial collapse of the intrathoracic portion of the tracheobronchial tree during forced expiration (which would not occur with the present test), by increased resistive factors in the chest wall or lung tissues, or by failure to exert maximal force. The finding of slightly increased airway resistance in patient 30 is not readily explained although it is possible that this slightly increased airway resistance might be the result of distortion of the airways as a result of the pregnancy; further studies must be done on a large group before any conclusions can be drawn.

No attempt will be made to correlate airway resistance measured by this test with maximal breathing capacity, timed vital capacity, or maximal expiratory flow rates, since these last named tests are "over-all" tests of mechanical factors during forced breathing and include many factors in addition to the specific airway resistance being measured here.

It appears that this method of measuring airway resistance alone has the following uses: a) Objective measurement of airway resistance in patients; it has the advantage of measuring one specific component of the mechanical factors in breathing, without the requirement of maximal respiratory effort on the part of the patient; b) Quantitative and objective evaluation of therapeutic procedures designed to relieve airway obstruction; c) Separate measurement of airway resistance so that tissue resistance can be determined as the difference between total resistance and airway resistance; d) Study of multiple physiological, pharmacological and environmental and pathological factors that may affect airway resistance.

SUMMARY

A new method is reported for the objective and specific measurement of airway resistance in human subjects. It requires the measurement of airflow and of alveolar pressure *during airflow;* the latter is measured by determining by means of a body plethysmograph the volume of compression and decompression of alveolar gas during expiration and inspiration.

Normal subjects tested by this method had a mean airway resistance of 1.5 cm. H_2O per liter per sec. (range 0.6 to 2.4) at a flow rate of 1 liter per second, panting. A preliminary study has been made of the airway resistance in 30 patients; the range of resistances was 0.6 to 10.8 cm. H_2O per liter per sec.

This method is thought to be applicable to measurement of airway resistance in patients, evaluation of therapeutic procedures designed to relieve airway obstruction, separation of airway resistance from tissue resistance, and study of multiple factors that may affect airway resistance.

REFERENCES

1. Rohrer, F., Der Strömungswiderstand in den menschlichen Atemwegen und der Einfluss der unregelmässigen Verzeweigung des Bronchialsystems auf den Atmungsverlauf in verschiedenen Lungenbezirken. Arch. f. d. ges. Physiol., 1915, **162**, 225.
2. von Neergaard, K., and Wirz, K., Über eine Methode zur Messung der Lungenelastizität am lebenden Menschen, insbesondere beim Emphysem. Ztschr. f. klin. Med., 1927, **105**, 35.
3. Bayliss, L. E., and Robertson, G. W., The visco-elastic properties of the lungs. Quart. J. Exper. Physiol., 1939, **29**, 27.
4. Fry, D. L., Ebert, R. V., Stead, W. W., and Brown, C. C., The mechanics of pulmonary ventilation in normal subjects and in patients with emphysema. Am. J. Med., 1954, **16**, 80.
5. McIlroy, M. B., Mead, J., Selverstone, N. J., and Radford, E. P., Measurement of lung tissue viscous resistance using gases of equal kinematic viscosity. J. Applied Physiol., 1955, **7**, 485.
6. von Neergaard, K., and Wirz, K., Die Messung der Strömungswiderstände in den Atemwegen des Menschen, insbesondere bei Asthma und Emphysem. Ztschr. f. klin. Med., 1927, **105**, 51.
7. Vuilleumier, P., Über eine Methode zur Messung des intraalveolären Druckes und der Strömungswiderstände in den Atemwegen des Mensches. Ztschr. f. klin. Med., 1944, **143**, 698.
8. Otis, A. B., Fenn, W. O., and Rahn, H., Mechanics of breathing in man. J. Applied Physiol., 1950, **2**, 592.
9. Mead, J., and Whittenberger, J. L., Evaluation of airway interruption technique as a method for measuring pulmonary air-flow resistance. J. Applied Physiol., 1954, **6**, 408.
10. Pflüger, E., Das Pneumonometer. Arch. f. d. ges. Physiol., 1882, **29**, 244.

11. Blair, H. A., Dern, R. J., and Bates, P. L., Measurement of volume of gas in the digestive tract. Am. J. Physiol., 1947, **149**, 688.
12. DuBois, A. B., Resistance to breathing measured by driving the chest at 6 cps. Federation Proc., 1953, **12**, 35.
13. DuBois, A. B., Brody, A. W., Lewis, D. H., and Burgess, B. F., Jr., Response of the chest wall, abdomen and diaphragm to forced oscillations of volume. Federation Proc., 1954, **13**, 38.
14. Nisell, O. I., and DuBois, A. B., Relationship between compliance and FRC of the lungs in cats, and measurement of resistance to breathing. Am. J. Physiol., 1954, **178**, 206.
15. DuBois, A. B., Botelho, S. Y., Bedell, G. N., Marshall, R., and Comroe, J. H., Jr., A rapid plethysmographic method for measuring thoracic gas volume: A comparison with a nitrogen washout method for measuring functional residual capacity in normal subjects. J. Clin. Invest., 1956, **35**, 322.
16. Bedell, G. N., Marshall, R., DuBois, A. B., and Harris, J. H., Measurement of the volume of gas in the gastro-intestinal tract. Values in normal subjects and ambulatory patients. J. Clin. Invest., 1956, **35**, 336.
17. Marshall, R., and DuBois, A. B., The measurement of the viscous resistance of the lung tissues in normal man. Clin. Sc., 1956.

27

Reprinted from *J. Clin. Invest.*, **30**(11), 1175, 1182–1184, 1187–1190 (1951)

MECHANICS OF AIRFLOW IN HEALTH AND IN EMPHYSEMA

By HOWARD DAYMAN

(From the Tuberculosis Service, Edward J. Meyer Memorial Hospital, Buffalo, N. Y.)

(Submitted for publication March 5, 1951; accepted August 13, 1951)

Essential manifestations of pulmonary emphysema are retarded expiratory airflow and incomplete expiration (1–3). These occur even though the patient makes a strenuous muscular effort to expel the vital capacity air as quickly and completely as possible. Inspiration is, by contrast, relatively unimpeded. The circumstances suggest the presence of expiratory obstruction, which is aggravated by increasing the expulsive force, in other words, a check valve type of obstruction. To determine whether such a mechanism exists we employed the method of Neergaard and Wirz (4) which, under suitable conditions, provides a continuous record of pleural pressure and rate of airflow. From these one may compute pulmonary pressure, by which we mean the pressure in the terminal air spaces; together with lung tension. The latter designates the net elastic recoil of the lungs, or "elastance" (5), expressed in centimeters of water pressure, under static conditions, at a particular lung volume. It represents the pressure required to maintain the lungs at that degree of distension when no air is passing in or out of the organs.

Relevant observations on the lungs at necropsy, and on the gross behavior of the major airways during forceful expiration were also included.

METHOD

As modified by us, the method is as follows: By means of a rubber mouth piece the subject breathes through a tube 30 cm. long and 2.5 cm. in diameter (Pneumotachygraph Figure 1). Within the lumen of the breathing tube are three bundles of thin brass tubing to prevent turbulence. Opposite small gaps between the bundles are side tubes to which short lengths of rubber tubing are attached. A cylindrical light bulb keeps the tube above body temperature to prevent condensation of moisture. An outer jacket enclosed both tube and bulb.

The difference in pressure between the two points where the side tubes are attached is a measure of the rate of airflow. This pressure difference is recorded by a differential tambour. The upper half of the tambour is of conventional shape, the lower half is provided with an airtight enclosure containing two glass windows. To the rubber membrane is attached an inverted aluminum fork bearing on its prongs a fine quartz fibre at the level of the window. The shadow of the cross hair with the beam of light is directed through a lens system against a vertical slit behind which electrocardiograph paper is being drawn at constant rate. When set up for actual use the natural frequency of the tambour is 3.4 complete cycles/sec. The resistance to breathing afforded by the airflow tube is negligible with rates up to 500 cc./sec. At faster rates it contributes a minor but measurable resistance. The exact resistance in the breathing tube is determined by having a subject breathe in and out through the tube at various rates while the pressure in the mouthpiece is being simultaneously measured by an optically recorded tambour. For a particular rate of airflow such

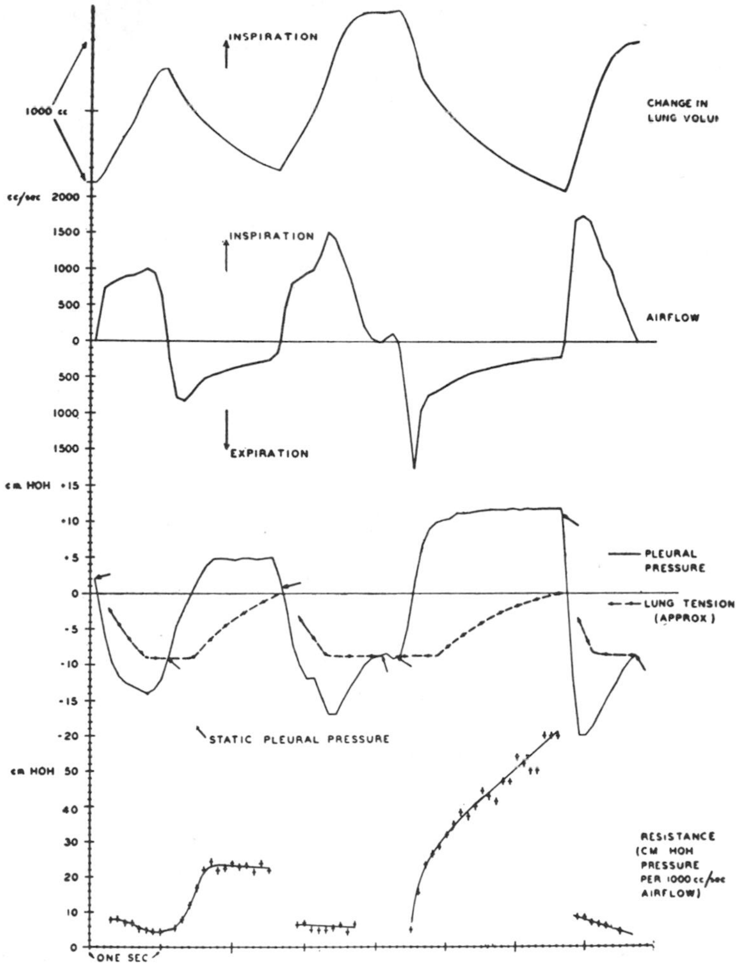

Fig. 7

pressure represents the resistance in the breathing tube itself, and in an actual experiment such a pressure is subtracted from the intrapulmonary pressure to calculate the resistance in the respiratory tract of the patient.

Pleural pressures were recorded by means of a simple tambour provided with a fork and cross hair, the shadow of the latter being cast on another strip of electrocardiograph paper wound on the same drum and marked with a synchronized timer. With a 14 gauge needle attached to the system the natural frequency of the tambour was 9 complete cycles/sec. The entire apparatus is conveniently managed by one operator.

[*Editor's Note:* Material has been omitted at this point.]

Advanced generalized obstructive emphysema

Case 8, G. B., male, age 41, a laborer, had since youth suffered from a severe chronic productive cough, wheezing and dyspnea. The symptoms were aggravated by frequent protracted attacks of acute bronchitis. For four years he had been unable to work because of dyspnea. The patient was well nourished, somewhat cyanotic, dyspneic on the slightest exertion, but not orthopneic. The chest was fixed in the inspiratory position. There were generalized expiratory rhonchi. The breath sounds were inaudible at rest and scarcely audible

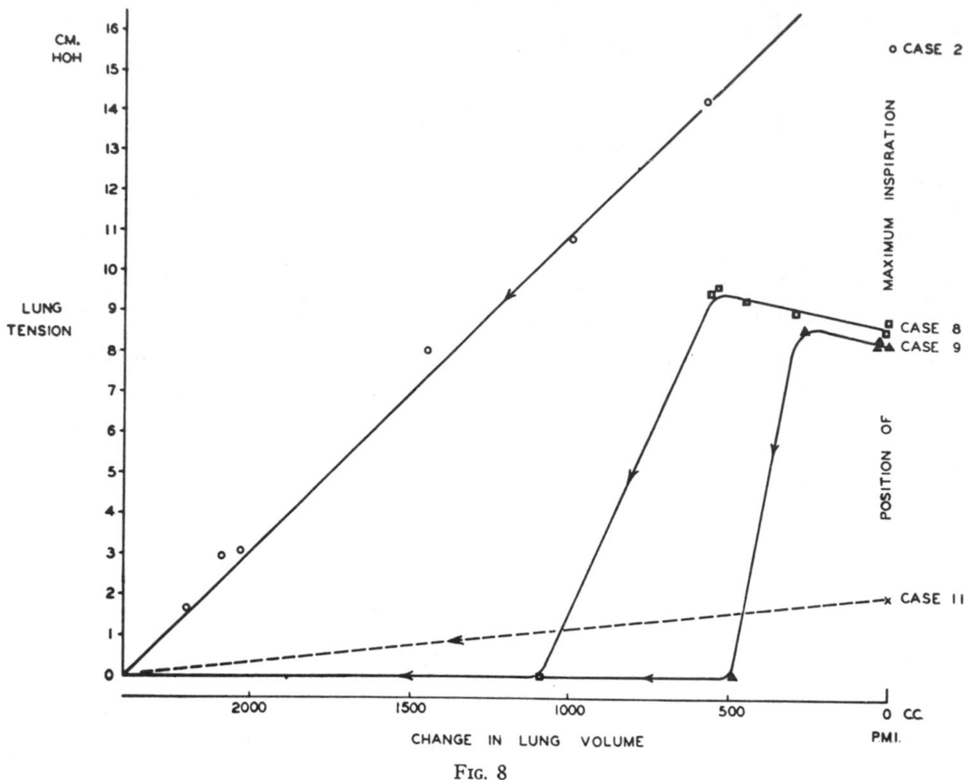

FIG. 8

with forced breathing. There was no evidence of cardiac or tuberculous disease. The estimated normal vital capacity was 5,000 cc. The test vital capacity was 2,100 cc. and the patient required ten seconds to expel this amount of air. The maximum minute ventilation was 32 L./min. The findings were typical of generalized bronchitis and advanced emphysema.

The patient developed a spontaneous pneumothorax on the left side and after the air had been almost entirely reabsorbed, the experiment was performed. The needle was inserted in the left fourth interspace. The data showed striking deviations from the normal (Figure 7).

Reasonably good rates of airflow occurred during inspiration and the rate could be augmented by greater effort though the resistance in the airways was clearly higher than normal. During gentle expiration a fair initial rate of airflow was obtained but the rate decreased despite a sustained positive pleural pressure. If expiration was forceful there was an initial good rate of airflow then a sudden decrease in rate. The decrease of airflow was more conspicuous the greater the effort to expel air. A pleural pressure of + 25 cm. HOH brought about rates of airflow in the range of only 200 to 300 cc./sec. As further evidence of the expiratory check valve mechanism in this case it was shown that a sustained positive pleural pressure of 11 to 12 cm. HOH failed to deflate the lungs much farther than a gentle effort (Figure 7).

Accurate measurement of pulmonary pressure was made difficult by the abnormal relationship between lung volume and lung tension (Figure 8). In the first place, expiration usually ended with a positive static pleural pressure. Since emphysema is characterized by a large residual air, and in this patient the lungs were visibly distended even at the end of expiration, we concluded that the positive static pressure was being exerted against a cushion of trapped intrapulmonary air. Release of such positive pleural pressure found lung tension to be zero at this lung size.

Inspiration was marked by a sudden rise of lung tension to about 9 cm. HOH where it remained to the point of maximum inspiration. This relationship between volume and tension is abnormal. In Figure 8 a normal relationship is illustrated for comparison. In this case of advanced emphysema, measuring from position of maximum inspiration, air could be expelled under satisfactory lung tension to the extent of about 800 cc. Thereafter lung tension fell quickly to zero. During such a period expiratory airflow suddenly shut off, déspite mounting, positive pleural pressure.

Derived from Figure 8, approximate lung tension curves were interpolated in Figure 7, and resistance determined. It is noteworthy that inspiration is relatively unimpeded while obstruction to expiration is extreme following the initial period. The terminal airflow can be regarded as mere leakage. The above findings can only be explained by an expiratory check valve mechanism.

[*Editor's Note:* Material has been omitted at this point.]

DISCUSSION

Laennec concluded that the essential lesion in emphysema was obstruction of the smaller airways. To explain why obstruction should lead to abnormal distention of the lungs, he asserted that the muscles of inspiration are more powerful than those of expiration, a view that is commonly held to this day. Nevertheless, greater force can be exerted against a column of mercury by expiratory effort than by inspiratory effort (11, 12), a point which we have verified. Moreover, in a tubular system, airflow should bear a more or less direct relationship to pressure, all else being constant; yet in emphysema expiratory airflow is not proportionately improved by greater effort. Greater force is met by greater resistance. Force, therefore, would be adequate were it not for the singular character of expiratory resistance to airflow.

Christie (2, 3) and others concluded that the essential disturbance in emphysema is a loss of pulmonary elasticity. Loss of elasticity could bring about expiratory impedance by a mechanism described below, but it is not the sole mechanism. The syndrome of relatively free inspiration, impeded expiration and increased residual air occurs in at least two conditions when elasticity is intact; during an acute paroxysm of asthma (13) and in lung distal to a local bronchial obstruction such as that resulting from tuberculous bronchitis. With release of the obstruction, the syndrome disappears. We, therefore, must seek explanation for ventilatory disturbance in emphysema in the extrinsic mechanical factors as they affect the calibre of the airways rather than inadequate expiratory force or loss of pulmonary elasticity *per se*.

Extrinsic force can have a decided effect on calibre of the airways. Momentary narrowing of the trachea as the glottis opens in the expulsive phase of a forceful cough, and occlusion of the trachea by herniation of the membranous portion during expiration in severe asthma are the evident results of a pronounced pressure gradient between the inside and outside of the airway. An unmistakable check valve mechanism is in effect.

Neergaard and Wirz attributed greater expiratory resistance to this mechanism, reasoning that the pressure in the parenchyma surrounding an airway would be greater than that within its lumen, thereby causing it to collapse (4). Our findings are in keeping with this theory but indicate that the operation of an expiratory check valve mechanism is subject to the interrelated factors of lung tension, pulmonary pressure, rate of airflow and intrinsic disease of the airways, in such a way as to minimize the obstruction in health and render it virtually absolute in certain forms of emphysema.

Consider first a hypothetical segment of normal lung at a moment of apnea with a pleural pressure of − 15 cm. HOH. All structures from the pleura to the hilum are part of a continuous elastic system; all, including the walls of the airways, are subject to the distending force of 15 cm. HOH; all are exerting an equivalent counter tension. Canalicular pressure is atmospheric.

Expiration is initiated by a rise of pleural pressure and an equivalent rise of pulmonary pressure. However, there is a descending canalicular pressure along the path of airflow and the force distending the airway becomes 15 cm. HOH minus the difference between parenchymal and canalicular pressure at a given point in the airway. Elastic equilibrium can be re-established by narrowing of .the airway and relaxation of its walls to the point of equal counter tension. The higher the pulmonary pressure the steeper the pressure gradient and the more the narrowing. Narrowing of the airway itself exaggerates the pressure gradient. Potentially a vicious circle is present.

Thus far we refer to passive narrowing of airways similar to diastolic arterial narrowing. Actual collapse at a given point in an airway could occur only if pulmonary pressure exceeded lung tension plus canalicular pressure at that point. Since pulmonary pressure is equal to the difference between lung tension and pleural pressure, the latter would have to be positive. Active expiratory effort, such as that occurring in coughing or sneezing, would be required. Passive expiration would be ineffective.

As the lung deflates lung tension decreases. This, itself, leads to passive narrowing of the airways. As lung tension approaches zero, pulmonary pressure can be maintained only by resorting to positive pleural pressure. Thus, decline of forces tending to maintain patency of the airways inevitably augments the forces tending to actively narrow them. The stage is set for expiratory check valve closure when expiration is carried to the point of zero lung tension.

Despite limitations imposed by the indirect method of measuring pulmonary pressure and lung tension the experimental findings in normal expiration agree with those postulated in the hypothetical segment. The general level of resistance to airflow in a given case is higher in expiration than inspiration, and is augmented by high pulmonary pressure. As lung tension diminishes the resistance tends to remain high despite declining pulmonary pressures. These changes, though slight, we regard as important indications of a potential check valve mechanism even in health.

Serious expiratory obstruction in health is averted, probably by the following mechanisms:

1. It is doubtful that pulmonary pressure is uniform from pleura to hilum. If it were, the air spaces near the hilum would deflate sooner than those at the periphery, thereby establishing a parenchymal gradient parallel to that in the airway. Such local deflation would, however, cause local decrease in lung tension.

2. The airways subjected to greatest stress in forceful expiration are armored against collapse by cartilage.

3. Resistance to airflow in the normal thoracic airways is slight and the pressure gradient thereby at a minimum. By measuring pharyngeal pressure it can be determined that most of the resistance to airflow in health is in the upper respiratory tract.

4. The healthy patient ventilates the lungs within a range of lung tension which permits adequate expiratory airflow without resort to positive pleural pressure. Thus Case 5 attained rates of 3,500 cc./sec. by passive recoil alone, surely enough for physiological needs, even in exercise. By positive expiratory effort a healthy man can attain rates of 10,000 cc./sec. or better, a remarkable achievement considering the complex structure of the lung, and one which is made possible only by the delicate balance of forces which maintain the calibre of the airways, of which the most important is lung tension.

There are two common disease conditions which can disturb this balance of forces: (*1*) intrinsic obstruction of the airways, (*2*) loss of lung tension.

1. Intrinsic obstruction of the airways: Regardless of the nature of the lesion, whether it be tumor, local inflammation, generalized bronchitis, or a paroxysm of asthma, an intrinsic lesion partially obstructing the airways produces two effects.

a. Fall of pressure along the course of the obstructed airway is more pronounced than normal.

b. Greater than normal pulmonary pressure is required to produce a given rate of airflow.

In turn, both circumstances predispose to check valve narrowing of the airway. It is understandable therefore, that if the degree of resistance is sufficient, expiratory impedance, premature arrest of expiration and increased residual air are common to all the above disease conditions. It is likewise apparent why a shift of the mediastinum in unilateral obstructive emphysema, due to a local bronchial lesion, is best elicited by a forceful expiratory effort. Closure of the bronchus at the site of such a lesion, *early* in expiration is described by Jackson (14). If bronchioles are the principal site of the obstruction, a similar closure would be anticipated in them.

In obstructive pulmonary disease two compensatory mechanisms may be employed: (*a*) The avoidance of rapid expiratory airflow, and (*b*) breathing so far as possible, within a range of high lung tension (13, 15). Both are employed during a paroxysm of asthma.

2. *Loss of lung tension:* In two forms of emphysema intrinsic obstruction of the airways may be slight or even absent, despite extreme pulmonary insufficiency with typical expiratory impedance and premature arrest. One form is a sequel to allergic asthma wherein the bronchial factor after many years has ceased but the patient suffers from sustained crippling emphysema which does not respond to adrenalin and is characterized at necropsy by advanced breakdown of the parenchyma. Case 11 is typical.

In such an instance sections along the bronchioles leave no doubt about the nature of the expiratory obstruction. The bronchioles are patent but their delicate structure, the tenuous remnants of parenchyma separated by gaping holes about their circumference and the evident loss of lung tension on actual measurement, presents a mechanical situation which can be likened to that of a leaky rubber valve from a basal metabolism apparatus. Such a valve-like bronchiole would conduct expiratory air under low external pressure but an attempt to increase airflow would inevitably lead to narrowing. Such bronchioles, unprotected by cartilage and unsupported by lung tension would be expected to close completely under pressure once any degree of narrowing occurs. With low or absent lung tension, shut-off of airflow typically becomes more sudden the greater the applied force (Cases 6, 8, 9). Furthermore the shut-off occurs under pressures which would be insufficient to materially collapse the major airways, again suggesting that the bronchiole is the site of the closure.

Intrinsic obstruction would, of course, increase the tendency of the unsupported bronchiole to collapse, but collapse would occur even in the absence of intrinsic obstruction provided sufficient pulmonary pressure is applied.

The second form of emphysema in which the unsupported bronchiole plays a part, regardless of intrinsic obstruction, is that complicating fibrosis of the lung, exemplified in conglomerate silicosis. Emphysema in these cases may be most severe, and without history of antecedent bronchial disease. Again, necropsy characteristically shows advanced breakdown of the parenchyma which must result in decreased lung tension and loss of bronchiolar support.

Pulmonary elasticity

Christie demonstrated the direct relationship between lung volume and lung tension in health, but in two cases of advanced emphysema lung tension increased proportionately at first, then as inflation continued, lung tension tended to level off. In the present study lung tension in four cases of advanced emphysema leveled off between 2 and 10 cm. HOH pressure. There can be no doubt that lung tension is decreased in these cases but we are not justified in saying that the remaining tissue in such lungs had necessarily lost elasticity. In the distension of hollow structures pressure measured in cm. of HOH does not directly express the stress nor does volume measure the strain. For example, the expression cm. HOH pressure means gm. per cm.^{2} The area over which this pressure is exerted, and therefore the total force, is unknown, but we do know that the area increases as the structure distends. In the distension of hollow spheres made of thin, good quality rubber, pressure rises to a peak (the "hump") and then levels off or slowly declines as inflation continues (16), a striking parallel to the curve in emphysema.

Since the essential features of emphysema may be present in lungs of normal tension, and loss of tension has been demonstrated only in advanced emphysema where breakdown of parenchyma is either demonstrated or would be expected, and since the tension/volume relationship in advanced emphysema does not necessarily indicate loss of elasticity, we are justified in concluding that the decreased tension is due to breakdown of the parenchyma, a disturbance of architecture, rather than a disturbance of elasticity. To the present there is no valid evidence that the remaining parenchyma of the emphysematous lung is inelastic.

CONCLUSIONS

1. The method of Neergaard and Wirz can be adapted to show the trends in pleural pressure, lung tension, airflow, pulmonary pressure, and resistance to airflow. Certain errors in the method are noted.

2. During expiration intrathoracic airways behave as check valves. A slight tendency in this direction is detectable even in health, serious obstruction being averted by a number of mechanical circumstances, the chief of which is adequate lung tension.

3. In advanced emphysema check valve obstruction becomes virtually absolute as expiration progresses to the point of zero lung tension.

4. Lung tension in advanced emphysema, measured in terms of cm. HOH, is reduced and does not bear a direct proportion to lung volume. This is probably the result of breakdown of the parenchyma and does not necessarily imply that the remaining parenchyma is inelastic. Such breakdown of parenchyma leaves the bronchioles unsupported and thereby vulnerable to expiratory check valve closure.

5. The tendency toward expiratory check valve closure is increased by high pulmonary pressure, intrinsic obstruction of intrathoracic airways, and low lung tension.

6. Application of the above principles can explain many of the ventilatory disturbances in obstructive pulmonary disease.

REFERENCES

1. Cournand, A., Richards, D. W., Jr., and Darling, R. C., Graphic tracings of respiration in study of pulmonary disease. Am. Rev. Tuberc., 1939, **40**, 487.
2. Christie, R. V., and McIntosh, C. A., The measurement of the intrapleural pressure in man and its significance. J. Clin. Invest., 1934, **13**, 279.
3. Christie, R. V., The elastic properties of the emphysematous lung and their clinical significance. J. Clin. Invest., 1934, **13**, 295.
4. Neergaard, K., and Wirz, K., Die Messung der Strömungswiderstände in den Atemwegen des Menschen insbesondere bei Asthma und Emphysem. Ztschr. f. klin. Med., 1927, **105**, 51.
5. Bayliss, L. E., and Robertson, G. W., Visco-elastic properties of the lungs. Quart. J .Exper. Physiol., 1939, **29**, 27.
6. West, H. F., Clinical studies on respiration; comparison of various standards for normal vital capacity of lungs. Arch. Int. Med., 1920, **25**, 306.
7. Gardner, L., Saranac Laboratory, personal communication.
8. Loeb, L. M., The etiology of emphysema. Arch. Int. Med., 1930, **45**, 464.
9. Alexander, H. L., Emphysema. Proc. Staff Meet., Mayo Clin., 1935, **10**, 377.
10. Lell, W. A., Bronchoscopy as an aid in the diagnosis and treatment of allergic pulmonary disease. Arch. Otolaryng., 1946, **43**, 49.
11. McLeod, J. J. R., Physiology in Modern Medicine, edited by Bard, P. C. V. Mosby Co., St. Louis, 1938, 8th Ed., 476.
12. Rahn, H., Otis, A. B., Chadwick, L. E., and Fenn, W. O., The pressure volume diagram of the thorax and lung. Am. J. Physiol., 1946, **146**, 161.
13. Baldwin, E., Bronchial asthma. Am. J. Med., 1946, **1**, 193.
14. Jackson, C. L., Bronchial obstruction. Diseases of the Chest, 1950, **17**, 125.
15. Prinzmetal, M., Relation of inspiratory distension of the lungs to emphysema. J. Allergy, 1934, **5**, 493.
16. Treloar, L. R. G., Stress strain data for vulcanized rubber. Rubber Chem. and Tech., 1945, **17**, 813.

28

Reprinted from *Bull. Johns Hopkins Hosp.*, **101**(6), 329–343 (1957)

MECHANISMS OF AIRWAY OBSTRUCTION

E. J. M. CAMPBELL[1], H. B. MARTIN[2], AND R. L. RILEY

Departments of Environmental Medicine and of Medicine, The Johns Hopkins University and Hospital

Received for publication July 25, 1957

INTRODUCTION

We have studied the effect of intrathoracic pressure on the resistance of the airways both because of its theoretical interest and in the hope that the findings may help to differentiate between the various mechanisms which contribute to the increased resistance to airflow in the asthma-bronchitis-emphysema group of conditions. Currently used tests of ventilatory function, such as the Maximum Breathing Capacity and various modifications of the Fast Vital Capacity provide good estimates of the severity of airway obstruction, but give little help in discriminating between the mechanisms causing the obstruction. Such discrimination is essential if progress is to be made in elucidating the basic mechanisms of obstructive disease, its pathogenesis and its response to treatment.

It is now generally recognized that the airways become wider in inspiration and narrower in expiration. This cyclic change tends to cause the airflow-resistance to be greater during expiration than during inspiration. In normal subjects this change in resistance is minimal during quiet breathing but during forced expiration and in emphysema it becomes very great (1).

One of the important factors involved in the changing diameter of the respiratory passages is the pressure difference across their walls; that is, the difference between the intraluminal pressure (P_L) in the airways and the intrathoracic pressure (P_T) surrounding them.[3] When an increased expiratory

This study was aided by a contract between the Office of Naval Research, Department of the Navy, and The Johns Hopkins University (NR 112-101); by funds provided under contract AF 18 (600)-435 with the USAF School of Aviation Medicine, Randolph Field, Texas; and by funds from research grant H 1929 from the National Institutes of Health.

[1] Comyns-Berkeley Fellow of Gonville and Caius College, Cambridge University and The Middlesex Hospital Medical School, London, England. Present address: The Middlesex Hospital, London W. 1, England.

[2] Fellow of the National Foundation for Infantile Paralysis.

[3] We have assumed that the intrathoracic pressure surrounding the alveoli is the same as that surrounding the respiratory passages and is equal to the intrapleural pressure. This assumption is reasonable when applied to normally functioning lungs but is not strictly valid in the presence of obstructive disease with variable amounts of air trapping in different parts of the lung. Within small (e.g. sub-segmental) units in which air trapping has occurred, the pressure surrounding the respiratory passages may be higher than in unobstructed regions because relatively non-compliant septa may prevent equalization of pressure throughout the lungs.

effort is made, the intrathoracic pressure and the rate of airflow both increase. The pressure in the terminal air spaces (alveolar pressure, P_{Alv}) equals the intrathoracic pressure plus an amount governed by the elastic recoil of the lung ($P_{Alv} = P_T + P_{El}{}^L$). The increased rate of airflow during an increased expiratory effort is associated with an increased pressure gradient (ΔP) between the alveoli and any point in the airways ($\Delta P = P_{Alv} - P_L$). Because of this pressure drop, the intraluminal pressure (P_L) does not increase as much as P_{Alv} or P_T. The possibility exists therefore that if a sufficiently great expiratory effort is made P_T may exceed the intraluminal pressure at some point in the airways and cause narrowing of the lumen.[4] This narrowing would increase the resistance.

During a forced expiratory effort, therefore, a level of intrathoracic pressure might be reached above which no further increase or even a decrease in flow rate might occur. Examination of the data of Fry *et al.* (2) and of Mead and Whittenberger (3) shows that such a decrease in flow rate does occur and suggests that the hypothesis outlined above may be valid. We term the intrathoracic pressure at which the maximum flow rate occurs the Maximum Effective Intrathoracic Pressure ($P_T{}^{Max\ Eff}$) and the corresponding flow the Maximum Expiratory Flow Rate ($\dot{V}_E{}^{Max}$).

We have attempted to measure the $P_T{}^{Max\ Eff}$ and the $\dot{V}_E{}^{Max}$ in normal subjects and in patients with obstructive disease.

METHODS

Three normal subjects, five patients with emphysema and three with asthma were studied (Table I). The group of patients with emphysema was specially selected to include only those whose history was dominated by progressive dyspnea. Those in whom asthma or bronchitis was a prominent feature were excluded. They were studied after the inhalation of bronchodilator (nebulized isuprel® 1:200 solution) in order to minimize bronchoconstriction. Our aim was to compare this group with the asthmatics who were studied during attacks and without the administration of bronchodilator. In the asthmatic patients the major disorder presumably was narrowing of the lumen of the air passages by increased bronchomotor tone, edema, mucus etc. The group of patients with asthma was selected to include only those who were free from exertional dyspnea between attacks, and in whom therefore, the structural changes of emphysema were presumably minimal.

Airflow was measured by means of a pneumotachometer containing a 325 mesh stainless steel screen. The pressure drop across the pneumotachometer screen was measured with a Statham differential pressure strain gauge transducer.

The pressure in the lower third of the esophagus (P_E) was measured by means of a thin walled balloon (12–16 cm. long) and a polythene tube of 1.5 mm. bore. These were prepared

[4] $P_L = P_{Alv} - \Delta P$; $P_L = P_T + P_{El}{}^L - \Delta P$. When $P_{El}{}^L = \Delta P$, P_L will equal P_T. With greater expiratory effort ΔP will increase without change in $P_{El}{}^L$, and P_L will therefore be less than P_T. When the intraluminal pressure (P_L) is less than the surrounding pressure (P_T), this pressure difference will tend to narrow the lumen. This reasoning and the underlying assumptions are further examined in the discussion.

TABLE I

Routine Ventilatory Findings

Subject	Diagnosis	Age	Height	Vital Capacity		One Sec. V. C.		Max. Breathing Capacity	
				Before broncho-dilator	After broncho-dilator	Before broncho-dilator	After broncho-dilator	Before broncho-dilator	After broncho-dilator
R. L. R.	Normal	44	69 ½	5240	—		—	163	—
E. J. M. C.	Normal	29	73	6030	—	5980	—	211	—
E. V.	Normal	32	72	6550	—	5610	—	199	—
E. B.	Emphysema	52	74 ½	2380	3080	890	1290	36	42
R. D.	Emphysema	66	61 ¼	1910	2360	900	1110	28	31
J. M.	Emphysema	43	66	1730	2040	800	1100	34	39
H. P.	Emphysema	67	65 ½	2400	2560	854	1033	34	45
R. T.	Emphysema	56	69	2670	2695	831	787	28	31
T. A.	Asthma	20	63 ½	1817	3300	695	2690	—	—
J. B.	Asthma	40	66 ½	3078	3975	1843	2335	42	56
G. C.	Asthma	22	65 ¾	763	3930	494	3772	—	104

in the manner recommended by Mead *et al.* (4). The pressure difference between the esophagus and the mouthpiece was measured with a Statham differential pressure strain gauge transducer. In recent years the esophageal pressure has been extensively used as an index of intrapleural and intrathoracic pressure. The limitations of the esophageal pressure in this respect have been examined by Cherniack *et al.* and by Mead and Gaensler (5, 6). It appears from their data that the esophageal pressure is a sufficiently good index of intrapleural pressure for the purposes of our study.

Tracings of airflow and esophageal-mouth differential pressure were recorded simultaneously by means of a Sanborn amplifying recorder. The recording paper was run at a speed of 100 mm/sec. All subjects were in the sitting position. The pneumotachometer was calibrated with a rotameter. The volume of air moved was determined by integration of the flow tracing.

The pressure required to overcome non-elastic resistance during quiet breathing was measured from the pressure-volume loop and plotted against the simultaneously recorded rate of flow to give a value for resistance. Resistance was measured in this way during inspiration at rates of airflow of 0.5–1 L/sec. Non-elastic resistance as determined in this manner includes lung tissue viscous resistance but is chiefly airflow resistance. (7)

The determination of $P_T^{Max\ Eff}$ presented additional problems. The lag of the esophageal balloon—strain gauge—recorder system on the pneumotachometer—strain gauge—recorder system was found to be less than 0.005 sec. However, it was found that there may be a delay in the response of the esophagus itself to rapid changes in intrathoracic pressure. This delay was measured as follows: The subject made a shallow short expiratory effort which produced a peaked record of flow and of esophageal pressure. The lag of the pressure peak on the flow peak was measured. This procedure was repeated a number of times and the mean value for the lag was used in measuring the $P_T^{Max\ Eff}$ as described below. The lag was found to vary between subjects within the range 0.01–0.05 sec. (normal subjects 0.01–0.03 sec.; patients with emphysema 0.01–0.05 sec.).

In one of the normal subjects, simultaneous mouth and esophageal pressure records were taken while he made short sharp expiratory efforts against a closed valve so that no airflow occurred. The lag of P_E in relation to mouth pressure was found to be the same as that ob-

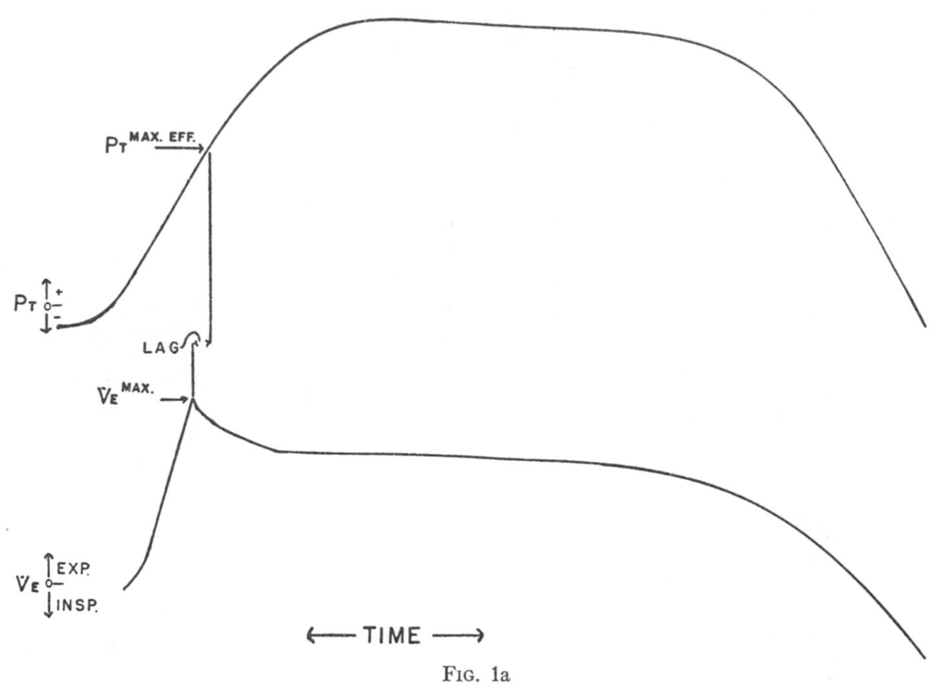
PT MAX. EFF.
PT + −
LAG
VE MAX.
VE EXP. INSP.
TIME

FIG. 1a

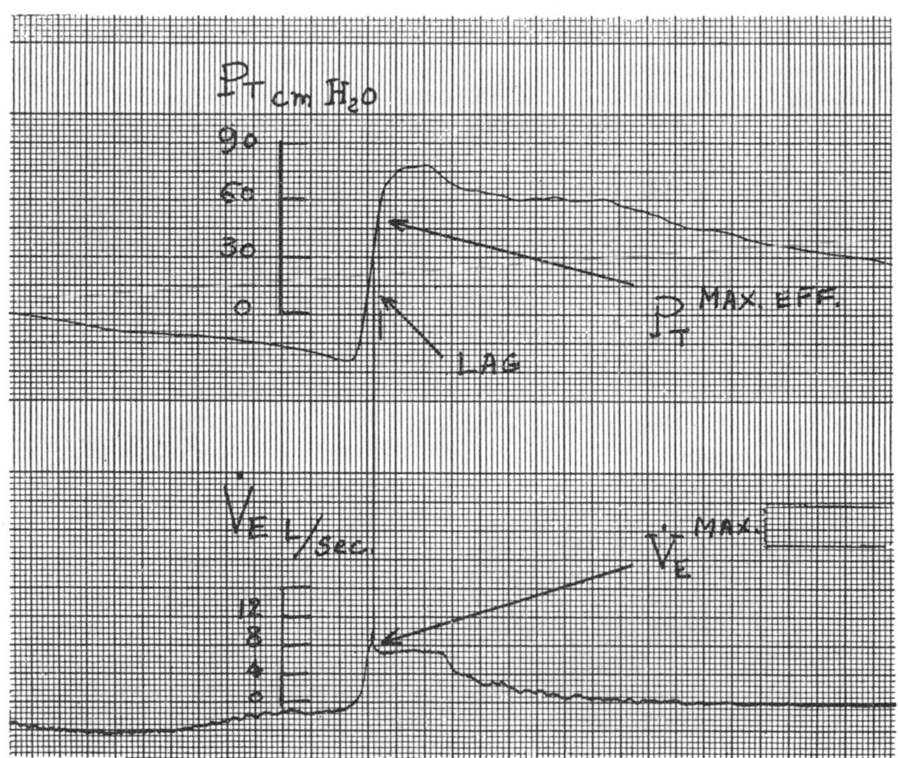
PT cm H2O
90
60
30
0
PT MAX. EFF.
LAG
VE L/sec.
VE MAX.
12
8
4
0

FIG. 1b

tained using the pneumotachometer and thus excluded errors in the determination of the lag due to airflow.

The subjects performed maximal expiratory efforts at two lung volumes, the resting respiratory level and at maximum inspiration. A drawing of the type of record obtained is shown in Figure 1A. Figure 1B is a photograph of a record taken subsequently with improved equipment. The peak flow rate was taken as maximum expiratory flow rate ($\dot{V}_E^{Max}$) and the simultaneous esophageal pressure (allowing for lag as described above) was taken as the $P_T^{Max\ Eff}$.

RESULTS

The data are recorded in Table II.

In the normal subjects the mean $P_T^{Max\ Eff}$ was 45 cm. H_2O at the resting respiratory level and 56 cm. H_2O at full inspiration. The mean value for $\dot{V}_E^{Max}$ was 5.4 L/sec. at the resting respiratory level and 10.6 L/sec. at full inspiration. Airflow resistance during quiet breathing was low, the mean value being 1.7 cm. H_2O/L/sec.

The findings in the patients with asthma and emphysema were strikingly different from normal and strikingly different from each other. Two of the patients with asthma were so distressed that $P_T^{Max\ Eff}$ and $\dot{V}_E^{Max}$ were only measured at the resting respiratory level. The mean value for $\dot{V}_E^{Max}$ in this group (0.82 L/sec.) at the resting respiratory level is very similar to that found in the patients with emphysema (0.96 L/sec.). There are, however, conspicuous differences between the two groups in the findings for resistance during quiet breathing and $P_T^{Max\ Eff}$. The mean resistance during quiet inspiration in the patients with asthma was 16.1 cm. H_2O/L/sec. whereas in the patients with emphysema it was only 6.6 cm. H_2O/L/sec. On the other hand, the mean $P_T^{Max\ Eff}$ at the resting respiratory level was 26 cm. H_2O in the patients with asthma and 9 cm. H_2O in those with emphysema. Only one of the patients with emphysema (E.B.) had a value for $P_T^{Max\ Eff}$ comparable with the normal or asthmatic subjects. At the time of study he had a mild respiratory infection with bronchitis and increased sputum production. In view of our subsequent findings and the theoretical analysis presented in the discussion it seems possible that this bronchitis contributed to the elevation of the $P_T^{Max\ Eff}$ above the values obtained in the other patients with emphysema.

Examination of Figure 1 shows that overestimation of the lag in the recording of esophageal pressure would lead to an overestimate of $P_T^{Max\ Eff}$ and vice versa. We have examined our records, taking both possibilities into consideration and find that, while the actual values quoted for $P_T^{Max\ Eff}$ may be slightly in error, they are sufficiently accurate to indicate without question a systematic difference between the three groups of subjects.

FIG. 1. Esophageal pressure (top tracing) and rate of airflow (bottom tracing) during a forced expiration. $P_T^{Max\ Eff}$: maximum effective expiratory pressure. $\dot{V}_E^{Max}$: maximum expiratory flow rate. A. Drawing of a typical record. B. Photograph of a record taken subequently with improved equipment (servo-spirometer, Custom Engineering and Development Co., St. Louis, Mo.). Paper speed = 50 mm. per second.

TABLE II

Pressure-Flow Data

Subject	Diagnosis	Resting Respiratory Level				Maximum Inspiratory Level				Flow Resistance During Quiet Inspiration cm H_2O/L/Sec.
		P_TMax Eff cm H_2O		$\dot{V}_E$Max L/Sec.		P_TMax Eff cm H_2O		$\dot{V}_E$Max L/Sec.		
		Mean	S.E.	Mean	S.E.	Mean	S.E.	Mean	S.E.	
R. L. R.	Normal	49.2	2.3	4.43	0.16	62.0	1.7	8.13	0.20	
E. J. M. C.	Normal	55.2	3.6	5.40	0.20	48.8	1.7	11.10	0.17	
E. V.	Normal	30.0	1.7	6.39	0.14	58.0	2.8	12.66	0.05	
Mean........		45.0		5.40		56.0		10.63		1.7
E. B.	Emphysema	24.0	1.7	1.06	0.04	35.5	1.9	2.73	0.39	
R. D.	Emphysema	4.3	0.5	0.66	0.05	6.0	0.7	1.35	0.01	
J. M.	Emphysema	8.5	1.3	0.58	0.06	25.0	3.5	2.08	0.10	
H. P.	Emphysema	7.0	1.0	1.26	0.17	18.0	2.7	3.18	0.05	
R. T.	Emphysema	2.5	0.5	1.26	0.09	6.0	1.2	2.37	0.02	
Mean........		9.0		0.96		18.0		2.34		6.6
T. A.	Asthma	35.0	3.7	0.79	0.04	—		3.17		
J. B.	Asthma	20.0	2.0	1.00	0.12	18.5	2.5	—	0.18	
G. C.	Asthma	21.5	1.0	0.66	0.08	—				
Mean........		26.0		0.82						16.1

DISCUSSION

Several observers (1, 2, 8, 9) have examined the increased resistance during expiration that is observed in patients with emphysema during quiet breathing or in normal subjects during forced breathing. They all conclude that this increase in resistance is due to compression of the intrapulmonary airways by intrathoracic pressure. Mead *et al.* (1) point out that direct observation of the bronchi at bronchoscopy and bronchography has shown narrowing to occur during forced expiratory efforts. However, the possibility must be considered that the decrease in flow rate immediately after reaching $\dot{V}_E^{Max}$ might be due to a sudden increase in turbulent flow at very high flow rates.

To investigate this possibility the relationship between P_T and $\dot{V}_E$ was studied in one of the normal subjects after a maximum inhalation of pure helium. Since helium has a higher kinematic viscosity than air it reduces the amount of turbulent flow in the airways, and since it has a lower density it decreases the resistance due to any given amount of turbulence. Therefore, for both reasons, helium would be expected to cause a marked reduction in airflow resistance at the level of $\dot{V}_E$ previously found to be maximal when breathing air. One would expect a marked reduction in P_T at this level of $\dot{V}_E$ if the decrease in flow rate at values of P_T above $P_T^{Max\ Eff}$ during air breathing were due to an increase in turbulent flow. The experimental findings were approximately the same with helium and with air, suggesting that turbulence is not a major factor determining $\dot{V}_E^{Max}$ and $P_T^{Max\ Eff}$. Indirectly this evidence supports the hypothesis that the increased resistance is due to narrowing of the airways.

The relationship between the data reported in this paper and the pressure-flow data reported by others is not obvious. Fry *et al.* (2) determined airflow velocity at increasing alveolar pressures in normal people and in emphysematous patients. The measurements were made at three different but constant lung volumes. In the emphysema group airflow velocity increased with increasing expiratory pressure until a maximal value was reached and remained essentially constant when expiratory pressure was further increased. These findings have been confirmed by Riley, Mani, Perti and Jain, using simplified techniques (10). They are likewise consistent with the findings of McDermott and McKerrow that maximal expiratory flow rate, as determined from a spirographic tracing, remains essentially unchanged when expiratory pressures in excess of the minimum required to achieve maximal flow are applied (11).

It is pertinent to ask whether the maximal airflow velocities found by the previously mentioned workers are the same as the $\dot{V}_E^{Max}$ values reported in this paper. In the work of Fry *et al.* airflow velocity was relatively constant prior to the instant at which the velocity measurement was made; in the work reported here, a sudden forced expiratory effort was made with very rapid acceleration to a peak velocity which was reached in a few hundredths of a second. The pressure relationships contributing to narrowing of the airways may not be the same in the two situations and the measured airflow velocities may therefore not be the same. On inspection of Fig. 1B it appears that our $\dot{V}_E^{Max}$ probably exceeds the maximum flow rates reported by others by the difference between the peak value and the plateau value on the velocity tracing.

What relationship does $P_T^{Max\ Eff}$ bear to the alveolar pressures reported by Fry *et al.* (2)? Let us assume that P_{El}^L can be estimated with reasonable accuracy and that it can be added to $P_T^{Max\ Eff}$ to give $P_{Alv}^{Max\ Eff}$. Would $P_{Alv}^{Max\ Eff}$ correspond to any specific point on a curve of P_{Alv} vs $\dot{V}_E$ as obtained by Fry *et al.*?

The curves of Fry *et al.* suggest that in patients with emphysema a constant maximum velocity is produced by any pressure in excess of a certain minimum, whereas in the present studies $\dot{V}_E^{Max}$ appeared to occur at a single specific pressure. Comparison of average results by the two methods indicates that $P_T^{Max\ Eff}$ in emphysema approximates the lowest pressure producing maximum velocity. The shape of the curve in Fig. 1B is consistent with this interpretation, as applied to the normal subject, if "maximum velocity" is taken to be the plateau value.

Theoretical Aspects

Numerous factors are involved in the change in caliber of the airways with breathing and a definitive analysis is impossible on the basis of present knowledge. From the following simplified analysis, however, certain semiquantitative conclusions can be drawn which are believed to be valid. We shall assume that a dynamic equilibrium between forces tending to open and close the airways occurs, permitting the airways momentarily to remain constant in size. The net pressure acting in an inward direction is the algebraic sum of the intrathoracic pressure (P_T), the pressure resulting from bronchomotor tone (P_{BM}), and the elastic recoil of the wall of the airway ($P_{El}{}^W$).[5] P_T, which is normally negative, is positive during forced expiration, and $P_{El}{}^W$ may be negative during forced expiration, indicating that the airways are resisting compression. The pressure acting in an outward direction is the intraluminal pressure (P_L). At any given position of the airway, whether narrowed or distended, these pressures balance, and the equality of inward and outward acting pressures can be expressed as an equation:

$$P_T + P_{BM} + P_{El}{}^W = P_L \qquad (1)$$

The more restricted expression which applies to the alveoli is:

$$P_T + P_{El}{}^L = P_{Alv} \qquad \text{(See page 330)} \qquad (2)$$

Here $P_{El}{}^W$ becomes $P_{El}{}^L$, P_L becomes P_{Alv}, and P_{BM} drops out.

In the static condition the transmural pressure difference across airway walls ($P_L - P_T$) is presumed to be the same as that across alveolar walls ($P_{Alv} - P_T$) and reflects the mean elastic tension of all the structures which make up the lung. Under dynamic conditions $P_{Alv} - P_T$ remains unchanged, because there is no flow of air through the alveoli, but $P_L - P_T$ may be grossly altered by changes in P_L related to the flow of air. The transmural pressure gradients resulting from inspiration are such as to expand the airways and may thereby cause high positive values of $P_{El}{}^W$. During forced expiration most of the airways have to resist compression and may develop highly negative values of $P_{El}{}^W$.

Each little segment of airway has its own pressure-volume curve which differs from the pressure-volume diagram of the lung as a whole. Such curves, recently obtained by Martin and Proctor for excised dog bronchi, show that airways of increasing size have the characteristic of offering increased resistance to both compression and distention (12). Larger airways require a higher collapsing pressure than small ones to produce the same proportional change in diameter. This characteristic is essential in preventing collapse of the larger airways during forced expiration.

When airways are subjected to various transmural pressures, each little segment responds according to its own pressure-volume curve, modified by the effect of bronchomotor tone if such be present. All airways will get smaller when the balance shifts in favor of the inward acting pressure, but the reduction

[5] The elastic recoil ($P_{El}{}^W$) is considered to include the narrowing tendency caused by surface tension.

in caliber may or may not be significant depending on the size of the transmural gradient and the size and stiffness of the airway. The following illustrations of pressure relationships during forced expiration will show the way these principles operate in the normal lung and in the presence of emphysematous and asthmatic changes.

In Figures 2, 3 and 4 the segment of airway nearest to the alveoli is considered to have no capacity to resist compression, but from this point to the trachea the stiffness of the airway steadily increases. The values of P_L differ in the three examples but always decrease progressively from the alveolus to the mouth. It is assumed in each case that the expiratory force provided by

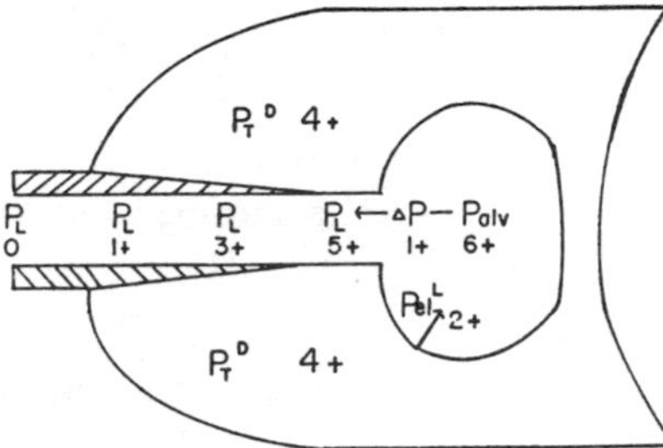

FIG. 2. Schematic diagram of some of the factors tending to open and close the airways during a forced expiration, in a normal lung.

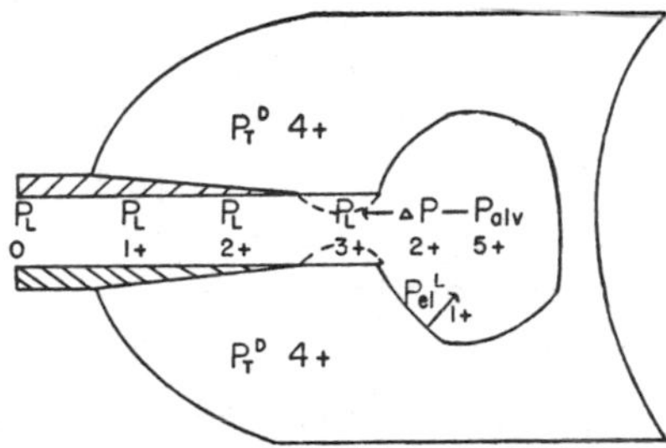

FIG. 3. Schematic diagram of some of the factors tending to open and close the airways during a forced expiration, in an emphysematous lung.

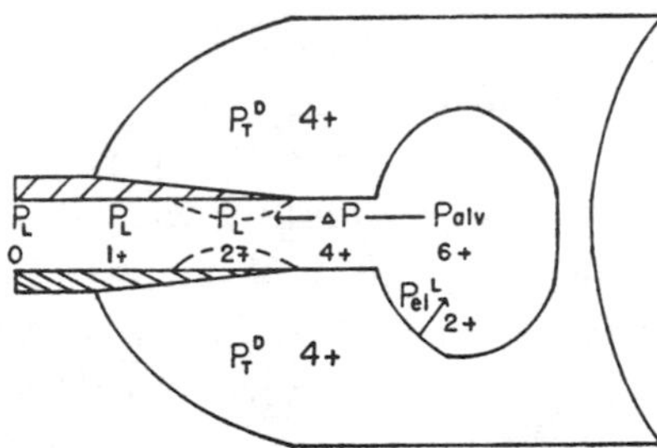

FIG. 4. Schematic diagram of some of the factors tending to open and close the airways during a forced expiration, in an asthmatic lung.

contraction of the muscles of expiration raises P_T^D[6] to 4+ above atmospheric. Figure 2 represents a normal lung in which the elastic recoil (P_{El}^L) increases the pressure within the alveolus by 2+. Alveolar pressure (P_{Alv}) therefore = $P_T^D + P_{El}^L = 4 + 2 = 6+$. In Figure 3, which represents an emphysematous lung, the elastic recoil is assumed to be only 1+ and $P_{Alv} = P_T^D + P_{El}^L = 4 + 1 = 5+$. In Figure 4, representing an asthmatic lung, the elastic recoil is assumed to have a normal value and $P_{Alv} = 6+$.

In Figure 2 the resistance in the segment of airway nearest the alveoli is so small that the pressure drop between the alveolar space and this point (ΔP) is only 1. P_L thus equals 5+. The pressure difference across the wall of the airway at this point, $P_L - P_T^D$, $= 5 - 4 = 1+$ in favor of P_L, the outward acting pressure. This tiny segment of airway, whose wall has no intrinsic rigidity with which to resist compression, will remain open because of the favorable transmural pressure relationships. Further downstream P_L falls below P_T^D indicating that the airway is compressed, but this part of the airway is larger and the wall more rigid so that collapsing pressures in the normal physiological range can be withstood without significant narrowing. It is known that the large airways do narrow appreciably when expiration is forced (13).

In the emphysematous lung (Fig. 3) more resistance in the segment of airway nearest the alveoli is assumed, and P_L in this segment therefore drops 2 below P_{Alv}. Note also that P_{Alv} is less than in the normal lung because of reduction in P_{El}^L. Since $P_L = P_{Alv} - \Delta P$, a reduction in P_{Alv} and an increase in ΔP both contribute to the lowering of P_L. In this instance the pressure difference across the wall of the airway, $P_L - P_T^D$, becomes $3 - 4$ or -1. This is the same as a pressure difference of +1 tending to narrow the airway. The segment of airway (perhaps an alveolar duct) having no ability to withstand compression, will be significantly narrowed or even completely collapsed by such a transmural gradient. Severe obstruction to the flow of air will result. In the larger airways the collapsing pressure increases and, if expiration were forced maximally (very high P_T^D), all the intrathoracic airways would probably be narrowed markedly. It is believed, however, for reasons which will be discussed below, that the segments of airway nearest the alveoli are the most vulnerable in emphysema.

In the asthmatic (Fig. 4) the middle sized airways are narrowed as a result of increased bronchomotor tone. The resulting increase in resistance increases the pressure drop, ΔP, in this segment of the airway. By thus lowering P_L to 2+ the transmural collapsing pressure is increased and further narrowing brought about. The very large airways are compressed as in emphysema but

[6] P_T^D is the symbol used to denote the intrathoracic pressure under dynamic conditions, i.e. when airflow is occurring.

are represented as patent in Figure 4 because the middle sized airways are believed to be the most vulnerable in asthma.

In reconstructing the chain of events suggested by these schematic drawings, it is important to realize that the sum total of inward acting and outward acting pressures cannot remain unbalanced. The lack of balance indicated in the figures refers to $P_L - P_T^D$ and represents the transmural pressure gradient which must be resisted by the wall of the airway. In order to balance equation 1, suitable values for P_{El}^W and P_{BM} must be inserted. Each segment of airway must widen or narrow until the point has been reached on its own peculiar pressure-volume curve where the necessary resistance to compression or distention becomes available.

Let us now analyze the data in Table II in an effort to estimate the value of P_{El}^W in the most vulnerable airway segments at the time of critical narrowing. By critical narrowing is meant narrowing of such a degree that airflow can no longer increase with further increase in expiratory pressure (P_T^D) because of a disproportionate increase in resistance. On inspection of Equation 1 it is apparent that of the four variables involved we have objective data regarding only one, namely P_T. When expiration is forced P_T must pass through $P_T^{Max\ Eff}$, and at $P_T^{Max\ Eff}$ critical narrowing occurs. Let us therefore rearrange Equation 1, substituting $P_T^{Max\ Eff}$ for P_T and adding primes to all the other symbols to indicate that now the specific values obtaining when $P_T = P_T^{Max\ Eff}$ are under consideration.

$$P_T^{Max\ Eff} + P_{BM}' + P_{El}^{W'} = P_L' \qquad (3)$$

One further substitution is desirable for algebraic convenience. Since a negative value of $P_{El}^{W'}$ indicates resistance of the airway wall to compression, this pressure can be thought of in the positive sense as acting in an outward direction. In order to introduce this idea in Equation 3, a new symbol, $P_{Out}^{W'}$ (pressure, outward, wall), will be used. By definition $P_{Out}^{W'} = -P_{El}^{W'}$. Equation 3 can now be rewritten as follows:

$$P_T^{Max\ Eff} + P_{BM}' = P_{Out}^{W'} + P_L' \quad \text{or}$$

$$P_{Out}^{W'} = P_T^{Max\ Eff} + P_{BM}' - P_L' \qquad (3a)$$

The problem of estimating $P_{El}^{W'}$ at the time of critical narrowing now becomes the problem of estimating $P_{Out}^{W'}$ when $P_T^{Max\ Eff}$ is known and rough estimates of P_L' and P_{BM}' are used.

In emphysema very low values for $P_T^{Max\ Eff}$ were found (Table II). P_{BM}' is also believed to have been low because resistance during quiet inspiration was relatively low and there was only minimal response to bronchodilators. The two positive factors on the right side of Equation 3a, $P_T^{Max\ Eff}$ and P_{BM}', were thus both low. We know little about P_L' except that it has a minus sign in front of it, indicating that it reduces the net value of the right side of Equation 3a. There seems little doubt, therefore, that $P_{Out}^{W'}$ was very low in the patients with emphysema. This implies that there was very little resistance to compression at the site of critical narrowing and suggests that the site of critical narrowing was probably in the very small airways.

$P_T^{Max\ Eff}$ was much higher in the asthmatics. Since these patients were suffering from severe bronchospasm, with high inspiratory resistance during quiet breathing and dramatic response to bronchodilators, there is every reason to believe that P_{BM}' was high. The factor, $-P_L'$, is elusive, but we do know the limits within which P_L' must lie. If critical narrowing occurred in the smallest airways, P_L' would have the highest possible value and this value could not exceed $P_T^{Max\ Eff}$ (see Fig. 4); if critical narrowing occurred in the largest intrathoracic airways, P_L' would have the lowest possible value and this could not be less than zero. A low value of P_L' would leave the net value of the right hand side of equation 3a very high in asthma, indicating a high value of $P_{Out}^{W'}$. If P_L' approximately equalled $P_T^{Max\ Eff}$, $P_{Out}^{W'}$ would approximately equal P_{BM}' and this would be the lowest possible value of $P_{Out}^{W'}$. In view of the fact that high bronchomotor tone is the predominant characteristic of the asthmatic state, it seems probable that even this minimal value of $P_{Out}^{W'}$ ($P_{Out}^{W'} = P_{BM}'$) would be considerably higher than the value of $P_{Out}^{W'}$ which was found to be typical of emphysema. This leads to the further deduction that critical narrowing occurred in more rigid, and hence larger, airways in the asthmatics.

$P_T^{Max\ Eff}$ was very high in the normal subjects and P_{BM}' was presumably low. P_L', which is unknown, must lie between the limits, $P_T^{Max\ Eff}$ and zero. Unfortunately in this case these limits are not helpful in estimating $P_{Out}^{W'}$, for when substituted for P_L' in equation 3a (assuming $P_{BM}' = 0$) the resulting values for $P_{Out}^{W'}$ range all the way from zero to $P_T^{Max\ Eff}$. It is apparent, therefore, that this analysis provides no information regarding the size of the airways which first narrow critically in normal people.

This attempt to make deductions based primarily on $P_T^{Max\ Eff}$ was stimulated by the fact that the experimental findings were strikingly different in the three groups studied. At the resting respiratory level average values for $P_T^{Max\ Eff}$ of the normal subjects, the asthmatics and the patients with emphysema were 45, 26 and 9 cm. of water, respectively. These differences are so great that failure to consider minor factors is not likely to cause a gross misinterpretation. Unfortunately sufficient evidence regarding three of the four major factors represented in equation 3a is lacking, but in spite of this, consideration of these factors has defined more sharply the problems involved in airway obstruction. It has become apparent, for example, that reduction in the elastic recoil of the lung as a whole (P_{El}^L) reduces not only the outward acting transmural gradient across the alveolar walls ($P_{Alv} - P_T$) but also the outward acting gradient at all points along the airways ($P_L - P_T$). A reduction in the outward acting gradient becomes an increase in the inward acting gradient during forced expiration. A reduction in the elastic recoil of the lung causes the inward acting gradient or collapsing effect associated with a given intrathoracic pressure to be applied more peripherally than it would be if the elastic recoil of the lung were normal. Thus a given collapsing pressure is applied to smaller airways which are less able to withstand compression. In addition to this elasticity factor which affects all segments of all intrathoracic airways, any abnormal resistance to airflow which is interposed at any point along the airways causes an abnormal decrease in P_L and hence, during forced expiration, an increase in the net inward acting pressure at all points between the resistance and the exit of the trachea from the thorax. Finally, a change in the structural characteristics of the airways might cause a given segment to narrow abnormally when subjected to a given amount of compression.

The values of $P_T^{Max\ Eff}$ and $\dot{V}_E^{Max}$ found at the maximum inspiratory level, though somewhat less consistent than at the resting respiratory level, showed sharp increases in the normal people and in the emphysematous patients (Table II). This is consistent with the concepts discussed above since the increase in lung volume at the maximum inspiratory level is associated with an increase in P_{El}^L and hence, for a given value of P_T^D, a decrease in the collapsing pressure affecting all the airways. For this reason critical narrowing is not caused by the values of $P_T^{Max\ Eff}$ found at the resting respiratory level. Higher values for intrathoracic pressure can be tolerated and higher velocities of air movement achieved before critical narrowing occurs. The increase in elastic recoil of the lung associated with the increased lung volume causes the collapsing effect of a given intrathoracic pressure to be applied to larger airways which are better able to withstand compression. This argument, when used in reverse, leads one to expect the small airways to become increasingly vulnerable as lung volume is reduced. We did in fact make a few observations in the normal subjects at lung volumes below the resting respiratory level and found $P_T^{Max\ Eff}$ markedly reduced. It is not unreasonable to suspect that there may be a critical lung volume above which the larger and more rigid walled airways are the site of first narrowing (the distal airways being kept patent by high P_{El}^L) and below which the distal airways are the site of first narrowing.

Throughout this discussion we have dealt with a single airway as though it provided an adequate model of the lung as a whole. This simplifying assumption probably causes no gross misinterpretation so long as the process under consideration is uniformly distributed in airways of the same size throughout the lungs. It is for this reason that patients selected for the study were as pure examples of asthma and emphysema as possible. The situation becomes too complicated for us to analyze when there is gross non-uniformity of the obstructive process in different parts of the lungs. Further difficulties arise when processes affecting both very small segments and larger segments of the airways exist simultaneously. If, for example, a patient with the typical findings of emphysema had an attack of bronchitis with narrowing of the larger airways, $P_T^{Max\ Eff}$ might increase and thereby mask the indication of an obstructive process in the very small airways. One of our patients (E. B.) probably exemplified this situation.

The Practical Distinction between Different Mechanisms of Airway Obstruction

Resistance during quiet inspiration

During quiet inspiration the pressure relationships are such as to maintain patency of the airways and hence an abnormal increase in resistance cannot be attributed to abnormalities of either P_{El}^L or P_{El}^W. Such factors as bronchospasm, inflammation, edema, secretions and angulation are therefore implicated. The change in resistance following the administration of a bronchodilator helps to distinguish between these factors.

$\dot{V}_E^{Max}$

The level of $\dot{V}_E^{Max}$ depends upon the sum total of all obstructive factors during forced expiration. Its value lies in providing a quantitative indication of the severity of the obstructive process without distinguishing between mechanisms.

$P_T^{Max\ Eff}$

This measurement, when taken in conjunction with qualitative estimates of P_{BM}' and limiting values of P_L', may be helpful in identifying the size of the airways in which critical narrowing first occurs.

ABSTRACT

When intrathoracic pressure (P_T^D) and rate of airflow are simultaneously recorded during a forced expiration, the rate of airflow rises to a maximum value and then decreases while P_T^D continues to rise. This observation suggests that there is a maximum effective intrathoracic pressure ($P_T^{Max\ Eff}$) associated with a maximum expiratory flow rate ($\dot{V}_E^{Max}$). If P_T^D rises above $P_T^{Max\ Eff}$ airway resistance increases disproportionately and flow rate decreases.

Using esophageal pressure to measure P_T and a pneumotachometer to measure $\dot{V}$, we determined $P_T^{Max\ Eff}$ and $\dot{V}_E^{Max}$ in normal subjects, in patients with diffuse emphysema and in patients with asthma. In both these diseases $\dot{V}_E^{Max}$ was found to be reduced. $P_T^{Max\ Eff}$ was markedly reduced in most of the cases of emphysema, moderately high in those with asthma and very high in the normal people.

Non-elastic resistance was also measured during quiet inspiration and found not to be increased in the patients with emphysema to a degree comparable with that found in the patients with asthma.

The physical basis of $P_T^{Max\ Eff}$ is discussed in terms of a simple mechanical model, and a mathematical analysis is presented from which it is deduced that critical narrowing first occurs in the very small airways in emphysema and in larger airways in asthma.

A plan for distinguishing between different mechanisms of airway obstruction is presented.

ACKNOWLEDGMENTS

We would like to thank Dr. L. E. Farhi, Dr. R. H. Shepard and Dr. A. B. Otis for much helpful criticism and discussion.

REFERENCES

1. Mead, J., Lindgren, I. and Gaensler, E. A.: The mechanical properties of the lungs in emphysema. J. Clin. Invest., 1955, **34:** 1005.
2. Fry, D. L., Ebert, R. V., Stead, W. W. and Brown, C. C.: The mechanics of pulmonary ventilation in normal subjects and in patients with emphysema. Am. J. Med., 1954, **16:** 80.
3. Mead, J. and Whittenberger, J. L.: Physical properties of human lungs measured during spontaneous respiration. J. Appl. Physiol., 1954, **5:** 779.
4. Mead, J., McIlroy, M. B., Selverstone, N. J. and Kriete, B. C.: Measurement of intra-esophageal pressure. J. Appl. Physiol., 1955, **7:** 491.
5. Cherniack, R. M., Farhi, L. E., Armstrong, B. W. and Proctor, D. F.: A comparison of esophageal and intrapleural pressure in man. J. Appl. Physiol., 1955, **8:** 203.
6. Mead, J. and Gaensler, E. A.: Comparison of intraesophageal and intrapleural pressures in subjects seated and supine. Fed. Proc., 1956, **15:** 127.
7. McIlroy, M. B., Mead, J., Selverstone, N. J. and Radford, E. P.: Measurement of lung tissue viscous resistance using gases of equal kinematic viscosity. J. Appl. Physiol., 1955, **7:** 485.
8. Neergaard, K. and Wirz, K.: Die Messung der Strömungswiderstände in den Atemwegen des Menschen insbesondere bei Asthma und Emphysem. Ztschr. klin. Med., 1927, **105:** 51.
9. Dayman, H.: Mechanics of airflow in health and in emphysema. J. Clin. Invest., 1951, **30:** 1175.
10. Riley, R. L., Mani, K. V., Perti, B. L. and Jain, S. K.: Unpublished data.
11. McDermott, M. and McKerrow, C. B.: The effect of external resistance on hyperventilation. Abstr. Brussels: XX Internat. Physiol. Congress, 1956, p. 628.
12. Martin, H. B. and Proctor, D. F.: Pressure-volume measurements on dog bronchi. Fed. Proc. (in press).
13. Ross, B. B., Gramiak, R. and Rahn, H.: The physical dynamics of the cough mechanism. J. Appl. Physiol. 1955, **8:** 264.

29

Reprinted by permission of the American Physiological Society from *J. Appl. Physiol.*, **13**(3), 331–336 (1958)

Relationship Between Maximum Expiratory Flow and Degree of Lung Inflation

ROBERT E. HYATT,[1] DONALD P. SCHILDER AND DONALD L. FRY.
From the Cardiopulmonary Laboratory of the Clinic of General Medicine and Experimental Therapeutics, National Heart Institute, National Institutes of Health, Bethesda, Maryland

ABSTRACT

HYATT, ROBERT E., DONALD P. SCHILDER AND DONALD L. FRY. *Relationship between maximum expiratory flow and degree of lung inflation.* J. Appl. Physiol. 13(3): 331–336. 1958.—There is a functional relationship between transpulmonary pressure, respiratory gas flow and degree of lung inflation. Over the upper half of the vital capacity the relationship between maximal expiratory flow and degree of inflation is effort-dependent. Over the lower half of the vital capacity this relationship is primarily determined by the physical properties of the lower airways and is termed the αFV curve. A simple, acceptably accurate method of obtaining the αFV curve is described, as well as data showing its reproducibility and essential independence of upper airway resistance. Preliminary data based on an empirical analysis of the curves in a group of normal, cardiac and emphysematous subjects is presented.

IT HAS BEEN SHOWN that a functional relationship exists between transpulmonary pressure,[2] respiratory gas flow and the degree of lung inflation (1). The relationship of these variables is most simply expressed in the form of a family of isovolume pressure-flow (PF) curves, each obtained at different degrees of lung inflation. Figure 1*a* shows four isovolume PF curves from a normal subject. The shape of each of the curves is different. Furthermore, the shape of the inspiratory part of the curve is different from that of the expiratory part. Inspiratory flow increases monotonically with decreasing pressure. Expiratory flow on PF *curves 1, 2* and *3* measured low in the vital capacity increases to the maxima,[3] *A*, *B* and *C* and then diminishes with increasing pressure. On PF curves high in the vital capacity (*curve 4*) expiratory flow maxima are not achieved, presumably because the subject cannot generate sufficient transpulmonary pressure. The shape of the isovolume PF curves will vary with changes in upper airway resistance and, hence, the value for transpulmonary pressure at the maximum[3] of a given isovolume PF curve will vary with such changes. On the other hand, theory would predict that the flow value at the maximum of a given PF curve will be relatively invariant and will depend essentially on the physical properties of the lower airway (2).

It, therefore, becomes important to study the relationship between the flow values occurring at the maxima of the isovolume PF curves and their corresponding volume values. The α-β segment, the solid portion of the curve in figure 1*b*, is a plot of the flow ordinates of the PF curve maxima against the volume at which the respective PF curve was obtained. As can be seen, one could extend the plot to PF curves that do not have true maxima, such as *curve 4*, by plotting the highest flow achieved, *point D*, against volume. This latter relationship forms the β-γ segment, the dashed portion of the curve. Thus, the entire curve in

Received for publication July 21, 1958.

[1] Present address: Cardiopulmonary Laboratory, Beckley Memorial Hospital, Beckley, W. Va.

[2] The difference between the pressure acting on the surface of the lung, as measured by the intra-esophageal pressure and the lateral mouthpiece pressure.

[3] Maxima will be defined as the points at which the slope of the tangent to the PF curve is zero. The slope must be positive to the left and negative to the right of this point.

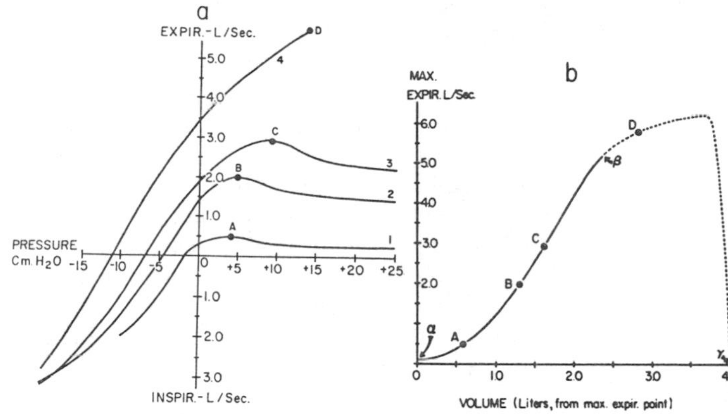

FIG. 1. *a*, Relationship of transpulmonary pressure and flow for a normal subject at different degrees of lung inflation. *Curves 1, 2, 3* and *4* were measured at 0.6, 1.2, 1.7 and 2.8 l., respectively, above the maximum expiratory point. *b*, A plot of maximal achievable expiratory flow against degree of lung inflation. Flow and volume *co-ordinates* of *points A, B, C* and *D* from fig. 1*a* are plotted as closed circles on this curve. α corresponds to maximum expiratory point and γ to maximum inspiratory point.

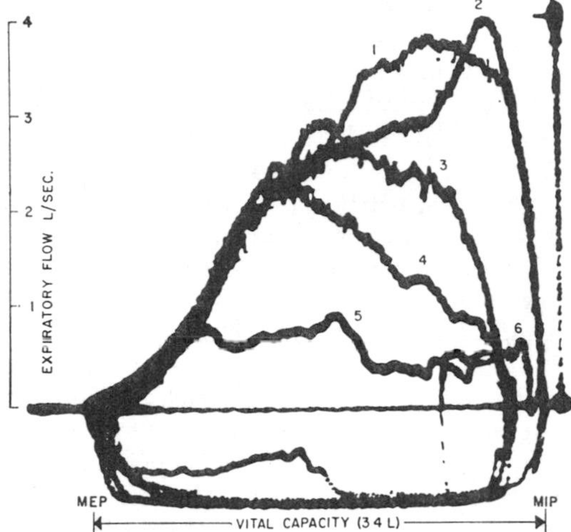

FIG. 2. Photograph of flow-volume loops of a normal subject from the oscilloscope face. MIP represents maximum inspiratory point and MEP, maximum expiratory point. The axes were placed on photograph at time of the study by zero controls of recorder.

figure 1*b* defines the maximal expiratory flow that this individual could attain at any volume in his vital capacity. The plot of the maximal achievable expiratory flow versus volume will be termed the flow-volume or FV curve. Since the β-γ segment is effort-dependent and is related to the dimensions and physical properties of the entire airway in a very complicated manner, its contour will not be constant. In sharp contrast, over approximately the lower half of the vital capacity, the maximal achievable expiratory flow theoretically bears a constant relationship to lung inflation that is uniquely determined by the physical properties of the lower respiratory tree and does not depend on maximal effort (2). This relationship is the α-β segment of the FV curve or the αFV curve. The purpose of this report is *a*) to describe a simple method of obtaining the αFV curve, *b*) to assess the validity of this simplified approach by comparing it with 'true' αFV curves constructed from isovolume PF curve maxima, *c*) to evaluate the effect of added upper airway resistance on the αFV curve and *d*) to present preliminary data on αFV curves obtained from normal, emphysematous and cardiac subjects.

METHODS

Respiratory gas flow was measured with a screen-type flowmeter utilizing a Statham P 97 differential strain gauge. The characteristics of this instrument are contained in a previous report (3). Volume was measured by sensing the position of the bell of a 6-liter spirometer with a potentiometer. The carbon dioxide canister was removed. Intrathoracic pressure was estimated from intra-esophageal pressure by a method previously described (4). All three variables were written simultaneously on a Sanborn model 67-1200 recorder. In addition, the flow signal was plotted on the *Y* axis of a DuMont type 304 A oscilloscope, while either spirometer volume or transpulmonary pressure could be displayed on the *X* axis. The display of the oscilloscope face was photographed with a DuMont type 2620 camera.

To obtain isovolume PF curves an adjustable microswitch was attached to the side of the spirometer and a lightweight pointer to the writing arm of the spirometer bell. The microswitch was in series with the spot 'intensity

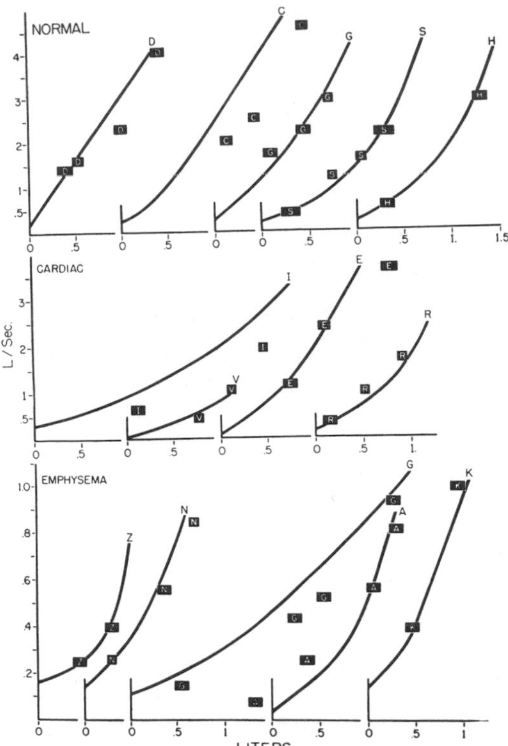

FIG. 3. Comparison of PF curve maxima and αFV curves. Letters identify data from each subject. *Solid curves* are envelopes obtained from flow-volume loops and *solid rectangles* are flow and volume *coordinates* of maxima from isovolume PF curves. The *ordinate* is maximal expiratory flow in l/sec. and the *abscissa* is volume in liters from maximal expiratory point.

control' circuit of the oscilloscope. Thus, when the microswitch was activated by the pointer, the spot simultaneously plotting pressure and flow would appear during the brief volume increment (approximately 120 ml) that the bell pointer and microswitch coincided. With noseclip in place the subject was connected to the spirometer-flowmeter system by a conventional mouthpiece. He was instructed to inspire to his maximal inspiratory point at which time the microswitch was adjusted to the volume position at which a PF curve was to be measured. The subject was then instructed to breathe in such a way that the pointer on the writing arm of the spirometer moved past the microswitch at increasingly greater rates in both the inspiratory and expiratory direction. One of the investigators looking through the camera watched the resulting plot on the long persistence oscilloscope face and 'coached' the subject so that missing segments in the PF curve could be filled in. During this period the shutter on the camera was open so that the continuous display was photographed. At the end of each isovolume PF curve determination the maximal inspiratory point was again recorded and found not to vary more than 150 ml from its initial value. This scheme made it possible to obtain within a few minutes several isovolume PF curves from which the flow ordinate of the maxima and the volume could be measured to construct a 'true' αFV curve.

Potentially one should be able to get the αFV curve directly by simultaneously plotting expiratory flow against volume and properly coaching the subject in his expiratory efforts to obtain maximal expiratory flow. This was done by simultaneously plotting the flowmeter output on the *Y* axis and the spirometer volume on the *X* axis of the oscilloscope. The subject was instructed to perform a series of expiratory breaths of nearly vital capacity volume. As the subject breathed, continuous flow-volume loops were traced on the oscilloscope face and were photographed one on the other. The investigator observing the oscilloscopic display could 'coach' the subject to exert varying degrees of expiratory effort. Figure 2 is the photograph of a typical experiment in a normal subject. The full range of inspiratory flow was not recorded. The indi-

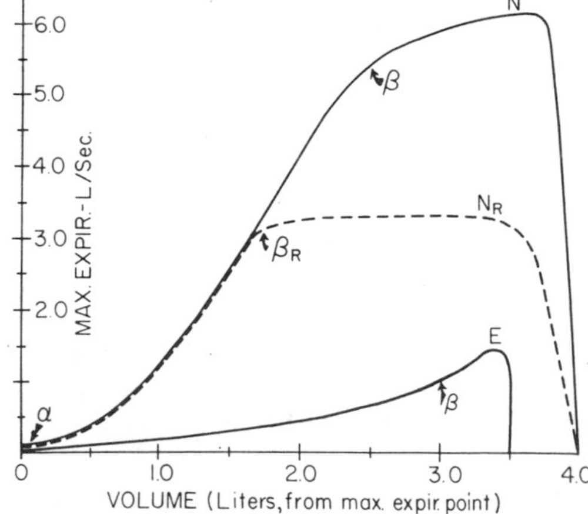

FIG. 4. *Curve N* is an FV curve from normal subject. *Curve N_R* is an FV curve from normal subject breathing against an increased external resistance. *Curve E* is from emphysematous subject.

vidual first performed two forced expiratory vital capacity maneuvers (*lines 1* and *2*). He was then 'coached' through three expirations (*lines 3, 4* and *5*) of lesser effort. As can be seen, these efforts all converge to follow a common path over the lower portion of the vital capacity, whereas a relaxed tidal volume breath (*line 6*) falls short of it. In general, three to four 'coached' expiratory efforts were sufficient to define this common path. The outer border of this path was taken to be the αFV curve, since by watching the plot it appeared to represent the greatest flow achievable at every volume over the lower portion of the vital capacity. In general, if the forced expiratory vital capacity was performed with sufficient effort, it was seen to fall below the αFV curve.

All the normal subjects had a negative cardiopulmonary history and had normal total and 1-second forced expiratory vital capacities. The emphysematous individuals had moderately severe to severe disease, as judged from clinical evaluation and from ventilatory studies. The cardiac subjects consisted of two individuals with intra-atrial septal defects with moderate exercise limitation, one young male with severe primary pulmonary hypertension and right ventricular hypertrophy and three individuals with rheumatic mitral valve disease.

RESULTS

The αFV curve obtained by the method described above was compared with the values of flow and volume at the maxima of isovolume PF curves obtained on the same day. The results of this comparison for five normal, four cardiac and five emphysematous subjects appear in figure 3. The solid curves are αFV curves obtained from flow-volume envelopes as seen in figure 2. The solid rectangles are the flow and volume ordinates of maxima taken from isovolume PF curves. The widths of the rectangles representing the maxima indicate the width of the microswitch volume increment. In most cases the maxima are seen to fall close to the experimental αFV curve. In some cases, such as *curve C* (normal), the maxima are seen to fall below, but parallel to, the experimental curve. The reasons for the other types of deviation that can be noted have not been established, but various possibilities will be discussed later. All problems considered, it is our opinion that the simple procedure of recording flow and volume simultaneously is a sufficiently accurate method for obtaining the αFV curve.

It is apparent that this simplified approach to measuring the αFV curve does not allow the precise location of the upper limit of the α-β segment, *point* β in figure *1b*. Obviously, the β point could only be located accurately by finding the degree of lung inflation at which the expiratory limbs of the isovolume PF curves begin to show maxima. In the five normal and four cardiac subjects the position of the β point was always found to be at a volume above the functional residual capacity. In the emphysematous subjects it was much higher in the vital capacity. Thus, only the FV curve over the lower one-third of the vital capacity was taken to represent the αFV curve.

As can be seen from figure 3, the αFV curve is not the same for all normal subjects. Furthermore, marked differences exist between the normal and the emphysematous subjects. This is illustrated in figure 4 where typical FV curves from these two groups are plotted on the same scale. Ultimately, it is hoped that mathematical analysis will permit precise quantification of these curves and also yield information about the basic physical properties of the lung. Since such an analysis is not yet available, a purely empirical approach has been adopted to permit some numerical evaluation of these curves. It was observed that the lower portion of the αFV curve could be fitted approximately by a simple exponential equation of the form:

$$q = Q_{max} 10^{-KV} \qquad (1)$$

where q is the flow in liters per second, arbitrarily restricted to the range of 0.2 to 1.0 l/sec., V the volume from the maximum inspiratory point expressed in liters, K the slope of the semi-log plot, and Q_{max} the zero volume (maximum inspiratory point) intercept of the semi-log plot. Curves from emphysematous

TABLE 1. CONSTANTS FOR THREE GROUPS OF SUBJECTS

	No. Subj.	Mean log Q_{max}	S.D.	Mean K	S.D.
Normals	35	4.45	1.13	1.30	0.36
Emphysema	8	0.71	0.44	0.77	0.31
Cardiac	6	1.95	0.37	1.08	0.43

Table 2. Constants for reproducibility and resistance study

	Control Period	Resistance Period
Mean log Q_{max}	4.79	4.85
Mean K	1.18	1.19

subjects generally form straight lines when plotted this way, while those from normals tend to form a slight curve to which a 'best' visual linear fit must be made. This method of analyzing these curves is subject to large variation and should be considered only as a temporary approach to the quantification of these curves. Subject to the foregoing, the constants K and Q_{max} may be used to characterize the αFV curve with no attempt at physical interpretation. Table 1 contains these constants for the group of normal, cardiac and emphysematous subjects. For convenience, the log of Q_{max} is used. Note that the mean log Q_{max} shows a wide separation between normal and emphysematous subjects. The cardiac subjects tend to fall between these extremes. The same separation, although not as great, holds for the mean K values.

Visual comparison of the curves of a given normal subject obtained at different times during the day or on different days suggested that the αFV curve was quite reproducible. The same was generally true for the cardiac individuals. Some variability of the curves obtained from the emphysematous subjects was noted and appeared to correlate with changes in clinical status.

The reproducibility of the αFV curve over a short period of time, as well as its independence from upper airway resistance was evaluated in a group of normal individuals. Five to six consecutive αFV curves were obtained in each of eight subjects over a 30-minute period. Two to three control curves were first recorded, then three curves were measured after the resistance of the patient-spirometer system had been increased 10-fold. On inspection, little or no difference could be detected between the lower parts of curves obtained with or without the added resistance, as is evident by comparison of *curve* N and N_R in figure 4. In addition, the empirical constants for all curves were determined and their mean values are presented in table 2. Statistically there was no significant difference between the mean log Q_{max} of the control and the resistance determinations. The same is true for the mean K values. These results demonstrate that the αFV curve is reproducible over a 30-minute period and is not significantly altered by increased upper airway resistance. On the other hand, small but significant increases in both log Q_{max} and K tended to occur following periods of high resistance breathing, presumably reflecting minor alterations in the properties of the lower airways secondary to the maneuver.

DISCUSSION

The shape of the αFV curve is uniquely determined by the physical properties of the lung below the carina (2). Therefore, the curve will be reproducible only to the extent that these properties remain constant. As will be shown in a subsequent paper (2), the elastic retractive stress of the lung parenchyma is one of the important factors controlling the shape of the curve. The elastic retractive stress at any given lung inflation depends not only on the degree of inflation but also on whether the volume is increasing or decreasing, on what the previous volume history has been (5) and on the frequency of respiration (6). The shape of the αFV curve will be reproducible only to the extent that the above can be controlled. Information based on studies done in this laboratory suggests that the compliance loop does become fairly reproducible if carried out over about the same volume excursions and over approximately the same time course. Although the time course of inspiration and of the β-γ segment of the FV curve can not be controlled by the simple flow versus volume method outlined, the volume excursions can be controlled. Thus, instructing the subject to approach the extremes of his vital capacity with each breath is an essential part of the method. If small volume excursions are used, a slightly differently shaped αFV curve will result, presumably related among other things to the change in compliance that occurs when one breathes repeatedly low in his vital capacity.

It is apparent that the volume and time course of breathing during measurement of the isovolume PF curves differed from that of the αFV curve. This fact, plus measurement error, probably explains the discrepancies noted in figure 3 between the experimental curve and the 'true' αFV curve constructed from the PF maxima.

The slight variations in the αFV curve that were noted from day to day and following periods of breathing against high resistance are most likely related to concomitant changes in the physical properties of the lung. Theoretically many things could change, including opening of previously plugged bronchioles, redistribution of blood and tissue fluid, change in bronchomotor tone and so on. Considering the number of variables involved one becomes impressed with the fact that the αFV curve is reproducible at all.

The foregoing discussion has dealt with variability intrinsic to the determinants of the αFV curve itself. Another type of variability is related to errors in attaining the αFV curve that are potentially avoidable. These errors are of two types, measurement errors and subject performance errors. Measurement errors could be lessened considerably by a better method of analysis and by improved instrumentation, particularly a recording system with greater resolution.

Subject performance errors are relatively easily recognized and avoided. The most common subject performance error is excessive expiratory effort. With excessive effort one develops transpulmonary pressure in excess of that required to reach the maximum flow at a given volume. This means that the subject is operating on the descending limbs of the expiratory PF curves. Referring to figure 1*a*, it can be seen that the flow recorded from the descending limb of a given isovolume PF curve will be lower than the flow ordinate of its maxima. Thus, excessive effort results in an underestimation of the maximal expiratory flow at a given volume over the α-β portion of the FV curve. This problem is most important in emphysematous subjects who readily develop extremely high transpulmonary pressures. It is, therefore, very important to coach these individuals to concentrate on slow, gentle expirations.

The second most common subject performance error is leaking air around the mouthpiece or noseclip. The third group of performance errors are represented by bursts of 'noise' on the flow tracing. These are presumably caused by the subject approximating his vocal cords or glottis during his expiratory efforts. The problem of leaks and 'noise' can generally be corrected by careful patient instruction.

Of the 50 normal subjects that have been studied to date there were 5 individuals in whom it was not possible to obtain an acceptable αFV curve. In these subjects the segment appearing to be the α-β segment was almost a vertical line and was not reproducible. There are several possible explanations for this finding. One is that these subjects had so little expiratory flow resistance that PF maxima either did not exist or occurred only at very low degrees of lung inflation. Hence, maximal flow over almost their entire vital capacity was effort-dependent. Another possibility, which seemed operative in three of the subjects, is that the individual involuntarily and repeatedly closed off his upper airway in such a manner as to limit his vital capacity in a variable way.

With certain precautions, the αFV curve *a*) may be relatively easily obtained, *b*) is essentially unaffected by wide variations in upper airway resistance, *c*) is reproducible and *d*) reflects properties of the lower airway as yet too complicated to analyze discreetly. Furthermore, it represents a simple, objective physiologic measurement that may be empirically quantified in a relatively reproducible way and may be used as a clinical index of lower airway and lung ventilatory mechanics.

The authors express their appreciation to Jean E. Caha and Raymond P. Kelly for valuable technical assistance.

REFERENCES

1. Fry, D. L., R. V. Ebert, W. W. Stead and C. C. Brown. *Am. J. Med.* 16: 80, 1954.
2. Fry, D. L. *Phys. Med. Biol.* In press.
3. Fry, D. L., R. E. Hyatt, C. B. McCall and A. J. Mallos. *J. Appl. Physiol.* 10: 210, 1957.
4. Fry, D. L., W. W. Stead, R. V. Ebert, R. I. Lubin and H. S. Wells. *J. Lab. & Clin. Med.* 40: 664, 1952.
5. Mead, J., J. L. Whittenberger and E. P. Radford, Jr. *J. Appl. Physiol.* 10: 191, 1957.
6. Otis, A. B., C. B. McKerrow, R. A. Bartlett, J. Mead, M. B. McIlroy, N. J. Selverstone and E. P. Radford, Jr. *J. Appl. Physiol.* 8: 427, 1956.

30

Reprinted from *Traité de Mécanique Céleste. Tome IV, 1807. Supplément à la Théorie de l'Action Capillaire*. N. Bowditch, trans., Vol. 4, Hilliard, Gray, Little & Wilkins, Boston 1829–1839, pp. 688–689, 1009, 1017

THEORY OF CAPILLARY ACTION

Pierre Simon de Laplace

Making use of this principle, I have determined the action of a fluid mass, terminated by a portion of a spherical concave or convex surface, upon a column situated within it, contained in an infinitely narrow canal, and directed towards the centre of that surface. By this action, I mean the pressure which the fluid, contained in the canal, would exert, by means of the attraction of the whole mass, upon a plane base situated within the canal, perpendicular to its sides, and at any sensible distance from the surface: this base being taken for unity, I shall show that this action is less or greater than if the surface were plane; *less* if the surface be *concave* [9275]; *greater* if the surface be *convex* [9276]. Its analytical expression is composed of two terms: the *first*, which is much greater than the *second* [9262*a*,*c*], denotes the action of a mass terminated by a plane surface; and *I think that upon this term depends the suspension of the mercury, in a barometrical tube, at a height two or three times greater than that which is produced by the pressure of the atmosphere; also the refractive power of diaphanous bodies, cohesion, and in general the chemical affinities. The second term denotes the part of the action, depending on the spherical form of the surface; or in other words, the action of the meniscus, included between that surface and the plane which touches it.* This action is to be added to, or subtracted from, the preceding one, according as the surface is convex or concave. It is inversely proportional to the radius of the spherical surface; for it is evident that the less this radius is, the greater will be the meniscus, near the point of contact. This second term produces the capillary action, which differs therefore from the chemical affinities corresponding to the first term.

From these results, relative to bodies terminated by sensible segments of a spherical surface, I have deduced this general theorem [9302]. "*In all the laws which render the attraction insensible at sensible distances, the action of a body terminated by a curve surface, upon an infinitely narrow interior canal, which is perpendicular to that surface, at any point whatever, is equal to the half sum of the actions upon the same canal, of two spheres which have the same radii as the greatest and the least radii of curvature of the surface at that point.*" By means of this theorem, and of the laws of the equilibrium of fluids,

[*Editor's Note:* References (four-place numbers in brackets) can be found in the original work.]

we can determine the figure which a fluid mass must have, when it is included within a vessel of a given figure, and acted upon by gravity. It depends upon an equation of partial differentials of the second order [9318], whose integral cannot be obtained by any known methods. If the figure be of revolution, this equation is reduced to common differentials [9324], and may be integrated by a very approximate method, when the surface is very small. By this means I shall prove that, in tubes of a very small diameter, the surface of the fluid will approximate the more towards the form of a spherical segment, as the diameter of the tube shall be decreased [9342, &c.].

[*Editor's Note:* Material has been omitted at this point.]

At the surface of a fluid, the attraction of the particles, modified by the curvature of the surface and of the sides of the vessel which contains it, produces the capillary attraction. Therefore these phenomena, and all those which chemistry presents, correspond to one and the same law, of which now there can be no doubt. Some philosophers have attributed the capillary phenomena to the adhesion of the fluid particles, either to each other, or to the sides of the vessels which contain them; but this cause is not sufficient to produce the effect. For, if we suppose the surface of water, contained in a glass tube, to be horizontal, and upon a level with that of the water in the vessel into which the tube is dipped by its lower end; the tenacity of the fluid, and its adhesion to the tube, would not curve this surface and render it concave. To produce that, it is necessary to suppose that there is an attraction in the upper part of the tube, which is not immediately in contact with the fluid.

[*Editor's Note:* Material has been omitted at this point.]

When I was occupied upon this subject, Mr. Thomas Young was likewise making upon it the ingenious researches which he has inserted in the Philosophical Transactions for the year 1805. In comparing, as Segner had done, the capillary action to the tension of a surface which would envelop the fluids, and applying to this force the known results of the tension of surfaces, he has discovered that it is necessary to notice the curvature of the fluid surfaces in two directions perpendicular to each other;

31

NEW NOTIONS ON A FUNDAMENTAL PRINCIPLE OF RESPIRATORY MECHANICS: THE RETRACTILE FORCE OF THE LUNG, DEPENDENT ON THE SURFACE TENSION IN THE ALVEOLI

K. v. Neergaard

This excerpt was translated by Rainer Arnhold, Kaiser Hospital, San Rafael, California, and Hans Hahn, North Senior Fellow, Cardiovascular Research Institute, University of California, San Francisco, from "Neue Auffassungen über einen Grundbegriff der Atemmechanik: Die Retraktionskraft der Lunge, abhängig von der Oberflächenspannung in den Alveolen," Z. Gesamte Exp. Med., ***66,*** *373–394 (1929)*

The investigations to be discussed are a continuation of clinical determinations of flow resistance and pulmonary elasticity carried out in human subjects with various diseases.[1]

The lung is probably unique among the tissues in its extraordinary ability to expand and retract. So far, this has been regarded as due to the elasticity of the tissue itself, and particularly that of the elastic fibers. Although attempts have recently been made to determine the elasticity of the elastic fibers directly with the aid of a micromanipulator (Redenz[2]), this does not prove that the entire retractility of lung can be attributed to these structures.

The opposite view is held by Sternberg,[3] who regards the elastic fiber as a rigid supporting structure resembling steel. The elastic fibers are stretched but show poor expansibility, that is, a high elasticity modulus. Similarly, Ranke[4] maintains that the elastic fibers in the aorta can only be straightened but cannot expand farther. The same indication is given by Müller's observation[5] that, in the expanded lung, the elastic fibers run straight, whereas in the relaxed lung they undulate. The various theories on the significance and value of the elastic fibers are still too diverse to give a satisfactory explanation of the striking expansibility of the lungs.

So far, one force has not been taken into account that definitely merits consideration in this context. This is *surface tension.* It is active at the boundary between alveolar epithelium and alveolar air. Wherever the surface of an aqueous solution touches upon a gaseous space, the influence of molecular attraction on the marginal layer of molecules gives rise to tensions in the solution that are described as surface tension. All the phenomena of capillary chemistry, the rise of liquids in fine capillaries, the pressure of soap bubbles, and numerous other phenomena, are based on surface tension. Considerable forces are involved which also play a role in other aspects of respiratory mechanics (as previously pointed out in the evaluation of the so-called adhesion of the pleural surface). The surface tension partly depends on the nature of the solution that constitutes the bordering medium and particularly on the curvature of the boundary. The smaller the radius of curvature, the stronger the force of surface tension, which is like a taut rubber membrane attempting to retract like a rubber balloon. Such deeply curved boundaries between fluid or an aqueous gel (the cellular membrane of the alveolar epithelium) and a gaseous space exist in countless numbers in the pulmonary alveoli. Ellenberger[6] long ago compared the alveolar wall to "an exceedingly delicate fluid lamella."

To visualize the mechanism even more clearly, one should imagine a thin capillary tube at the end of which a soap bubble has been blown. As soon as blowing is discontinued and the inside of the soap bubble is allowed to communicate with the atmosphere via the capillary, the bubble immediately becomes smaller and retracts owing to the influence of surface tension. The smaller the diameter of the capillary in this situation and the smaller the radius of curvature of the bubble, the more rapid and more energetic the retraction. Such small bubbles, which communicate with the atmosphere via narrow capillaries, can be compared to the alveoli of a lung.

In view of the almost complete saturation of expired air with water vapor, we can imagine the alveolar epithelium as covered by a thin film of fluid. The surface tension attempts to make the alveoli smaller, and therefore exerts an influence in the same direction as the retractive force of the entire lung. There can be no doubt, therefore, about its *qualitative* significance, but the quantitative aspects are not known.

There exists a method of measuring surface tension, described by Jäger[7] and especially used by Kobler[8] (under Zangger) and Czapek[9] for biological purposes, in which a capillary is immersed in the fluid to be examined. This capillary is connected with a level glass and a manometer. Measurement is made of the pressure required to displace the fluid from the capillary, just sufficient to push air bubbles out of the lower end. Using this sample model, we can now try to quantitate surface tension. Let the capillary correspond to the respiratory bronchiole or alveolar duct and the bubble to the alveolus.

The mathematical relationship pertaining to this process has been established by Schrödinger,[10] among others, as

$$\alpha = \frac{r}{2}p\left(1 - \frac{2}{3}\frac{\rho r}{p} - \frac{1}{6}\frac{\rho^2 r^2}{p^2}\right)$$

where α = surface tension in dynes, r = capillary radius in centimeters, p = air pressure at the time of detachment of the bubble in dynes cm^2, and ρ = density of the fluid.

To evaluate the function of surface tension, the value of p must be found. The magnitude of the intraalveolar pressure that corresponds to the retractile force under static conditions is what we are trying to find.

$$p = \frac{\alpha}{r} + \frac{1}{3} r \rho \pm \frac{1}{2r} \qquad \sqrt{\frac{1}{3}\left(\frac{10}{3}\rho^2 r^4 + 12\sigma^2 + 8r^2\rho\alpha\right)}$$

Regarding anatomical conditions and units, we refer to publications by Felix,[11] Dräser,[12] Rohrer,[13] Aeby,[14] Hüfner,[15] Vierordt tables, and especially to Marcus,[16] Loeschke,[17] and Husten.[18]

By introducing mean anatomical data to cgs units, that is, $r = 1.5 \times 10^{-2}$ cm, $\rho = 1.03$ dynes, and $\alpha = 60$ dynes, the equation can be considerably simplified because several members are eliminated.

$$p \sim \frac{2\alpha}{r} \text{ Dyn}$$

When converted to the conventional unit of pleural pressure (cm H_2O), the value obtained for p is 8 cm H_2O.

Some time ago, using the most accurate method so far employed in a human subject, I found a static mean pressure of 5.6 cm; thus, the agreement with the rough estimate is good.

EXPERIMENTAL METHOD

In any case, the quantitative aspect of surface tension merits full consideration, and our task was to design an experimental setup permitting quantitative analysis of the contribution of surface tension to the total retractile force. An attempt to increase the accuracy of our theoretical reasoning will be discussed later. I shall first report on our experiments.

To measure the influence of surface tension on retractility, the total retractile force must first be measured by known methods; that is, the so-called elasticity curve in relation to lung volume must be obtained. Since it is impossible to measure surface tension by itself independent of tissue elasticity, our only alternative was to eliminate surface tension in a second series of determinations, thus measuring tissue elasticity separately. The difference between total retraction and the retraction remaining after elimination of surface tension is a measure of surface tension at the same lung volume.

To eliminate surface tension, the lungs had to be filled with a fluid down to the alveoli to remove the effect of the air–tissue interface. Replacement of air by fluid was not immediately possible, because of the small size of the bronchioli. To overcome this difficulty, the lung was completely filled with pure CO_2 by the method of Rohrer and Wirz; the CO_2 was then replaced by a diluted barium hydroxide solution, which absorbs CO_2 and penetrates into the remotest alveoli. Determination of retraction on air and fluid filling, taking into account the lung volume, indicates that retractility is mainly due to surface tension. Barium, however, has a toxic effect on tissues, giving rise to hemolysis and interstitial edema. It was therefore necessary to find a fluid that met optimal physiological requirements. Calcium hydroxide was also tried as CO_2 absorbent. Although its solubility is so poor that its chemical CO_2 binding capacity is insufficient, a test showed that, because of the good solubility of CO_2 in water, the two processes together are sufficient to ensure complete absorption of CO_2 from the lungs. By the addition of suitable electrolytes, the ion concentrations were made to resemble those of a Tyrode solution as closely as possible. Edema, however, could not be completely avoided. In order to adjust the oncotic pressure, gum arabic was added to the solution as it is to intravenous infusions in clinical work. The solution was still far too alkaline, but as a result of CO_2 filling of the lung, calcium carbonate was formed, which with the excess CO_2, constituted a buffer solution that came close to the requirement of a physiological H-ion concentration. To eliminate even this uncertainty in H-ion concentration and the possible objection that the CO_2 filling and the Ca-ion concentration might alter the elastic characteristics of the tissue, *the lung was finally emptied of air by a pressure difference method and then immediately filled with an isotonic gum solution.* By the addition of about 7 percent gum arabic to the Tyrode solution, the oncotic pressure was adjusted so that no edema occurred. The solution thus obtained met physiological requirements to a very high degree. Immediately after sacrificing the test animals, we ligated the trachea so as to avoid collapse when removing the lung. The trachea, or the main bronchus in tests with only one lung, was mounted on a support in a glass vessel. The water jet pump then acted simultaneously on the bronchus and the space between

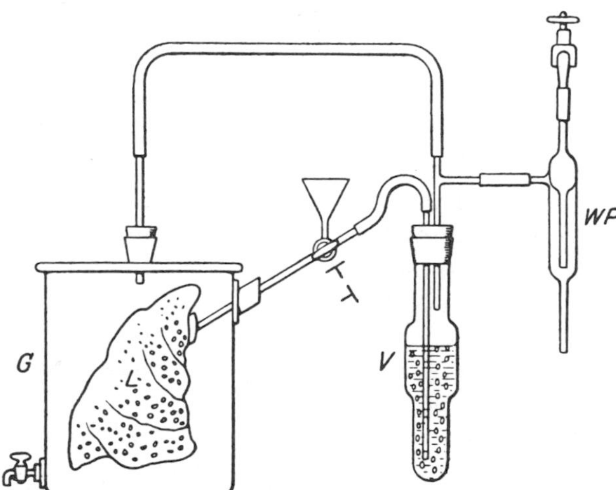

Figure 1 Apparatus for evacuation of air from the lung. *G* = glass vessel; *L* = lung, the main bronchus of which has an airtight connection with the lateral support; *V* = water valve to obtain a difference between intrapleural and extrapleural pressure; *WP* = water jet pump. Between *WP* and *V*, a mercury manometer is used to determine total retraction on filling with air. (Reproduced from *Z. Gesamte Exp. Med.*, **66,** 377 (1929); copyright © 1929 by Springer-Verlag, Berlin.)

lung and vessel wall. By means of a water seal in the connection between the pump and bronchus, the pressure outside the lung in the glass vessel was kept constantly at 8–10 cm H_2O more negative than the intrabronchial pressure. This ensured good expansion of the lung. As a result, all alveoli were in free communication with the bronchial tree until evacuation was complete. Whereas otherwise adhesion of the smallest air passages prevented suction drainage of air from the alveoli, this was feasible without difficulty when the lung was expanded. Because the difference between intrapulmonary and extrapulmonary pressure was within the physiological range all the time, any straining or rupture of tissue was avoided despite gradual complete evacuation. After obtaining a vacuum corresponding to the water vapor tension of the tissue, the lung could be filled with the physiological electrolyte–gum solution through a funnel.

Unfortunately, it was impossible to fill the lung *in situ* in the animal because the vacuum immediately sucked blood into the lung. When the lung was rapidly processed, the postmortem changes in elasticity were not so great as to be of significance.

Every test was divided into two parts. First, the elasticity curve had to be plotted under ordinary conditions, that is, with the lung air-filled. The volume at various phases of expansion was determined by filling the glass vessel with a physiological electrolyte solution. The lung was weighed and the initial volume determined with the main bronchus or trachea closed. The volume was derived as the difference between the capacity of the empty vessel and the volume of physiological electrolyte solution for which there was room beside the lung. Taking into account the specific weight of the empty lung (1.056 according to Vierordt), it was possible to calculate the initial quantity of air in the lung from the weight and from the difference between initial volume and reduced weight. The lung was then filled with the maximum quantity of air in order to avoid partial atelectasis and to ensure equal expansion. For this filling, the desired quantity of electrolyte solution was simply drained from the glass vessel and the lung inflated until the glass vessel was filled up to the upper support. Below the upper support a wire net prevented air bubbles from being trapped. Before determination of pressure, the water was drained to prevent the hydrostatic pressure from superimposing itself on the retraction pressure. Step by step, by gradual release of the air in the lung, the retraction curve was then obtained for inspiration and expiration. The smoothness of the curve constituted a very good criterion for the correctness of the test and the freshness of the specimen. If the specimen was not sufficiently fresh, kinking readily occurred and individual points could be far off.

In this conventional method of obtaining an elasticity curve, a slight error was sometimes unavoidable. The weight of the lung parenchyma was added to the retractility proper. This error is included in all elasticity curves made so far from isolated organs but has not hitherto been accounted for; it can probably only be eliminated when the inflated lung is placed in a medium that has the same specific weight, which also has to be variable. The error has been calculated by Rohrer[13] but is so small that it can be neglected.

After the elasticity curve was obtained in the air-filled lung, the second part of the test followed: evacuation and filling with the gum–electrolyte solution via a funnel. For this purpose the tap below the funnel was only partially opened, so as to avoid alveolar ruptures as a result of too rapid inflow. Air bubbles had to be prevented from entering. In obtaining the elasticity curve of the filled lung, the lung weight had to be taken into account; that is, the space between lung and vessel had to be filled as well so that there was no measurable hydrostatic pressure difference. When the alveoli were well filled, the lung looked glassy; an incision made after completion of the test released a clear fluid without air bubbles; this was confirmed by histological examination.

The results of the tests are shown in the curves. The ordinate gives the retraction pressure in cm H_2O; the abscissa shows the total volume of one lung. As examples of numerous tests with similar results, only two are presented. Tests with fresh human lungs* showed similar features. But since this material is never as fresh as that obtained in animal experiments, irregular curves are more likely to occur.

From a comparative physiological point of view, we shall mention interesting differences between the lungs of different species. The ram has lungs that are abundant in tissue relative to their volume, are rather firm, and have a relatively limited range of expansion. Dogs, on the other hand, have lungs that are very large in proportion to the animal's size, with a low specific weight and a strikingly wide range of expansion. The surface area is large compared to the small tissue mass and, unlike the ram's, the dog's lungs seem well adapted to the animal's considerable mobility. Other characteristics are found in porcine lungs, in between the extremes described above. The human lung resembles the canine lung but does not quite reach the latter's perfect elasticity and economy of design.

The upper curve (Figure 2, curve *a*) shows the total retraction on filling with air. In the lower range of expansion, up to about three times the volume of the collapsed lung, the curve is almost linear in accordance with Cloetta's[19] findings; when greater demands on elasticity are made, a slight kink is seen, which indicates a relatively accelerated increase of retraction. The lower curve, *b*, shows retraction characteristics of the inflated lung after eliminating surface tension. Of course, the entire retractility is not based on surface tension; the parenchyma has to have elasticity of its own even if we disregard a special elasticity of the elastic fibers and simply imagine the tissue as a homogeneous gel. After the elimination of surface tension, the remaining retraction must be ascribed to true tissue elasticity. In swine, ram, dog, and human lung

* I am indebted to Prof. v. Meyenburg, for supplying this material.

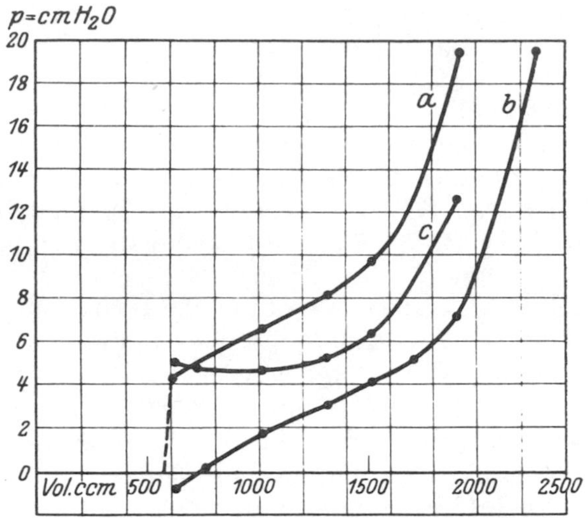

Figure 2 Left porcine lung. Weight 239 g. (*a*) Total retraction at air filling; (*b*) tissue elasticity following elimination of surface tension; (*c*) retractility based on surface tension only. (Reproduced from *Z. Gesamte Exp. Med.*, **66,** 379 (1929); copyright © by 1929 Springer-Verlag, Berlin.)

alike, and without significant difference with different methods of filling, our experiments systematically show the important fact that tissue elasticity regularly reached the zero point much earlier than would correspond to the collapsed lung volume. *As far as one can estimate from the retraction pressures so far measured, the true tissue elasticity reaches its limits somewhere near the position of end expiration.* This is also indicated by a test with a lung from a 20-year-old human subject. The true tissue elasticity reached its zero point at 3400 ml. According to Rohrer,[13] normal lung volume at end-expiration is 2800 ml. Adding 600 ml for tissue volume in accordance with weight, we reach a volume of 3400 ml; that is, the two values agree. Indeed, it is difficult to see why the lung should still be under pressure below its smallest physiological volume. More exact determination of the zero point of tissue elasticity in its relation to lung volume is impossible because determining the position of end-expiration requires active cooperation of the subject. The volume of the lung in a cadaver is no substitute for this value, because the state of expansion of cadaver lungs does not agree with any physiological state of expansion.

In the lower range, the linearity of tissue elasticity is even more ideal than that of total retraction. Only upon increased stretch to maximum physiological values does it show a disproportionate increase. Another very interesting feature is that true tissue elasticity after elimination of surface tension may even reach a negative value, which is a linear continuation of the positive part of the curve (Figure 2, curve *b*). This means that the lung tissue can be compressed like a sponge and tries to return to the position of relaxation even from this state. In the above-mentioned human test, in which the tissue elasticity for both lungs together reached the zero point at a volume of 3400 ml, negative values were seen, which at 2670 ml reached −0.8 cm. If the total retractile force consists of these two major components, surface retraction and true tissue elasticity, then the significance of surface tension can only be determined as the difference between the two curves. The middle curve, *c,* shows the values thus determined for surface tension alone. *In all states of expansion, therefore, surface tension is a bigger part of total retraction than tissue elasticity.* There is no parallelism, however, because the contribution of surface tension is particularly marked near maximum expiration, whereas in the midrange it is only two to three times bigger than that of tissue elasticity.

For surface tension alone, the relation between volume and pressure is not linear; the pressure increases disproportionately with increasing pulmonary expansion. As will be demonstrated, this is to be expected theoretically. In the lower range where normal respiration takes place, surface tension is much less dependent on volume than tissue elasticity. It remains almost constant over a wide range, and occasionally even shows a very striking increase as the lung approaches the collapsed state (Figure 2, curve *c*). Retraction by surface tension alone can thus be greater than total retraction. This remarkable finding is explained by the above-mentioned negative values (negative in the sense of the test arrangement) of tissue elasticity. The compressed tissue antagonizes surface retraction and thus reduces total retraction.

This approximately constant influence of surface tension over the tidal range can be regarded, teleologically, as exceedingly valuable for respiratory economy. As I have demonstrated in a previous publication[1] on flow resistances in the respiratory tract, resistance rapidly increases with increasing flow rates; retractility, which shows minimum variability over a considerable range of expansion, therefore ensures a more constant rate of flow, displacing a larger volume of air in the same time with relatively small effort. But, we cannot explain from our experiments why surface tension remains relatively constant at end-expiration or even goes up a little; that will only become clear later from theoretical considerations.

Figure 3 shows essentially the same behavior in a canine lung except that curve *a* (total retraction) is somewhat steeper and shows a more even curvature, without an abrupt increase. Curve *b* of tissue elasticity is linear despite the large lung volume, which is four times the collapsed volume. In this case, too, tissue elasticity becomes zero at 580 ml, that is, long before the lung reaches the collapsed state at 280 ml. Curve *c* of surface tension is also slightly steeper but again shows a reduced decrease in the lower range. The contribution of surface tension to total retraction is again two to three times bigger than that of tissue elasticity.

The objection may be raised that, as a result of friction of the gum–

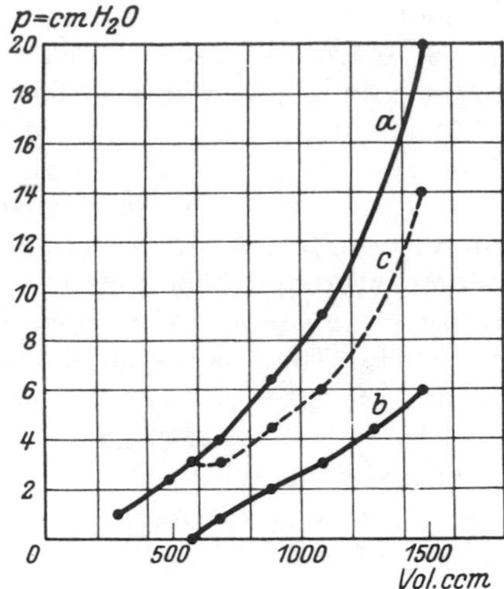

Figure 3 Left canine lung. Weight 130 g. Curves *a, b,* and *c* as in Figure 2. (Reproduced from *Z. Gesamte Exp. Med.,* **66,** 381 (1929); copyright © 1929 by Springer-Verlag, Berlin.)

electrolyte solution, which has a much higher viscosity than air, curve *b* is erroneous. This objection would be justified if we were measuring dynamic processes such as flow resistances. This paper is only concerned with static forces, however, and dynamic factors play no role. Also, when we determined retraction in fluid-filled lungs, equilibrium was established within a few seconds. This means that movement of air was unimpaired in the time available, which was also unlimited.

The question might then be raised as to why, in testing the influence of surface tension, surface-active substances such as those used in inhalation were not added to the air used for inflation, instead of using a fluid for filling. Such a procedure would be ineffective. To begin with, the concentration that can be reached in this way is completely uncontrollable; thus a quantitative study of the influence of surface tension would be impossible. Second, it might be very difficult to achieve a high enough concentration of surface-active substances in the alveoli. Their efficacy considerably diminishes with dilution. It is moreover probable, as will be shown, that the surface tension in the alveoli is naturally very low, so that it is questionable whether one can obtain further reduction with a diluted surface-active substance applied from outside. Third, even if these difficulties could be overcome, surface-active substances are known to be toxic and would cause severe damage to the tissue, thus causing incalculable changes in the true tissue elasticity. In spite of these considerations, I did some experiments along these lines in the following way: after evacuation of the lung using the pressure difference procedure, the lung was once again filled with air previously saturated in a washing flask with a mixture of chloroform and amyl alcohol.

In another test, an exceedingly fine spray of this fluid was applied to the lung with an inhalation apparatus. A mixture of equal parts of chloroform and amyl alcohol has a surface tension of $\alpha = 27.3$ dynes/cm, determined by Lenard's bow method.[20] Upon hundredfold dilution with water (a higher concentration on the surface of the alveoli can probably not be reached by the inhalation method), it was already equal to 48 dynes/cm. In both cases a slight decrease in total retraction was seen in the experiment, which for the above-mentioned reason warranted no quantitative conclusions.

Another possible objection to this test arrangement should be mentioned. We do not know the magnitude of surface tension in the alveoli. The value for serum amounts to about 60–65 dynes; the lowest value for a biological fluid, as far as we know, is about 50 (for bile); water at 16°C is known to have a surface tension of 73 dynes/cm. In the gum–electrolyte solution used for filling, I found it to be 55 dynes. No method of measuring the intraalveolar surface tension has so far been developed. To obtain an estimate of this value, I have used the Gibbs–Thomson rule that such surface-active substances as are involved would accumulate both at the lung surface and in an aqueous extract obtained from the pulmonary parenchyma. In such extracts I found unexpectedly low values of 35–41 dynes, according to the most accurate measurement of the surface tension with the above-mentioned Lenard method. From a physicochemical point of view, it would be understandable that surface-active substances gradually accumulate at the alveolar surface. It is also conceivable that this would be useful for the respiratory mechanism because without it pulmonary retraction might become so great as to interfere with adequate expansion. In the course of extraction, however, cells are destroyed, and determinations in extracts are certainly not reliable. For comparison, therefore, I used the same method (20 g of lung ground up with 30 g of quartz sand, extracted with 20 ml of 0.9 percent NaCl and suction filtered through porcelain) to prepare extracts from muscle, spleen, liver, and heart; in these, values found were regularly higher (47–53 dynes).

The question was then studied from yet another angle; the surface tension of the gum–electrolyte solution was measured before filling and after drainage from the lung. Surface-active soluble substances are likely to enter the gum solution when they are accumulated at the boundary. In one case we found a smaller value than in the lung extract, but not in the other tests. The question, therefore, remains to be answered.

According to Freundlich,[21] the surface tension at the contact surface of two nonmixing fluids, which is difficult to measure directly, approximates the difference in surface tension between the two components as measured against air. The uncertainty about our results, arising from the fact that we do not know the exact surface tension in the alveoli, cannot therefore be fundamental, because the surface tension of the gum solution is very low, and that in the alveoli must also be very low, that is, at the lower biological limit. The difference which possibly exists is reduced even further by the fact that we are dealing with aqueous solutions, so that mixing at the boundary surface is probable, which would neutralize tension differences. Therefore, the error cannot be great; it is probably less than individual and species differences. Our main findings and their order of magnitude remain unchanged; nevertheless, the question should be further investigated.

THEORY

The theoretical aspects must now be considered in some detail because they further our understanding, afford valuable information for future experiments, and also confirm the relations established. My starting point was the Schrödinger equation. But further consideration showed that this equation does not apply to the conditions in the lung without conversion. It gives the relations at the time of maximum demands on surface tension, at which surface tension fails and the bubble detaches itself. Such a maximum demand on surface tension, however, would be incompatible with life. Moreover, pressure and radius are reciprocally related, and the surface tension should assume the highest values at expiration and the lowest at inspiration; this would be contrary to respiratory mechanics and especially to the experimental data.

Let us recall the Jäger method.[7] It is not the detachment of the bubble that is comparable with the situation in the lungs, but the process at the *onset* of the Jäger test, *because with gradual increase in pressure in the capillaries a small bubble will first swell out and grow as the pressure increases.* Here we have a direct relation between pressure and bubble volume, analogous to the process in respiration and without maximum demands on surface tension. If the capillary has a constant radius (Figure 4, r), what can be said about the dimensions and especially the radii as the pressure increases? At a low pressure, the bubble forms a shallow bulge, the segment of a circle with a large radius R_1. With increasing pressure, the volume of the bubble increases, but the radius R_2 is smaller. The bubble is now the relatively larger segment of a small circle. The radius of the bubble finally equals the radius of the capillary (i.e., the bubble has become a hemisphere). *In a similar way, we could imagine that the alveoli in the lungs represent segments of spheres with a smaller volume but larger radius during expiration and with a larger volume but smaller radius during inspiration.*

These relations have not so far been submitted to physical study, and I must thank Prof. Scherrer of Zurich Federal Technological College for his help and interest in this investigation.

We wish to establish the relation between the volume (V) of the al-

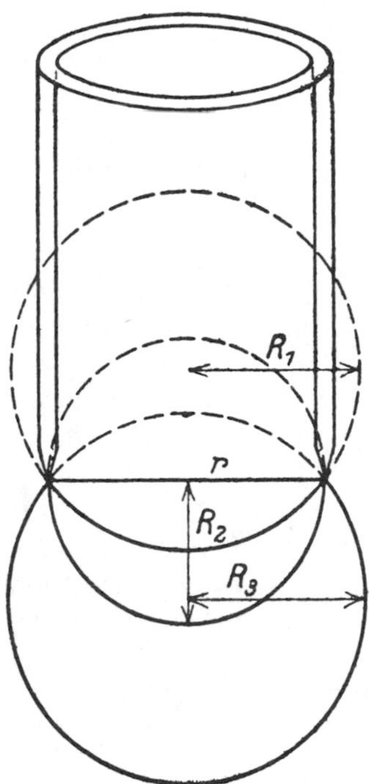

Figure 4 Diagram of the relation between capillary radius r and the radii of a bubble (R_1, R_2, R_3) at increasing intracapillary pressure. (Reproduced from *Z. Gesamte Exp. Med.*, **66,** 384 (1929); copyright © 1929 by Springer-Verlag, Berlin.)

veoli, imagined as the segment of a sphere, and the retraction pressure (p)at a given surface tension (α) and a given radius of the alveolar base or segment of a sphere (r). The relation, therefore, is a four-dimensional one.

The volume of the segment is

$$V = \frac{\pi}{3} h^2(3R - h)$$

To eliminate h (height of segment) and R (its radius of curvature), which are unknown, h is substituted for by the following equation, based on the Pythagorean rule,

$$h = R - \sqrt{R^2 - r^2}$$

(r = radius of capillary or alveolar base), and R is substituted for by the equation between surface tension, radius, and pressure:

$$R = \frac{2\alpha}{p}$$

Thus, we find

$$V_{I} = \frac{\pi}{3}\left(\frac{2\alpha}{p} - \sqrt{\frac{4\alpha^2}{p^2} - r^2}\right)\left(\frac{4\alpha}{p} + \sqrt{\frac{4\alpha^2}{p^2} - r^2}\right) \qquad (1)^*$$

$$V_{II} = \frac{\pi}{3}\left(\frac{2\alpha}{p} + \sqrt{\frac{4\alpha^2}{p^2} - r^2}\right)\left(\frac{4\alpha}{p} - \sqrt{\frac{4\alpha^2}{p^2} - r^2}\right) \qquad (2)^*$$

The pressure initially increases with an increasing volume of the segment according to Equation I; it reaches its maximum when capillary radius and bubble radius are equal, and then shows a reciprocal relation in which the pressure decreases despite increasing volume. For physiological conditions, we remain within the range of Equation I; that is, the alveoli are smaller than a hemisphere and, with increasing expansion, approach the hemisphere form. It follows from the application of this equation that in deep inspiration we are probably very near the maximum possible surface tension, and upon further expansion run risk of entering the range of the second equation, with decreasing tension despite further increasing volume (i.e., in very unfavorable conditions). It is entirely possible that we do, in fact, enter the range of the second equation in some pathological conditions, but this remains to be proved. For example, overexpansion and increase of the radius of curvature can lead to a decrease in retraction caused by surface tension and impede the return to a normal position, in the same way as this may be provoked by overstretching an elastic band. The physical mechanism, however, is fundamentally different. The numerous possible pathological and clinical correlates will be discussed in subsequent publications.

In this paper, it is sufficient to discuss briefly the graphic relationship between retraction pressure and lung volume. According to previous views on true tissue elasticity, this relationship is linear as long as the limit of perfect elasticity is not exceeded. This also applies to the new view on the remaining true tissue elasticity. With regard to the surface tension component, the relationship is demonstrated in Scherrer's Equation 1. As this gives no graphic representation of the curve, the various p values and corresponding volumes have been calculated and plotted in the graph shown in Figure 5. For this purpose, we assumed $\alpha = 50$ and $r = 1.10^{-2}$. This curve is approximately linear in its middle part; with increased expansion the pressure decreases slightly, while in the lower range it rapidly falls to zero. Compared with the experimental curves, which are plotted the same way, the theoretical curve (r being constant) shows the opposite curvature, with the concavity pointing downward. The explanation of this apparent paradox lies in the fact that, during alveolar expansion, alveolar ducts and therefore the alveolar bases also expand so that r is changed. If, for example, r is reduced on relaxation, then p becomes relatively larger; that is, the curve concavity points

* *Editor's Note:* Errors in Neergaard's Equations 1 and 2 are corrected here.

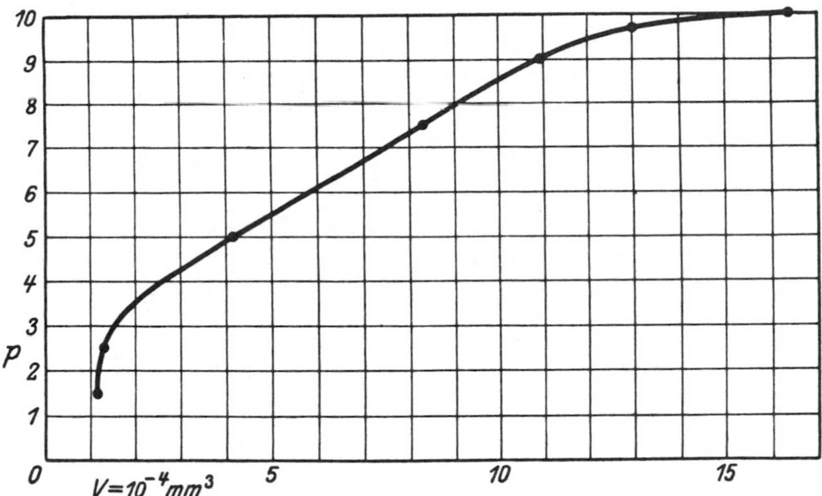

Figure 5 Relation between volume (V) and retraction pressure (p) calculated at constant values of α and r. (Reproduced from *Z. Gesamte Exp. Med.*, **66**, 386 (1929); copyright © 1929 by Springer-Verlag, Berlin.)

upward. This phenomenon will be discussed in detail later. The interrelations between volume, surface tension, radius of the alveolar base, and pressure are exceedingly complicated; as the equation shows, the curve shown in Figure 5 only holds for a specific case with specific values of r and α. By changing the interrelations between the various values, the character of the curve can be altered considerably. Since we do not know enough at the present time about the anatomy, it seems useless to extend the theory.

Regarding the relationship between pressure and volume change, at first only the change in alveolar volume need be considered. However, the sum of alveolar volumes is only part of the total lung volume because of the dead space of the afferent air passages. What this space comprises in our specific case we do not know. It probably extends very far into the periphery, because it must be presumed that, despite some fluctuations of the luminal width of the respiratory bronchioli and alveolar ducts, they are far less pronounced than the volume changes in the alveoli proper. In this case the dead space would be a considerable part of the total lung volume, which should be added as an approximately constant value to the curve of the alveolar volume fluctuations.

To make the matter clearer, the graph in Figure 6 shows the dependence of volume on surface tension at constant values of p and r; it will be understood that the graph shows the smallest volumes at high surface tension as a result of increasing retraction, and vice versa. The relation is not linear; as the surface tension decreases, the volume shows a relatively smaller increase.

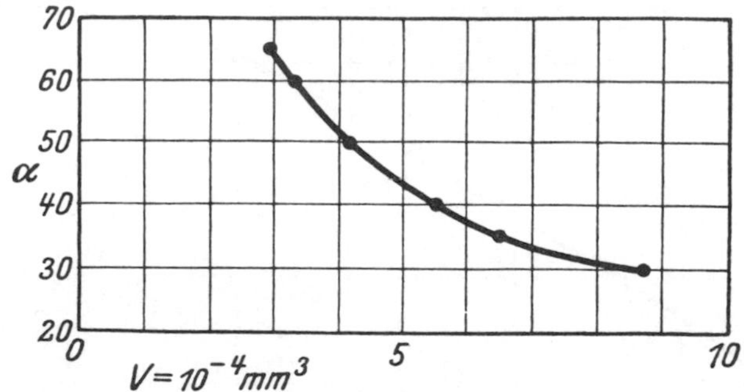

Figure 6 Dependence of the volume (V) on the varying surface tension at a constant value of p (5 cm) and r (10^{-2} cm). (Reproduced from *Z. Gesamte Exp. Med.*, **66**, 389 (1929); copyright © 1929 by Springer-Verlag, Berlin.)

As an example, in Equation I we shall give p a value of 7 cm H_2O = 6860 dynes, $\alpha = 60$ dynes, and $r = 1.7 \times 10^{-2}$ cm, which is at the upper limit of anatomical measurements; we then find that the volume of an alveolus is 0.0074 cm^3. In the literature, we find the volume of an alveolus quoted as 0.007–0.008 cm^3. Thus, the calculated value and the experimental data agree well. In one experiment we found the surface tension to exert a retraction pressure of $p = 6.5$ at mid-lung volume.

As another example, let us give r the smaller and probably more correct value of 0.014 cm, $\alpha = 50$, and $p = 7$; the volume of the alveolus imagined as the segment of a sphere is then 0.00347. Zuntz[22] quotes this volume as 0.00414. Bearing in mind the exceedingly complicated nature of the morphological relations in the lungs, the agreement between theoretical calculation, based on acceptance of a very simple model, and the values measured is excellent. The differences are probably due to lack of information on anatomical data. The uncertainty in this respect is based chiefly on the value for r. At first we substituted for this the diameter of the respiratory bronchiole, which is partly supplied with alveoli, or the diameter of the alveolar duct, which has about the same width. The critical factor is the ring that constitutes the boundary between alveolus and alveolar duct; the significance of this ring is indicated by the histologically verified dense network of elastic fibers and the sphincter-like musculature at this site (Müller[5]). Although the other anatomical data are already inadequate for our purpose in that they neglect functional aspects, particularly the relationship to lung volume, they are completely insufficient when it comes to the question of the diameter of this ring. The equation presumes that the bubble has a flat, smooth base; biologically, this is not the case, because the ring is not in one plane but attaches laterally to the alveolar duct, which has about the same diameter as the alveolus. The alveolar base is therefore cylindrically curved, like a glass bubble blown out of the side of a test tube.

The prospects of obtaining measurements adequate to these requirements and of adapting the equation to the variable cylindrical curvature of the alveolar duct are poor for the time being; the question may therefore be approached from yet another point of view, which has the advantage of greater descriptiveness.

For the above-mentioned Scherrer equation, the known relation $p = 2\alpha/R$ was used, in which p and α have the significance indicated, while R represents the radius of curvature of the alveolus. Since its derivation leads over nicely to the dynamic relationships, and also confirms the above considerations, it may be briefly discussed here.*

The work performed to enlarge the alveoli against surface tension can be expressed (1) as a change in surface work,

$$\text{surface tension} \times \text{change of surface} = \alpha \times dO$$

or (2) as a change in the volume work,

$$\text{pressure} \times \text{change in volume} = p \times dV$$

From this we obtain

$$\alpha \times dO = p \times dV$$

and consequently

$$p = \alpha \frac{dO}{dV} \text{ dynes/cm}^2$$

Now

$$O = 4\pi R^2 \qquad V = \frac{4}{3}\pi R^3$$

from which we differentiate†

$$dO = 8\pi R\, dR \qquad\qquad dV = 4\pi R^2\, dR$$

$$\frac{dO}{dV} = \frac{8\pi R}{4\pi R^2} = \frac{2}{R}$$

$$p = \frac{2\alpha}{R}$$

If we give the diameter the values used above, 0.28 or 0.34 mm, we obtain $p = 7$ or 5.75 cm H_2O; this is in good agreement with what has so far been discussed. These values apply at a surface tension of $\alpha = 50$. It need hardly be pointed out that this term, despite its superficial similarity, has another meaning than that derived from the Schrödinger equation at the beginning of this paper, in which r represented the radius of

* For this I am indebted to Dr. M. Kleiber of the Federal Technological College.
† *Editor's Note:* Errors in Neergaard's equations are corrected here.

the capillary or the ring. *Apart from the magnitude of surface tension, only the radius of curvature of the alveoli is important for the retraction exerted by surface tension.* That is the important conclusion from this derivation. We are reminded of the well-known school example of a T-shaped tube, with two soap bubbles of unequal size at the two ends. When the two bubbles are in open communication at constant pressure, the *smaller* bubble with the smaller radius, and consequently larger surface retraction, contracts, pressing air into the larger bubble. In reality, the alveoli are of course not completely regular segments of spheres; they are more or less unequally curved in different planes. We therefore have to substitute the mean Gaussian curvature

$$K = \frac{1}{R_1} + \frac{1}{R_2}$$

in which R_1 and R_2 constitute the smallest and largest radius of curvature of the segment of the sphere. For surface retraction we derive from this the more exact equation

$$p = \alpha \times \left(\frac{1}{R_1} + \frac{1}{R_2}\right)$$

Of course, the term derived can also be used by substituting for p the values found in experiments. In an animal experiment, assuming a surface tension of 50, we found radii of curvature of 0.4, 0.3, and 0.17 mm at small, medium, and large lung volumes, respectively.

The chief advantage of this theoretical version, however, is its descriptiveness. Shape and size of the ring, diameter of the alveolar duct, and respiratory bronchiole become completely subordinate. During inspiration the alveolus further protrudes from its relatively firm ring of elastic fibers, as schematically shown in Figure 4. Thus, the volume of the alveolus and therefore the volume of the lung increases, while the radius of curvature of the alveolus decreases as the hemisphere form is approached; consequently, retraction caused by surface tension increases. During expiration the reverse process occurs; the alveolus becomes flatter and the radius of curvature increases; retraction, according to experience, diminishes. The question remains, as has been pointed out, whether the shape and size of the ring, alveolar duct, and respiratory bronchiole take any part at all in the volume changes. In a previous report on the determination of flow resistance *in vivo,*[1] the results indicated that, as a result of dynamic intrapulmonary pressure differences, during inspiration there is dilatation, and during expiration, compression of the smallest air passages, which are not made rigid by cartilage. In a similar way it may be possible to interpret the above-mentioned striking fact that the curve of surface tension (Figure 2) in the lower range at first runs horizontally, and finally surface tension even increases. In the lower range of expansion, therefore, a reduction in alveolar duct volume seems to be produced not only dynamically but also statically. As a result, the base of the alveolus, the ring, must also be reduced in size. When the rings are reduced in size, however, the radii of the alveoli rapidly decrease, even without a change in volume; that is, the retraction from surface tension increases again, as shown in the curve in question.

Husten[18] emphasized that the alveolar ducts and the bases of the alveoli are surrounded not only by strong elastic fibers, but also by a highly developed musculature. Müller[5] even speaks of sphincter-like rings; these may be of greater importance in respiration than has so far been taken into account. It seems highly likely that this musculature plays a role in the suspected narrowing of the alveolar bases and the consequent increase in surface tension in the lower volume range. It is also possible that in this range nervous regulation counteracts too large a drop in retraction pressure. This would have very important physiological implications.

After what has been said, it is not unnatural to compare the lung with soap foam. Yet this comparison is a poor one, and it very clearly indicates the special biological features of the lungs. In soap foam, the separate bubbles are no longer spheres or sphere segments but, because of the compliance of the liquid medium of which they consist, they are in contact with one another in the smooth planes of a polyhedron. From the above-mentioned relation between radius of curvature and surface tension pressure, it follows that in these soap bubbles a significant positive pressure can no longer exist. If in the lungs the alveoli also formed a polyhedric pattern, surface tension would no longer count as the most important component of pulmonary retraction. Sections and casts of lungs show, however, that no polyhedric arrangement or formation of saddle-shaped minimal planes exists. There must be something, therefore, to prevent the alveoli from forming such patterns. The "something" can only be the resistance of the tissue to deformation. The cells or the tissue structure has its own form and cannot be stretched to form membranes like a soap solution.

Despite Moissejeff's[23] view to the contrary, we are inclined to accept the view of Sternberg[3] and Ranke[4] that the elasticity of the elastic fiber is much less than is usually assumed; these fibers rather should be regarded as a rigid, steel-like structure of struts, comparable to the metal frame of an airship. After these investigations of the significance of surface tension, it is no longer necessary to attribute special elastic forces to the tissue. On the contrary, the comparison with soap bubbles shows the importance of tissue resistance to deformation of a structure necessary for normal function. Anyone who has experienced the forces required to reexpand an only partially collapsed lung, in which the walls of the smaller air passages have fallen together, will understand the importance of structured supports. At least with regard to the lungs, Sternberg's comparison of the elastic fibers to a steel-like framework deserves close attention.

A number of consequences of this new concept of pulmonary retraction will be briefly discussed.

It has been pointed out that the presence of smooth musculature in the rings and alveolar walls, which presumably has some function, opens up the possibility that the retractile force could be altered via nervous pathways. Contraction of these muscles changes the radius of alveolar curvature. In this way the retractility of the lungs could change rapidly.

Surface tension is known to be changed by H-ion. *The H-ion concentration* in the alveoli is determined by the CO_2 pressure, which changes continuously and must therefore lead to transient changes in the retractility of the lungs. Since, according to Frey,[24] the surface tension of blood serum is lowered by H-ions, the retraction pressure during expiration would be reduced and that during inspiration increased if this observation also applied to the alveoli (which is probably but has not been demonstrated). The extent of this influence on surface tension retraction remains to be established.

For completeness, mention must be made of the fact that, with increasing temperature, the surface tension decreases in all fluids, including colloids; in the latter, this decrease is greater than in pure dispersion aids (Ostwald[25]). For example, the surface tension of a 2 percent arabic gum solution decreases by 6 percent between 0 and 17°C, and that of a 2 percent gelatin solution by 9.5 percent. In physiological conditions, changes in temperature can hardly play a significant role.

An entirely different consequence of the new point of view concerns *the question of pulmonary elasticity in neonates.* According to current views, no elastic tension exists during intrauterine life. It is believed to develop once the neonate is extrauterine by the thorax growing more rapidly than the lungs, as a result of which the lungs attain their tension. That the tissue is probably not under tension before the first breath is very likely according to what has been said. Because surface tension likewise plays no role in the atelectatic lung, it is understandable that the first inspiration, despite considerable effort of the respiratory muscles, is not sufficient to achieve full expansion of the atelectatic lungs. As Haag[26] has demonstrated, this requires days, and atelectatic islets persist for some time, because the considerable force of surface tension, which later will constitute the major factor in pulmonary retraction, *inhibits* the first expansion of the lungs. It is even probable that the surface tension is a counteracting force that provokes maximum inspiratory efforts. After expansion of the lungs, it is probable that both the surface-tension component and the tissue component of lung retraction take up their functions. However, all these aspects have to be investigated experimentally.

The most important results obtained can be roughly summarized as follows. The so-called pulmonary elasticity, one of the fundamental principles of respiratory mechanics, has so far been axiomatically ascribed to the elasticity of the elastic fibers. The following findings are arguments against this concept.

1. *The total retraction of the lungs consists of two components; the more important component is the action of surface tension; true tissue elasticity is less important.* The quantitatively most significant part of the total retraction of the lungs is due to surface tension at the boundary between alveolar epithelium and alveolar air.

2. The significance of surface tension for pulmonary retraction can be *experimentally* verified by plotting elasticity curves of animals and human lungs before and after elimination of surface tension. Elimination of surface tension is achieved by filling the lung with a physiological solution of gum and electrolytes using different negative pressures. As a result, the boundary between alveolar epithelium and alveolar air is limited. The retraction that exists after filling must be ascribed to tissue elasticity.

3. Measurements show that, depending on the state of expansion, *retraction due to surface tension is about two to three times larger than that caused by true tissue elasticity.*

True tissue elasticity is approximately linear throughout the physiological volume range. *Long before a state of collapse is reached, it leads to relaxation* (this happens close to end-expiration). Upon continued volume reduction, tissue tension may change sign owing to compression.

The difference between total retraction and the component of true tissue elasticity makes it possible to plot the curve of the apparent elastic effect of surface tension. With decreasing expansion, it initially shows a steep decline; it then remains almost constant, and may increase again in extreme expiratory positions.

It is possible that the surface tension of the alveoli is reduced compared to other physiological solutions, according to the Gibbs–Thomson law, by the accumulation of surface-active substances.

4. In addition to experimental evidence, a theoretical substantiation is presented, based on laws of surface tension and anatomical conditions. In various ways, values of surface-tension action are calculated, which agree very closely with the experimental findings. *Retraction* as a result of surface tension is *a function of the radius of curvature of the alveoli.* During expiration, the alveoli are flat spherical segments with a relatively large radius, that is, relatively slight surface retraction. At maximum inspiration, the alveoli approach a hemisphere with minimum radius but greater surface tension. An evaluation of the curves, taking into account the theory, indicates that in the lower range volume reduction in the alveolar ducts is added to alveolar reduction. The investigations would seem to confirm Sternberg's conception of elastic fibers as a supporting structure.

By recognition of the great significance of a physicochemical force—

surface tension—as one of the fundamental principles in pulmonary mechanics, a vitally important force has been transferred from purely morphological consideration to functional evaluation.

5. There is the *possibility of brief transient changes in the retractility of the lungs.* By a nervous mechanism, the sphincter-like smooth musculature at the bases of the alveoli and the alveolar septa may change the curvature of the alveoli and thus surface tension. Also, retractility can be increased or decreased by fluctuations in the H-ion concentration of the alveoli (CO_2 pressure).

6. The consequences in terms of pulmonary elasticity in *neonates* are discussed. In this respect, too, surface tension in the alveoli is of vital importance.

REFERENCES

1. Neergaard and Wirz: *Z. Klin. Med., 105,* 35, 51 (1927); Neergaard: *Beitr. Klin. Tbk., 65,* 476 (1927).
2. Redenz: *Z. Zellforsch., 4,* 611 (1927).
3. Sternberg: *Virchows Arch., 245* (1925).
4. Ranke: *Beitr. Pathol. Anat., 73* (1925) and *75* (1926).
5. Müller, Jos.: Diss., Giessen, 1906.
6. Ellenberger: *Vergleichende Physiologie der Haussäugetiere,* Bd. 2. 1890.
7. Jäger: *Wiener Berichte, 105,* 425 (1896), and *108,* 1516 (1899).
8. Kobler: Inaug.-Diss., Zürich, 1908.
9. Czapek, Fr.: *Über eine Methode zur direkten Bestimmung der Oberflächenspannung der Plasmahaut von Pflanzenzellen.* Jena, 1911.
10. Schrödinger: *Ann. Physik., 46,* 413 (1915).
11. Felix: In Sauerbruch: *Chirurgie der Brustorgane,* Bd. 1, Teil 1, 3. Aufl.
12. Dräser: *Z. Exp. Med., 26,* 223 (1922).
13. Rohrer: *Handbuch der normalen und pathologischen Physiologie II.* Berlin, 1925.
14. Aeby: *Bronchialbaum der Menschen und Säugetiere,* 1880.
15. Hüfner: *Arch. Physiol.,* 1890.
16. *Morphologisches Jahrbuch,* Bd. *59,* S. 561. 1928.
17. Loeschke: *Beitr. Pathol. Anat., 68,* 213 (1921).
18. Husten: *Beitr. Pathol. Anat., 68,* 496 (1921).
19. Cloetta: *Pflügers Arch., 152,* 339 (1913).
20. Lenard: *Ann. Physik., 74,* 381 (1924).
21. Freundlich: *Capillarchemie 2.* Aufl., 1922.
22. Zuntz: In *Herrmann's Handbuch der Physiologie,* Bd. *4,* 2. Teil, S. 90. 1882, Z. *Exp. Med., 66.*
23. Moissejeff: *Z. Exp. Med., 59,* 344 (1928).
24. Frey, W.: *Transvaal Med. J.,* August 1908.
25. Ostwald, Wo.: *Grundriss der Kolloidchemie,* 1921.
26. Haag: Diss. Bern, 1917.

32

Reprinted from *Lancet,* **266,** 1099, 1101 (1954)

THE PULMONARY ALVEOLAR MUCOID FILM AND THE PNEUMONOCYTES

Charles C. Macklin
M.D., Ph.D., D.Sc. Western Ontario, F.R.S.C.
FORMERLY RESEARCH PROFESSOR OF HISTOLOGY, UNIVERSITY OF WESTERN ONTARIO, LONDON, CANADA

Does a thin watery mucoid film provide a surface for the air spaces of the lung? Since all exposed areas of the endodermal tracts, alimentary and respiratory, are covered by a layer of mucus, it might be argued, a priori, that such a film, though of submicroscopic thickness (Frey-Wyssling 1953a) and in a much modified aqueous state, should overlie the attenuated epithelium (Low 1952, 1953) of the lung alveoli.

[*Editor's Note:* Material has been omitted at this point.]

The pneumonocytes are the characteristic cells of the lung, and are assumed to be of endodermal origin. They have also been called niche cells, septal cells, epicytes, alveolar epithelial cells, &c. The list is a long one, and it is high time that we had a suitable term for universal adoption. All the current names have drawbacks. The vague designation "alveolar cells" (Bertalanffy and Leblond 1953) has least to commend it, for there are many kinds of alveoli and they may contain many kinds of cells. "Pneumonocyte," a translation into Greek of the French term "la cellule pulmonaire" (Bratianu and Guerriero 1930) has all the advantages and none of the disadvantages.

[*Editor's Note:* Material has been omitted at this point.]

Organology

This concept of the derivation of the alveolar mucoid lining assigns an exocrine glandular function to the granular pneumonocytes. Brodersen (1933) regarded them as secretory cells. The collective mass of the granular pneumonocytes constitutes a diffuse organ within the lung, whose volume in man has been estimated to equal that of the spleen (von Hayek 1942) but whose modus operandi, though often speculated on, remains in many ways a mystery. In human lungs it would manufacture a mucoid film which, if it could be pieced together as a continuous sheet, would measure as much as 100 sq. m. (von Hayek 1942). If it were even 0·2 μ thick, its volume would be 20 c.cm. Such a mucoid film would lie upon an attenuated epithelium as recently interpreted by Low (1952, 1953) from electron micrographs (see figure), or possibly a layer of specialised connective tissue, as conceived, for instance, by Leblond and Bertalanffy (1951). We may postulate that it would be cohesive, flexible, and viscous. Phase-contrast microscopy seems to show that it wrinkles minutely when the wall is contracted. It transmits silver-nitrate molecules, which become segregated in the underlying silver lines. It would, of course, be readily penetrable by the molecules of oxygen and carbon dioxide (Terry 1945), and must retain its integrity and proportional water content under the high water-vapour tension of the alveolar air. It may be causally related to the myelin figures (Leathes 1925) which are seen by phase-contrast microscopy to emerge in great abundance from the surfaces of the alveolar walls in sections of fresh lung mounted in water or in physiological saline solution, for they are generated in hydrophilic material (Frey-Wyssling 1953b). It may have something to do with the inhibition of bubble formation, for in life no air-bubbles are normally formed in the alveoli. If they were so formed, in quantity, the effect would be disastrous. They are often seen after death. The mucoid film may be responsible for the maintenance of constancy in the surface tension of the alveolar wall (Macklin 1946)—a matter of paramount importance. After complete and prolonged collapse of the lung, such as that produced by Loosli et al. (1949), the mucoid film may prevent adhesion of the alveolar walls, which would be expected if the approximated surfaces were formed of naked connective tissue. In œdematous thickening of the alveolar walls it may help to retain the augmented contents, and thus would be functionally represented in specimens such as those illustrated by Short (1950). In lungs of mice subjected while alive to drastic intrabronchial decompression (Macklin 1953a) I have noted that the extravasated blood in certain swollen walls that have been broken down interiorly is confined on either side by a thin layer that corresponds to that described and figured by Short. The alveolar wall should not be looked on merely as a capillary plexus. The capillaries occupy the *milieu interne*, but are supported on either side by an independent confining layer of relatively stable character that has a fluid mobile air surface, the mucoid film. These confining layers persist after the capillaries have been broken down; and it is between these layers that the growing rays of adenomata, such as those of urethanised mice, infiltrate.

REFERENCES

Bertalanffy, F. D., Leblond, C. P. (1953) *Anat. Rec.* **115,** 515.
Bratianu, S., Guerriero, C. (1930) *Arch. Anat., Strasbourg,* **11,** 423.
Brodersen, J. (1933) *Z. mikr.-anat. Forsch.* **32,** 73.
Frey-Wyssling, A. (1953a) Submicroscopic Morphology. London; p. 2.
———. (1953b) *Ibid,* p. 55.
Leathes, J. B. (1925) *Lancet,* i, 957.
Leblond, C. P., Bertalanffy, F. C. (1951) *Canad. Med. Ass. J.* **65,** 263.
Loosli, C. G., Adams, W. E., Thornton, T. M. jun. (1949) *Anat. Rec.* **105,** 697.
Low, F. N. (1952) *Ibid,* **113,** 437.
———. (1953) *Ibid,* **117,** 241.
Macklin, C. C., (1946) *Trans. roy. Soc. Can.* **49,** 93.
———. (1953a) *Anat. Rec.,* **115,** 343.
Short, R. H. D. (1950) *Phil. Trans.* **235,** 35.
Terry, R. J. (1945) *Anat. Rec.* **91,** 302.
von Hayek, H. (1942) *Anat. Anz.* **93,** 149.

33

Reprinted from Nature (Lond.), **175,** 1125–1126 (June 1955)

Properties, Function and Origin of the Alveolar Lining Layer

In acute lung œdema in the rabbit, fluid and foam are found in the trachea. This foam has an altogether peculiar property, in that it is unaffected by silicone anti-foams ; these rapidly destroy the foams produced by shaking œdema fluid or blood serum with air. Equally stable foam is found in the bronchi of an animal the respiratory movements of which have been paralysed and into the trachea of which a mixture of oxygen and ammonia gas has been insufflated for one or two hours ; similar foams are obtained from healthy lung by cutting and squeezing under water, or after introduction of saline into the trachea. The stability of such foams is due to an insoluble surface layer on the bubbles ; this layer can be attacked by pancreatin or by trypsin.

Œdema foam is thus not produced by agitation of the œdema fluid with air during respiration ; it can only have been formed by air originally contained in the fine air spaces of the lung being broken up into bubbles and afterwards expelled into the bronchi and trachea. The lining layer of the bubbles cannot have come from the œdema fluid, and must therefore have formed the original lining layer of the fine air spaces. By drying and weighing samples of the foam of known bubble-size distribution, the thickness of the layer (assuming density 1·3) has been found to be about 50 A.

In air-saturated water, bubbles (say 40μ in diameter) from foam from the lung usually remain unchanged in size for long periods (60 min.), whereas similar bubbles from serum and other foams, owing to their internal excess pressure, dissolve and disappear within a few minutes. The surface tension of the lung bubbles is therefore zero ; or, to put this another way, the surface pressure of the layer is equal to the surface tension of the underlying liquid.

Published calculations[1] on the pressure balance between the lung capillaries and the alveoli have disregarded the surface tension at the sharply curved, and probably moist, alveolar wall. If the surface tension were that of an ordinary liquid, enough suction would be exerted to fill the alveoli with a transudate from the capillaries. Means for keeping the surface tension low must therefore be part of the design of the lung. It is thus evident that the alveoli are lined with an insoluble protein layer which can abolish the tension of the alveolar surface.

40-μ bubbles squeezed from a fragment of the artificially inflated lung of a mature fœtal rabbit (within a few seconds of inflation) and kept in air-saturated saline usually contract by about 30 per cent in diameter and then remain stable. The layer is therefore initially formed by rapid surface adsorption from a substance already present in the fœtal lung. It probably matures somewhat during the first few hours after birth. A layer is likewise rapidly formed when an adult lung which has been consolidated is re-expanded.

By none of the many methods tried have small bubbles stable in air-saturated saline been regularly produced from blood or from amniotic fluid. The layer is thus not formed from either of these liquids, or from a transudate from the blood. Such bubbles have been formed from nasal (but not, so far, from tracheal) mucus; they are easily formed from a solution of an extract of hog gastric mucosa ('gastric mucin'), and from this solution also a foam resistant to silicone anti-foams has been prepared. These findings suggest that a layer of some form of mucus[2], secreted in the depths of the lung, is the source of the insoluble alveolar lining layer.

This communication is published by permission of the Chief Scientist, Ministry of Supply.

R. E. PATTLE

Ministry of Supply,
Chemical Defence Experimental Establishment,
Porton, Wilts.
March 3.

[1] Drinker, C. K., "Pulmonary Oedema and Inflammation", 26 (Harv. Univ. Press, Cambridge, Mass., 1950). Courtice, F. C., and Korner, P. I., *Aust. J. Exp. Biol. and Med. Sci.*, 30, 511 (1952).

[2] Macklin, C. C., *Lancet*, i, 1099 (1954).

34

Reprinted from *Proc. Soc. Exp. Biol. Med.*, **95**, 170–172 (1957)

SURFACE TENSION OF LUNG EXTRACTS

John A. Clements

Directorate of Medical Research, Chemical Warfare Laboratories, Army Chemical Center, Maryland

Von Neergaard described the important role played by surface forces in the recoil of the lungs and made measurements of surface tension in lung extracts(1). Recently, Radford and his coworkers repeated and extended von Neergaard's experiments, again calling attention to the importance of surface tension in the static pressure-volume characteristics of the lungs(2) and pointing out the need for proper determination of the surface tension of the lung lining. In the interim Radford used the so-called static tension of serum (50 dynes cm) in interpreting his results, assuming the surface to be thermodynamically reversible. From microscopic study of air bubbles squeezed from lung slices Pattle(3) concluded that the pulmonary alveoli are lined with mucoprotein (suggested previously on the basis of histochemical evidence by Macklin(4)) and that this material reduced the surface tension to less than 1 dyne per cm. In the last year Brown(8) repeated Radford's experiments and by assuming the lung to be composed of many identical hemispherical units computed surface tension from the pressure-volume data. The tension-area relationship so derived is similar to that of bubbles of nasal mucus, but depends upon an assumed

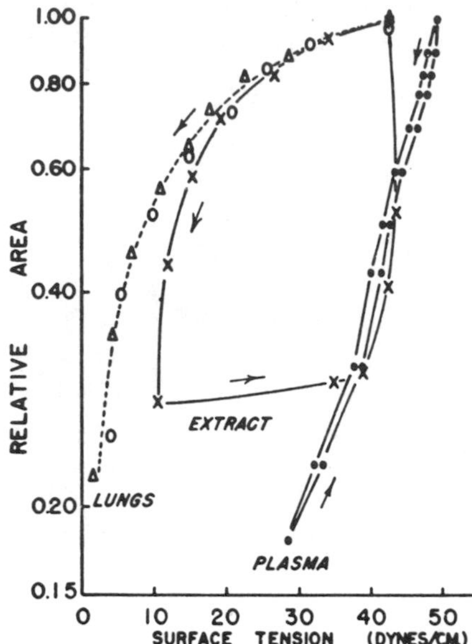

FIG. 1. Variation of surface tension with surface area. Upper curve (lungs) calculated on the basis of relative area from Brown's data. Large loop constructed from measurements on lung extract in Wilhelmy balance. Narrow loop constructed from measurements on blood plasma in Wilhelmy balance.

area-volume function ($A = KV^{2/3}$) which is not acceptable if the lung units deviate significantly from the mean radius. In addition Brown's calculations did not correct for the tendency of the units to close off above zero volume as the transpulmonary pressure is reduced. To obtain more direct evidence bearing on the above points, we have studied the tension-area behavior of lung-derived surfaces, using modifications of the Langmuir-Adam film balance and the Wilhelmy balance (5). Surfaces of the following fluids were examined: a. normal saline (0.85% NaCl) after it had been used to inflate degassed lungs via the trachea; b. mince of whole lungs in normal saline, filtered through loosely-packed cotton; c. normal saline, to which slices of lung parenchyme had been touched. These were prepared from rat, cat, and dog lungs.

Results. The results were similar in all cases. A typical tension-area plot is shown in Fig. 1. This figure demonstrates that the tension of the lung-derived surface varied from 46 to 10 dynes cm as its area was changed, and further that the surface exhibited extreme hysteresis, although 80 minutes was used for the compression-expansion cycle. The same pattern was obtained when the cycle was repeated. Thus, the mechanical behavior of the surface was far from reversible, within the duration of most pressure-volume measurements on lungs.

The coefficient of compressibility $\left(\frac{1}{A}\frac{dA}{d\gamma}\right)$ of these surfaces ranges from 0.010 to 0.025 cm/dyne at the higher tensions, agreeing well with Brown's values. This characteristic of the surface has a stabilizing influence and might be called an "anti-atelectasis factor." At lower tension the surface compressibility rises and closure of lung units becomes probable. It is in this range that Brown's data depart from the extract data, signalling trapping of gas within the lungs(6).

We have examined Pattle's conclusion that the surface tension of his "alveolar bubbles" (about 40 μ diameter) and hence of the pulmonary alveoli was less than 1 dyne cm. While repeating his experiments we found that lung bubbles which were "stable" in static air-saturated saline, dissolved slowly when the saline continuously perfused the microscope chamber. Determining increments of hydrostatic pressure necessary to double the instantaneous rates of solution permitted calculation of the surface tension of the bubbles. Although the method was crude, it gave values from 10 to 15 dynes cm. Bubbles of the same diameter prepared in an air-saturated soap solution having a surface tension of 27 dynes cm dissolved rapidly. The transfer coefficients were 9.3×10^{-5} and 1.7×10^{-3} cc/cm^2 -atm.-sec., respectively. Taking the difference of the reciprocals we estimated the specific diffusion resistance of the lung bubble surfaces at 1.0×10^4 sec cm; this is much higher than the specific resistance of compressed films of 18- to 20-carbon fatty acids to water diffusion found by Archer and LaMer(7). Thus the slow solution of the lung bubbles appears due mainly to the diffusion characteristics of the surface. Calculation shows that if this surface existed in the lungs, it would more than account for the diffusion resistance at rest. Measurement of the relationship between surface pressure and diffusion resistance of lung-derived films is indicated.

Summary. Saline-extractable surface-active material has been found in the lungs of rat, cat, and dog. This material, probably mucoprotein, imparts large hysteresis and characteristic elasticity to the fluid surface. Its effect on lung mechanics has been studied. Its possible influence on diffusion across the alveolar barrier remains to be elucidated.

1. von Neergaard, K., *Z. f. d. ges. exp. Med.,* 1929, v66, 373.
2. Radford, E. P., Jr., Proc. Soc. Exp. Biol. and Med., 1954, v87, 58.
3. Pattle, R. E., *Nature,* 1955, v175, 1125.
4. Macklin, C. C., *Lancet,* 1954, v266, 1099.
5. Adam, N. K., *The Physics and Chemistry of Surfaces,* 3rd Ed. (1941, Oxford Univ. Press, London)
6. Clements, J. A., *A. J. Physiol.,* 1956, v187, 592.
7. Archer, R. J., and LaMer, V. K., *Ann. N. Y. Acad. Sci.,* 1954, v58, 807.
8. Brown, E. S., Proc. Soc. Exp. Biol. and Med., 1957, v95, 168.

Received March 4, 1957. P.S.E.B.M., 1957, v95.

35

Reprinted from *Proc. R. Soc. Lond.*, **B148**, 217–218, 220–221, 222–224, 226, 229–231, 232, 233–234, 236, 238–240 (1958)

Properties, function, and origin of the alveolar lining layer

By R. E. Pattle

Chemical Defence Experimental Establishment, Porton, Wiltshire

The properties of foam and bubbles arising in the lung have been studied, and evidence has been obtained as to the nature of the alveolar lining.

In acute lung oedema, whether accompanied by respiratory movement or not, foam is found in the trachea; it is unaffected by chemical anti-foams, which rapidly destroy the foam formed by shaking oedema fluid with air. A method for obtaining similar foam from excised lung is described.

In air-saturated water, bubbles 40 μ in diameter, obtained from the lung, may be stable for hours, while ordinary bubbles of this size contract and disappear in a few minutes under the influence of surface tension. From observations of these and also from measurements of sessile bubbles, it is shown that their surface tension may be less than 0·06 dyn/cm. The 'stability ratio' of such bubbles is defined.

They are stabilized by a layer of insoluble protein about 50 Å thick, and it is shown that this can only have had its origin as the original lining of the alveoli of the lungs.

If the sharply curved alveolar surface had a surface tension as great as that of blood serum, there would be produced a negative pressure which would draw a transudate from the blood into the alveoli. The lining layer prevents this by reducing the surface tension to nearly zero.

From observations on bubbles obtained from the lung under various conditions, it is shown that the lining layer is produced by surface adsorption from a substance (the lung lining substance) present as a jelly or slime lining the small air spaces. In the guinea-pig it develops only late in foetal life. Its peculiar surface properties are not present in blood or in tracheal mucus; it is therefore a specialized secretion and not a transudate from the blood.

Methods for preparing atelectatic lung *in vitro* and for obtaining a solution of the lung lining substance are described.

From gastric mucin, which has properties somewhat similar to those of the lung lining substance, a foam highly resistant to anti-foams has been prepared.

The possible origin and pathological significance of the lung lining are discussed.

1. Introduction

The anatomical nature of the alveolar lining has long been a matter of controversy; in particular the existence or otherwise of an alveolar epithelium has been much discussed (Short 1950; Bertalanffy & Le Blond 1956). The question of what intervenes between the solid wall of the alveolus and the contained air has received less attention. Macklin (1954) on histological grounds suggests that the alveolus is lined with a layer of mucus.

That the alveolar surface may have peculiar properties suggests itself when the pressure balance between the blood and the alveoli is considered. Drinker (1950), for instance, sets the osmotic pressure of the plasma proteins (25 to 30 mm Hg) against the sum of the pressure (10 mm Hg) in the alveolar vessels and the net negative intrathoracic pressure (10 mm Hg) due to breathing movements on the other. This leaves a balance of 5 to 10 mm Hg in favour of the alveolus remaining dry. Courtice & Korner (1952) make similar calculations. But there is a fourth factor which must, in the absence of good cause to the contrary, be assumed to influence the distribution of liquid between blood and alveoli. This is the effect of surface tension in causing a porous body to soak up liquid. The pressure needed to keep a liquid of surface tension γ out of a narrow tube of radius a whose walls are wetted by the liquid is given by $(2\gamma/a)$. If we put $\gamma = 55$ dyn/cm (the value given by du Noüy (1926) for blood serum), the curved surface of an alveolus of diameter 40 μ will produce a pressure difference across the interface of 41 mm Hg. This is more than enough to wipe out the balance in favour of dryness shown in the calculations of Drinker (1950); Sarnoff & Berglund (1952), showed that a pressure rise of the order of 20 mm Hg in the left auricle of a dog produced pulmonary oedema, and found rapid transudation into a perfused lung when the blood pressure was raised to 50 mm Hg.

These figures suggest that if the surface tension of the alveolar wall were that of a normal liquid, the alveoli would fill with a transudate from the blood. One might expect therefore that a substance capable of reducing surface tension would be present in the alveolus.

Insects possess tracheas 1 μ or less in diameter which periodically fill with and are emptied of liquid. Here surface forces would produce negative pressures of the order of two atmospheres, and examination of the surface properties of the tracheas might give evidence as to how these pressures are sustained.

[*Editor's Note:* Material has been omitted at this point.]

3. Properties of the bubble lining layer

(a) *Its insoluble, solid, and air-permeable character*

When a sample of tracheal foam is shaken gently with distilled water, so that the bubbles pass below the water surface, it remains unbroken. It can be washed in this way with several changes of water, and still retains its resistance to antifoams. When a bubble from the foam is immersed in air-free water, viewing under the microscope shows that the air dissolves and a just visible 'ghost' of irregular shape is left.

These observations show that the bubbles are lined with, and owe their peculiar properties to, a layer of a solid substance insoluble in water and freely permeable to air.

(b) *Its high surface activity*

If the bubbles are washed in pure or dilute 'Teepol' (an anionic detergent) and the latter is then washed away with water, the foam is still unaffected by antifoams. 'Teepol' will displace many other substances (such as saponin and albumen) from liquid surfaces; the behaviour of the tracheal bubbles shows that their lining is highly surface-active.

(c) Protein nature of the bubble surface layer

Some evidence has been obtained in support of the natural expectation that the bubble lining layer would consist of protein.

Samples of the foam agitated and incubated at 37° C for 4 h with pancreatin or trypsin either disappeared or, at the end of the period, were easily destroyed by octyl alcohol. Samples similarly agitated and incubated without addition of enzyme did not disappear during the treatment and were unaffected by octyl alcohol after it.

Again, anti-foams such as oleic acid, which are not protein precipitants, but rapidly destroy albumen or peptone foams (Pattle 1950) have no effect on tracheal foam. The latter is, however, destroyed slowly by a strong solution of mercuric chloride, or by amyl alcohol, and rapidly by lower alcohols. It is also slowly destroyed when ether vapour is poured on it. All these latter substances are protein precipitants.

Neither ferric chloride in 10 % solution nor octyl alcohol will destroy the foam, but foam treated with ferric chloride for a few seconds can be destroyed by octyl alcohol. The same effect is found with other combinations of a protein precipitant with a surface-active anti-foam. This suggests that the ferric chloride first denatures the surface layer of the bubbles, and that the layer is then removed by the octyl alcohol. Observations of small submerged bubbles (§ 5(*c*), p. 228) show that their surface tension is raised by protein precipitants.

[*Editor's Note:* Material has been omitted at this point.]

4. The very low surface tension of bubbles from tracheal foam

(a) Stability of submerged bubbles

Resistance to anti-foams is usually associated with low surface tension. Attempts to measure by a capillary tube method the tension of a surface obtained by breaking tracheal foam *in vacuo* were not successful. It was therefore decided to observe under the microscope the decay of bubbles in various liquids which were in equilibrium with the atmosphere.

When an ordinary small bubble is situated in a liquid saturated with gas at atmospheric pressure, the gas contained in it gradually dissolves, because surface tension gives it an internal pressure greater than atmospheric, and gas diffuses from the surface layer of the liquid to the bulk liquid. The rate of solution is higher the greater the surface tension. This may be observed if a drop of liquid, with a few bubbles, is placed on a microscope slide. This slide is then inverted over another slide provided with a hollow; the drop thus hangs in the hollow, and the bubbles can be watched through the upper slide. To prevent evaporation the two slides may be sealed together with a drop of water. A number of liquids were examined by this means. In each experiment an isolated bubble, $50\,\mu$ or less in diameter was chosen and its diameter was measured, by means of a graticule in the microscope eyepiece, at suitable intervals of time.

Figure 1, curve 1, shows how a bubble 50 μ in diameter in oxalated guinea-pig blood contracted over a period of about 10 min, to 20 μ; after this, extinction took place in less than a minute. Many other liquids (see § 10(*b*), p. 237), showed similar behaviour. Bubbles from saline or from pure water (figure 1, curve 2) disappeared more rapidly.

The behaviour of bubbles from the tracheal foam of an animal with lung oedema was totally different. One such bubble was placed in 1 % Teepol and was observed for 105 min; its diameter fell from 21 to 20 μ in the first 10 min (figure 1, curve 3) and then remained constant. Another remained in pure water at a diameter of 12 μ for 64 min, the lifetime of a bubble of this diameter formed from 1 % Teepol being less than half a minute. The bubbles from oedema foam remained perfectly circular in horizontal section, showing that positive surface tension was or had been

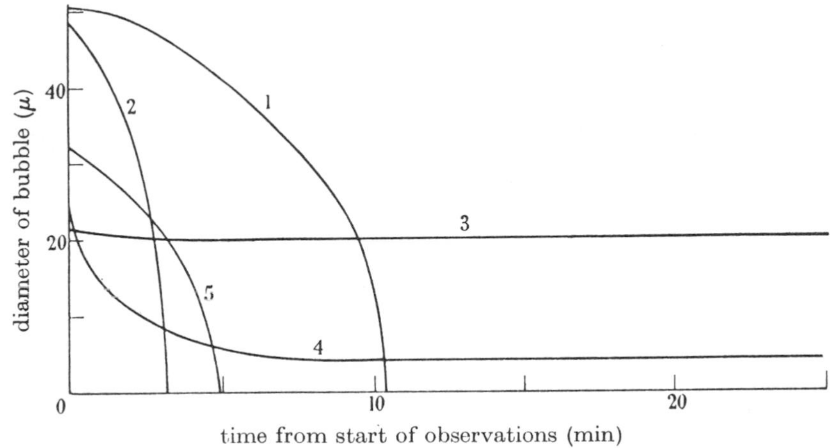

FIGURE 1. Time-course of contraction of bubbles (in air-saturated liquid except curve 5). Curve 1. Oxalated whole guinea-pig blood. Curve 2. Distilled water. Curve 3. Bubble from the trachea of a rabbit suffering from acute lung oedema; transferred to water for observation. Curve 4. 0·25 % gelatin solution; prominent 'ghost'. Curve 5. Bubble from oedema foam transferred to partially de-aerated water. Prominent 'ghost' remained.

at work. By squeezing a fragment of lung into a drop of water, stable bubbles down to 1 μ in diameter may be obtained.

Occasionally in a foam made from a solution a bubble became stable after much contraction. A bubble from 0·25 % gelatin solution contracted normally down to a diameter of 10 μ (figure 1, curve 4). Contraction then slowed, and a bubble 4 μ in diameter, surrounded by a prominent 'ghost', remained. The difference between this type of stability and that of bubbles from the lung is discussed in § 4(*d*), p. 226.

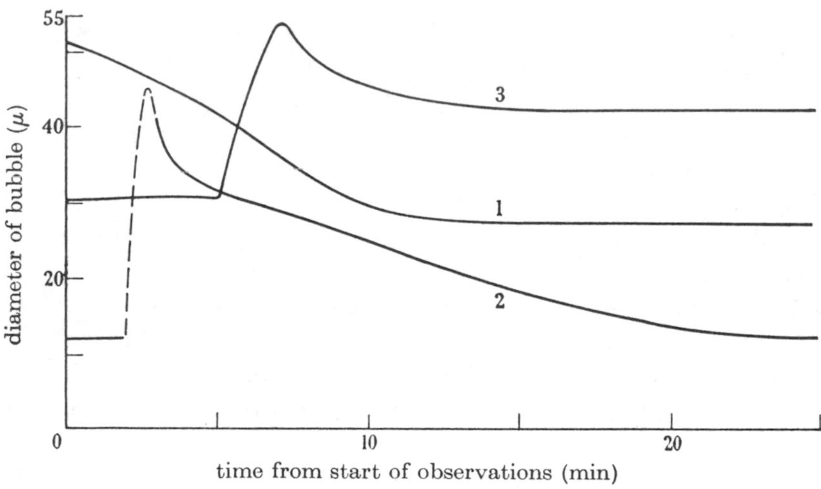

FIGURE 2. Time-course of contraction of bubbles in air-saturated liquids. Curve 1. Bubble of stability ratio 0·26 squeezed from slice of guinea-pig lung. Curve 2. Stable bubble from slice of lung, expanded by heat during the third minute, and later resuming its original diameter. Curve 3. Stable bubble from slice of lung, expanded by heat after 5 min, and later becoming stable at a greater diameter.

(*b*) *Estimation of their surface tension*

A bubble in an air-saturated liquid contracts more rapidly the greater its surface tension. Epstein & Plesset (1950) have derived an equation for the lifetime of an isolated bubble of a single gas when (as in the cases with which we are dealing) contraction is slow enough for a steady state of diffusion from the bubble to be established. The lifetime of a bubble lying under a slide will be longer than that of an isolated bubble; a correction factor (1/ln 2 or 1·44) can be derived from the mathematically analogous case of the electrostatic capacity of two similar charged spheres in contact (Russell 1925). Equation (41) in the paper of Epstein & Plesset (1950) can then be written

$$T = (pr^3 + 2\gamma r^2)/(6D\lambda\gamma \ln 2), \tag{1}$$

where T is the lifetime of a bubble of radius r in a liquid of surface tension γ saturated with gas at the atmospheric pressure p. D is the diffusion coefficient of dissolved gas, and λ the ratio of its concentration to the density of the gas in equilibrium with it.

Several factors make reproducible measurements of the contraction times of air bubbles in ordinary liquids difficult; local supersaturation, caused by neighbouring bubbles, and the fact that oxygen is more soluble than nitrogen, are two of these.

In pure water (the only liquid in which D is known for dissolved gases) small bubbles are difficult to produce; they are much more easily formed in aqueous solutions of surface tension either higher or lower than that of the pure liquid. (The cause of this phenomenon is at present obscure.)

Observations have been made on air bubbles contracting from 24 to 16 μ in diameter in solutions of ethyl and amyl alcohols. None of the bubbles had neighbours nearer than 200 μ. The times obtained were some 25 % greater than those calculated from equation (1) using values of D and λ appropriate to nitrogen in pure water.

Under the circumstances, such experiments seem suitable only for indicating the order of magnitude of the surface tension and not for its measurement.

The bubble of figure 1, curve 3 (20 μ in diameter) cannot possibly have contracted by more than 1·5 μ in the last 90 of the 105 min for which it was observed. It can, therefore, be assumed that the composition of its contained gas was constant; and, as its neighbours were also stable, that local supersaturation was negligible. Inserting in equation (1) the values of D and λ appropriate for air, and calculating the value of γ for which a bubble of diameter 21·5 μ has a lifetime 90 min greater than that of one of diameter 20 μ, we obtain as an upper limit to the surface tension

$$\gamma = 0{\cdot}026 \text{ dyn/cm}.$$

The true surface tension may well have been much smaller.

[*Editor's Note:* Material has been omitted at this point.]

(e) *Criteria of the presence of true surface layer in stable bubbles*

There are, as discussed above, various possible causes of bubble stability, and one cannot assume that because a bubble is stable it has a surface layer like that found in foam from the lung. In particular, a criterion is needed which can be applied to distinguish between stability due to a surface layer and stability due to the bubble being embedded in jelly. A bubble (such as the one in gelatin solution, whose behaviour is described in § 4 (*a*), p. 223, and in figure 1, curve 4) may contract by as much as tenfold in diameter and attain stability only when it is surrounded by a prominent 'ghost' larger than itself. Such bubbles are visibly embedded in a solid mass, and their stability should be ascribed to stresses in this mass rather than to a true surface layer.

For the same reason, the formation of stable bubbles from substances which are not true liquids (nasal mucus, for instance) is no proof of the presence of a substance resembling that of the lung lining. Nor does the fact that bubbles in mucus sometimes collapse much more slowly than similar bubbles in true liquids necessarily mean that the surface tension of mucus is very low; its effects may be counteracted by stresses in the surrounding medium.

If, however, stable bubbles can move independently when in close proximity, and are not surrounded by 'ghosts' of thickness comparable with their radii, it will be inferred that their stability is due to the existence of a true surface layer which counteracts the forces of surface tension.

[*Editor's Note:* Material has been omitted at this point.]

6. Origin of the bubble lining layer from that of the alveoli

In the experiments described in § 2(*d*), p. 219, large numbers of bubbles with diameters from 500 down to 20 μ were produced with the lungs at rest. They could not have had their origin in large air masses broken up by respiratory movement, and must therefore have come from a situation where there was already a body of air having a surface large in relation to its volume. This situation could only have been the fine air spaces of the lung. The evidence suggests that the oedema foam was formed by the air in these spaces being broken up into bubbles and expelled into the bronchi by ingress of oedema fluid into the alveoli and bronchioles. The following argument shows that the lining layer of the bubbles must consist of the original lining layer of the fine air spaces.

Consider a small air space in the lung cut off by a plug of liquid from the atmosphere, and suppose that further liquid attempts to enter the air space either (as in adrenaline or phosgene oedema) through the walls of the space or (as when saline is introduced into the trachea) by seeping between the solid wall and the contained gas. The layer originally next to the gas may be liquid (with or without an insoluble surface film) or it may be solid.

If the layer originally next to the gas is liquid, and the added liquid has a surface-active constituent, this constituent may displace the original surface layer of the liquid lining of the alveolus. If, however, there is no such surface-active constituent, any insoluble surface layer originally present will be retained on the interface between liquid and gas, and will eventually form the lining layer of the bubble or bubbles formed by the air. The fact that oedema fluid and saline have surfaces different in character from those found in the bubbles produced in acute lung oedema, or after instillation of saline in the trachea, shows that the surface layer of these bubbles cannot have been formed from these liquids, but must have been present in the alveolus before they were added.

If the layer originally next to the gas is solid, and no liquid intervenes between it and the solid wall of the alveolus, the added liquid will part the gas from the solid. The original surface layer will then either remain attached to the solid wall (as it would, for instance, if the air space were lined with paraffin wax), the new surface layer being formed entirely from the liquid or from substances dissolved in it; or it will strip off from the solid and continue as a surface layer on the liquid. (Adam & Jessop (1925) found that the surface layer of a mass of cetyl alcohol, solidified under water so that the —CH_2OH groups faced outwards, stripped off and remained attached to the water surface when the solid was removed from the water.) Once the gas is detached from the solid, either with or without the surface layer thereof, the resulting bubble (unless it passes into another liquid phase, makes contact with another solid, unites with another bubble, etc.) can only acquire a surface layer from the liquid, and can only get rid of its surface layer if the latter dissolves in the liquid.

The surface layer of tracheal foam bubbles is insoluble, and the surface layer of bubbles formed by shaking oedema fluid with air has quite different properties from that of tracheal foam bubbles. These facts show that the bubbles of tracheal foam must have brought their surface layer from the place where they were last in contact with a solid, or with a liquid having a highly insoluble surface layer. This place could only be a small air space in the lung.

The lining of the bubbles of lung oedema foam must therefore be derived from that of the small air spaces of the lung.

The question of the relative areas of the bubble surface layer and of the lung lining layer from which it is derived will be discussed in § 8, p. 233. It may be noted that the values found (table 1, p. 221) for the specific surface of tracheal foam are of the same order as the value (310 sq.cm/ml., Lovatt Evans 1952) usually accepted for the ratio of lung surface to lung air content).

It has therefore been shown that the alveoli are lined with a layer which is capable of reducing the surface tension to nearly zero, and this explains why the surface tension of the sharply curved alveolar wall does not draw liquid from the blood into the alveoli.

7. Methods for studying the lung lining layer

(a) *Definition of the stability ratio* (s.r.)

It is here convenient to introduce the concept of the *stability ratio* of a bubble or surface. This will be defined as the inverse of the ratio of the area of the surface (or surface area of the bubble) to that which it must attain in order for the surface tension to be reduced to nearly zero. For instance, if a spherical bubble of diameter d_1 contracts and remains stable at a diameter d_2, its stability ratio before contraction will be given by d_2^2/d_1^2. Figure 2, curve 1, shows the contraction of a bubble initially of stability ratio 0·26.

Bubbles more than 52 μ in diameter contract rather slowly, while those initially less than 36 μ in diameter are liable to have contracted somewhat between the time at which they were formed (e.g. by expulsion from a slice of lung) and the time at which their initial diameters were recorded. It was therefore decided to use only bubbles initially between 36 and 52 μ in diameter for stability ratio measurements, and where an s.r. is quoted it refers to a bubble initially in this size-range.

Bubbles squeezed from a slice of lung may have any s.r. between zero and unity, and where possible large batches of bubbles have been studied. Usually there were between twenty-two and twenty-seven bubbles in each batch.

As explained in § 4 (*e*), p. 226, stability in bubbles which have contracted a great deal may be due to mechanical support of the bubble surface of a dense 'ghost'. Where the s.r. is less than 0·01, therefore, stability does not imply the presence of a substance similar to that which lines the lung.

(b) *Investigation of bubbles*

It is shown above that the alveoli of the lung are lined with a layer of insoluble protein, about 50 Å in thickness, which is capable of reducing the surface tension to nearly zero; and that this layer probably has the function of preventing liquid from being sucked from the small blood vessels of the lung by surface forces.

The question now arises of how, and from what the layer is formed. It is therefore necessary to find some means of gauging the completeness of the layer in a given specimen of lung.

If a particular lung never gives rise to bubbles which can attain stability, it may be supposed that no lining layer is present. If, however, stable bubbles are obtained from two lungs, it is difficult (as described below) to make a comparison; and in practice most of the lungs examined (either foetal or adult), either have lining layers indistinguishable by our methods from that of normal adult lungs, or cannot be shown to have any lining layer at all.

A simple method for obtaining bubbles from lung is to squeeze a small slice into a drop of water. To obtain a large series of s.r.'s of bubbles from normal lung, for instance, an animal was killed with urethane. The lungs were excised and were then allowed to collapse, as a cut slice would in any event collapse to an unknown degree. A slice about 1 mm across was cut from the lung and was transferred to a drop of water hanging from a microscope slide. It was then squeezed with forceps so that bubbles were expelled, and was removed from the drop. This slide was placed over another slide with a hollow, and bubbles were watched in the hanging drop as already described. A sketch of the microscope field was drawn and the initial sizes of some of the bubbles were marked in. The contraction of these bubbles was watched and their final stable diameter was noted about 30 min after the start of observations. From the initial and final diameters the stability ratio of each bubble was calculated, and a series of s.r.'s was obtained which could be compared with series of s.r.'s from other sources.

[*Editor's Note:* Material has been omitted at this point.]

Bubbles can also be obtained from lung by causing lung oedema in the animal, by instilling saline into the trachea during life, or by forcing saline into the excised lung. In these cases, foam escapes from the lungs into the trachea. The s.r. of bubbles obtained from normal lung in such ways is uniformly high; for instance, the mean s.r. of five bubbles from the trachea of a mouse drowned in physiological saline was 0·984. The mode of formation of such bubbles is probably much simpler than that of those formed by cutting and squeezing; there may be only a simple contraction of the lining layer as a cut-off body of air assumes spherical form.

[*Editor's Note:* Material has been omitted at this point.]

8. The lining layer in normal lungs and in insect tracheas

To investigate any possible change in the lining layer of the lung after death, a rabbit was killed with urethane and its lungs were excised and allowed to deflate. Slices were then cut at intervals over a period of 83 min and bubbles were squeezed from them. The mean s.r. of twenty-seven bubbles was 0·788.

After the lung had been stored at room temperature (20° C) for 24 h, a further series of twenty-seven bubbles was obtained. The mean s.r. was 0·733.

There is no significant difference between the two series; there is therefore no evidence of any change in the lining layer over the 24 h.

The mean s.r. of sixty-four bubbles similarly obtained from deflated guinea-pig lungs was 0·753, and of fifty-eight bubbles from mouse lung was 0·858. The difference between the two series was statistically significant, but is not considered evidence of a real difference between the lining layers. The smaller size of the mouse alveolus, for instance, may be its cause. Bubbles squeezed from rat lung or from the lung of a pigeon resemble those from the other species.

When saline was forced into excised guinea-pig lungs through the trachea, fourteen out of twenty-five bubbles obtained had s.r. unity, and the mean s.r. was 0·967. Six bubbles from the trachea of a rabbit in which lung oedema had been induced by injection of adrenaline had a mean s.r. of 0·99.

From the fact that bubbles formed by injection of saline into a lung have an almost complete coating of surface layer (s.r. nearly unity), deductions can be made as to the actual s.r. of the lung lining *in vivo*. If we assume that a body of air trapped in the lung forms a spherical bubble without change in volume the ratio of the surface areas of the original body of air and the bubble will depend on the shape of the former. For instance, a cylinder of radius a and length $4a$, with hemispherical ends, will form a sphere after a reduction in surface area of 16 %. On any reasonable assumption about the initial shape of the air bodies values of 20 % or less are obtained; and so, as the stability ratio of the spheres formed is found to be close to unity, the stability ratio of the original lung lining layer must have been 0·8 or more.

The fact that the sharply curved alveolar surface does not draw oedema fluid from the blood into the alveolus is itself strong evidence that the surface has no tendency to contract. Further evidence was obtained as follows.

A parallel-sided slice of lung, its cut sides being at right angles to the direction of the bronchi, was weighted and sunk in saline. Very few bubbles rose from it. When acetone as added to the saline, copious bubbles were evolved. By contrast, a glass capillary, although it may be of apparently uniform diameter, placed in saline, expels its contained air in the form of bubbles from its wider end. This suggests that the surface tension of the lung lining is nearly zero, and that the acetone, by denaturing the lining layer, raises the surface tension and causes expulsion of bubbles.

On the evidence available, therefore, it appears that the stability ratio of the normal lung lining *in vivo* is nearly unity.

The effect of respiratory movements on the lining layer is discussed in § 9 (*a*), p. 235.

Eleven bubbles squeezed from a slice of frog lung had a mean s.r. of 0·797. This shows the presence of a lining layer which can abolish surface tension; there is no evidence that it differs from that of mammalian lung.

Bubbles squeezed from the head, thorax and abdomen of a bluebottle (*Calliphora*), however, never attained stability. As they contracted they assumed irregular non-spherical shapes and then suddenly became circular in cross-section. Contraction to a non-spherical shape then began again. A lining layer of the kind found in lung is therefore absent from the trachea of this insect.

[*Editor's Note:* Material has been omitted at this point.]

(*b*) *Lungs of foetal and new-born animals*

Two species were used to investigate the growth of the lining layer when the lungs are first inflated—the rabbit, which is blind and hairless at birth, and the relatively much more mature guinea-pig.

Full-term foetuses were obtained by caesarean section. The lungs were excised and inflated by means of a blunt hypodermic needle passed down the trachea. Slices were cut and squeezed 15 s after inflation. The mean s.r. of twelve bubbles from foetal rabbit lung was 0·572, and of twenty-five from foetal guinea-pig lung was 0·724. There is thus no evidence that the lining layers so formed differed in any way from the lining layers of either normal or recently re-expanded adult lung. Foetal lung which had been soaked in cyanide possessed the same properties. These lungs were not investigated by injection of water or by plucking; but as far as can be deduced from the results obtained by cutting and squeezing, the process by which lining layer is formed when foetal lung is expanded is identical with that in adult atelectatic lung.

Two series of experiments were carried out by the cutting and squeezing method on the lungs of new-born animals obtained by caesarean section. No difference could be demonstrated between the lungs of a rabbit which had breathed for 3 min (ten bubbles, mean s.r. 0·777), those of a guinea-pig which had inspired twelve times before being killed (seventeen bubbles, mean s.r. 0·700), and normal lung.

There is therefore present in the mature foetal lung a substance which is capable of forming a lining layer, and this layer is similar in its formation and final properties to that of adult lung. As in adult lung, alternate stretching and relaxation of the lung tissues during respiration will help to make the lining layer complete provided that the ground substance is present.

Bubbles were also obtained by inflating artificially the lungs of two premature guinea-pig foetuses.

One, 7 weeks from conception, was hairless and its eyes were closed. Of seven bubbles obtained, only one became stable (s.r. = 0·059; mean of 7, 0·0084).

The other, 8 weeks from conception, had its eyes open and fur was beginning to grow. Nine out of eighteen bubbles became stable after much contraction (mean of 18, s.r. 0·00983).

As explained in § 4 (*e*), p. 226, stability after such extensive contraction does not imply the presence of substance similar to that found in adult lung.

These experiments show that the substance from which the lining layer forms is absent, or almost absent, in the guinea-pig at a late stage in foetal life, although, externally, the 8-week foetus appeared more mature than a full-term baby rabbit.

[*Editor's Note:* Material has been omitted at this point.]

11. Discussion

It is clearly essential to the life of a being with a highly convoluted lung that the tendency of the air-lung interface to contract should be reduced. A substance which can do this seems to have appeared early in vertebrate evolution. The fact that a dipterous insect can keep tracheas 1 μ or less in diameter free from liquid, but does not appear to possess a substance with the properties of the alveolar lining, suggests that in this insect active secretion of water through a cellular membrane may take place.

The insoluble layer of high surface pressure, which can reduce the net surface tension to nearly zero, is formed by surface adsorption from a substance present in the lung. Further work is needed to elucidate the nature of this substance. It must be of very high molecular weight, as otherwise it would interfere with the osmotic balance between the blood and the alveoli. Its resistance to denaturation by heat suggests that it is a conjugated protein rather than a simple protein. No substance of known composition has so far been found to have similar surface properties; such a substance exists in gastric mucin, but does not appear to be one of the identified constituents thereof.

Macklin (1954) has on histological grounds postulated a layer of mucus lining the alveoli; he suggests that its function is in some way concerned with surface tension. The present findings, if we identify the alveolar lining substance with the material of his mucous layer, confirm his hypothesis. As blood never forms stable bubbles, the alveolar lining substance cannot be a transudate from the blood. Tracheal mucus does not possess the distinctive surface properties of the alveolar lining substance. The latter must therefore be secreted in the depths of the lung, below the level at which the ciliated epithelium terminates; for otherwise it would be swept upwards and appear in tracheal mucus. Apart from this, the present findings give no clue as to its anatomical origin. Attempts to localize the lining layer or its source histologically have not so far succeeded. Macklin suggests that the granular pneumonocytes secrete a mucous layer in the alveolus.

Macklin considers the alveolar mucin to be a watery fluid. That watery fluids, such as that found in the foetal trachea, or the solution obtained by forcing saline into the lung and incubating, can to some extent display the correct properties, has been shown here. The facts that the liquid squeezed from a collapsed lung does not form stable bubbles, that the surface properties of bubbles formed from oedema fluid are irregular, and that surface active material, capable of forming fresh surface layer, is sometimes found adhering to bubbles squeezed from the lung, suggest that, at least in the adult animal, the alveolar lining substance has the character of a jelly which is dispersed in water only with difficulty.

The question naturally arises of what pathological conditions, if any, are due to absence of the lung lining layer. In adrenaline and phosgene oedema the layer is intact.

If a pathological process were to inhibit the formation of the lining substance, the re-expansion of collapsed lung *in vivo* would be hindered. It might likewise be hindered if a liquid—inhaled amniotic fluid for instance—were to overlay the lining substance and prevent its reaching the air-liquid interface; formation of the insoluble surface layer would thus be inhibited. Conversely, excess secretion of the lining substance might build up an effective barrier between blood and air.

The finding that the lung lining substance appears only late in the foetal life of the guinea-pig suggests that absence of the lining substance may sometimes be one of the difficulties with which a premature baby has to contend; such a defect may possibly play a part in causing some cases of atelectasis neonatorum. The appearance of a hyaline membrane might possibly be due either to a defective lining layer causing transudation from the blood or to excessive secretion of lining substance. These matters need experimental investigation.

The author is grateful for the assistance of Mr J. A. G. Edginton in these experiments; to Mr S. Callaway for advice on the preparation of the manuscript; to Dr P. J. Lawther and Dr P. C. Elmes for specimens of blood from clinical cases; and to Mr F. Burgess for the histological work.

Acknowledgement is made to the Controller of H.M. Stationery Office for permission to publish this paper.

References

Adam, N. K. & Jessop, G. 1925 *J. Chem. Soc.* **127**, 1863.

Courtice, F. C. & Korner, P. I. 1952 *Aust. J. Exp. Biol. Med. Sci.* **30**, 511.

Bertalanffy, F. D. & Leblond, C. P. 1955 *Lancet*, **269**, 1365.

Drinker, C. K. 1950 *Pulmonary oedema and inflammation*, pp. 25–26. Cambridge, Mass: Harvard University Press.

du Noüy, P. L. 1926 *Surface equilibria of colloids*, p. 56. New York: Reinhold.

Epstein, P. S. & Plesset, M. S. 1950 *J. Chem. Phys.* **18**, 1505.

Fisher, R. A. & Yates, F. 1953 *Statistical tables for biological agricultural and medical research*, p. 76, 4th ed. Edinburgh: Oliver and Boyd.
Gibbons, R. A., Morgan, W. T. J. & Gibbons, M. 1955 *Biochem. J.* **60**, 428.
Kaplan, J. G. & Fraser, M. J. 1952 *Biochem. biophys. Acta*, **9**, 585.
Laqueur, E. & de Vries Reilingh, D. 1920 *Dtsch. arch. klin. med.* **130**, 310.
Lovatt Evans, C. 1952 *Principles of human physiology*, pp. 722, 746, 11th ed. London: J. and A. Churchill.
Macklin, C. C. 1954 *Lancet*, **266**, 1099.
Mitchell, J. S. 1937 *Trans. Faraday Soc.* **33**, 1129.
Nickerson, M. & Curry, C. F. 1952 *J. Pharmacol.* **114**, 138.
Pattle, R. E. 1950 *J. Soc. Chem. Ind., Lond.* **69**, 363.
Pattle, R. E. 1955 *Nature, Lond.* **175**, 1125.
Pattle, R. E. 1956 *J. Path. Bact.* **72**, 203.
Porter, A. W. 1933 *Phil. Mag.* (7) **15**, 163.
Radford, E. P. 1954 *Proc. Soc. Exp. Biol., N.Y.* **87**, 58.
Rosenbluth, M. B., Epstein, F. H. & Feldman, D. J. 1952 *Proc. Soc. Exp. Biol., N.Y.* **80**, 691.
Russell, A. 1925 *Proc. Phys. Soc. Lond.* **37**, 282.
Sarnoff, S. J. & Berglund, E. 1952 *Amer. J. Physiol.* **170**, 558; **171**, 238.
Short, R. H. D. 1950 *Phil. Trans.* B, **235**, 35.
von Neergard, K. 1929 *Z. ges. exp. Med.* **66**, 273.

36

Reprinted from *A.M.A. J. Dis. Child.*, **97**, 517–523 (May 1959)

Surface Properties in Relation to Atelectasis and Hyaline Membrane Disease

MARY ELLEN AVERY, M.D., and JERE MEAD, M.D., Boston

Recent observations suggest that a low surface tension may be an important attribute of the lining of the air passages of the lung.[1-4] The purpose of this paper is to present evidence that the material responsible for such a low surface tension is absent in the lungs of infants under 1,100-1,200 gm. and in those dying with hyaline membrane disease. The role of this deficiency in the pathogenesis of the disease is considered.

Surface tension operates so as to minimize the area of the surface. In the lungs, where the internal surface (the alveolar lining) is curved concave to the airway, the tendency of the surface to become smaller promotes collapse. Although the forces not only of surface tension but also of the elastic tissue tend to collapse the lungs, their behavior differs in one important respect. When the lung contains only a small volume of air, the elastic recoil of the tissue is diminished, that is, the less the tissues are stretched, the less are the elastic stresses. In contrast, the contribution of surface tension to the retractive force of the lung is increased. Thus, as the air spaces become smaller and more sharply curved, the "mechanical advantage" of surface tension may be thought of as increasing, promoting the tendency to collapse. Since the air spaces are not uniform in size and are all connected to the airway, the smaller, more sharply curved ones tend to empty their contents into the larger. A high surface tension would favor this phenomenon and predispose to atelectasis, whereas a low surface tension would be a stabilizing influence, diminishing the tendency to collapse. For example, if an alveolus can be thought of as a partial sphere with a radius of 40μ and a surface tension equal to that of plasma (55 dynes/cm.), pressure difference would be 20.5 mm. Hg between the inside and outside of the sphere.* This is the pressure tending to collapse the alveolus. If, however, it had the same radius but a surface tension of only 5 dynes/cm., the pressure tending to collapse it would be 1.86 mm. Hg.

Pattle, and more recently Clements and Brown have focused their attention on the magnitude of the surface tension within the lung. Pattle,[1,2] noting the stability of foam and bubbles arising from the lung, concluded that their surface tension must

Submitted for publication Dec. 3, 1958.

This work was supported in part by a special traineeship (BT-259) (C1) from the National Institute of Neurological Diseases and Blindness, U. S. Public Health Service.

From the Department of Physiology, Harvard School of Public Health, and the Newborn Service, Boston Lying-In Hospital. Research Fellow in Pediatrics, Harvard Medical School (Dr. Avery). Associate Professor of Physiology, Harvard School of Public Health (Dr. Mead).

* This is in accord with the LaPlace relationship, $P=2T/r$, where P is the pressure across the wall of the sphere; T is surface tension, and r is the radius of the sphere.

be extremely low. On the basis of measurements which showed that these bubbles were more stable than those produced from plasma or transudates, he deduced that the bubbles from the lung were lined by a material which he thought was derived from the internal surface of the lung. He suggested that absence of this material in the lungs of premature infants might play a role in atelectasis neonatorum and hyaline membrane disease.

Clements [3] and Brown [4] demonstrated that the tension of a surface film derived from the lung was not a constant value; when the surface was stretched the tension was relatively high (40 dynes/cm.), but when the surface area was decreased the tension fell to 10 dynes/cm. These workers first pointed out that such a reduction in surface tension during deflation of the lung would tend to stabilize the air spaces by permitting them to remain open at low lung volumes.

It must be noted that the measurements made by Pattle and Clements and Brown were on material derived from the lung, and not on the alveolar surface itself. Pattle's assumption was that the material lining the internal surface of the lung would also cover small bubbles expressed from its cut surface. Clements and Brown assumed that if a portion of lung were cut in small pieces and stirred with saline, the most surface-active material in the mixture would seek the surface where its tension could be measured. None of these workers knows the precise chemical nature of the surface film studied. However, the observation that the films can be altered by incubation with trypsin and pancreatin suggests that they are at least in part protein.

For the study of the surface behavior of proteins, the classical methods employing a capillary tube or a platinum ring are inadequate since they record only a single value. The surface tension of protein films changes when the area of the surface is changed. Film balances such as the Langmuir-Wilhelmy type used by Clements permit measurements of surface tension as a function of changes in surface area.[5] The dependency of tension on area is an important elastic-like property of protein films. In surface films obtained from lungs the change in tension is not a constant value, but continues to change in time. It is presumed that in addition to elastic behavior there is a time-dependent viscous component, which produces this lag in response, termed hysteresis.[6] Thus the films derived from the lung behave as if they were viscoelastic entities.

Despite the lack of direct measurements of surface tension at the alveolar-air interface, the low values obtained by Pattle and Clements and Brown with indirect methods would account for the stability of an alveolus at end-expiration. If then the prevention of atelectasis depends on the presence of a material with a very low surface tension lining the air spaces, it seemed attractive to examine the lungs of small premature infants and those dying with hyaline membrane disease for this material. In these infants there is always some atelectasis. The absence of a low surface tension in extracts of their lungs would support the theory put forward by Pattle and Clements and Brown, and at the same time explain the predisposition of these infants to atelectasis.

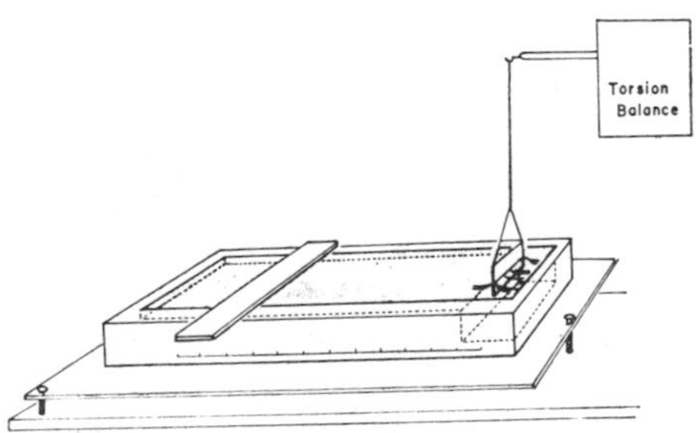

Fig. 1.—The dimensions of the trough are 15×7.5×1.7 cm. outside, 11.8×5×1 cm. inside. At one end is a well 5×1.5×1.3 cm. to permit submersion of the stirrup for a zero reference point. The trough is filled so that barrier touches the surface (65 ml.). A centimeter scale is attached to one side to permit measurement of the area where the barrier is moved. The metal plate under the trough is supported by three screws to permit leveling.

Methods

The method to be described is similar to that used by Clements. The film balance is shown in Figure 1. The trough is constructed of a single block of polytetrafluoroethylene (Teflon).† (This has the advantage over paraffin-coated troughs in that it is less wettable than paraffin, chemically inert, and provides a surface which is easy to clean.) A thin, frosted platinum strip or "stirrup" is partially submerged in the fluid. The force of surface tension, pulling down on the wettable stirrup,‡ is measured on a torsion balance with attached transducer through a direct-writing oscillograph.

Four grams of lung was cut into pieces approximately 2 by 5 mm. and diluted with 65 ml. of 0.85% saline. The mixture was stirred vigorously for about five minutes, filtered through gauze, and poured into the trough. The surface was "aged" one hour before testing. To change the area of the surface, a Teflon strip (11.3 cm. $\times$ 2.2 cm. $\times$ 0.3 cm.) under a heavy brass bar used as a barrier, was moved once a minute in 1 cm. steps, starting from the end of the trough opposite the stirrup and approaching 0.5 cm. from the stirrup (15% of the original area). The precedure was reversed to extend the film.

A change in surface area was promptly followed by a maximal change in tension, which decreased with time. By the end of one minute at tensions above 20 to 30 dynes per centimeter about 90% of the change has taken place.

At lower tensions the surface appeared irregular and occasionally had whitish linear streaks parallel to the barrier. This easily recognizable change was considered a "gelling" of the film. When this occurred the initial and one-minute readings were nearly the same, and the tension remained constant even on further compression of the surface. Thus there seemed to be a lower limiting tension, often about 5 dynes/cm. At lower tensions when the film did not "gel," the surface tended to creep over the edge of the trough, gradually extending the area so that the one-minute readings had no meaning in terms of tension at a given area. When this happened only the initial value was recorded. (The initial readings at all areas are called dynamic values. The one-minute readings are called quasistatic values.)

The possible influence of concentration of tissue on the results was studied by using 0.5 gm. of lung per 65 ml. of saline and 20 gm. of lung per 65 ml. of saline. The highest and lowest tensions recorded were the same. No attempt was made to establish the minimal amount of tissue needed. Four grams per 65 ml. was the concentration used in these experiments because of convenience in handling this amount.

The possibility that the age of the tissue after death would alter the surface behavior was investigated because the samples of human lungs were obtained at different times post mortem. Therefore samples of dog lung were studied immediately after the animal was killed, and after either refrigeration or freezing for as long as six days. Within these limits there was no significant change in the results obtained.

Temperature changes, within the range of 70 to 101 F and changes in pH of the substrate by addition of HCl and NaOH to a range of pH 1-pH 11 did not influence the surface tension-area relationship. Most of the measurements of the human lungs were made at temperatures between 75 and 85 F, while the pH of the filtered lung extracts was usually 6.5 to 7.0.

Results

The relationship of surface tension to area as measured on the film balance, is shown in Figure 2. Here the path of changing tension with decreasing area is on the left, and the tension with increasing area is on the right side of each plot. The solid lines connect the points obtained immediately after moving the barrier. The inner dotted lines connect the points recorded after one minute at the same area.

These curves differ from the one published by Clements in that they show a steeper slope at the beginning of compres-

† Dupont registered trade-mark.

‡ One correction necessary when using a partially submerged stirrup is for buoyancy. With a very thin platinum strip, this is almost negligible. It can be measured by recording the tension of a known solution with the stirrup at different depths. If subsequent measurements are made at a given depth, the contribution of buoyancy is known.

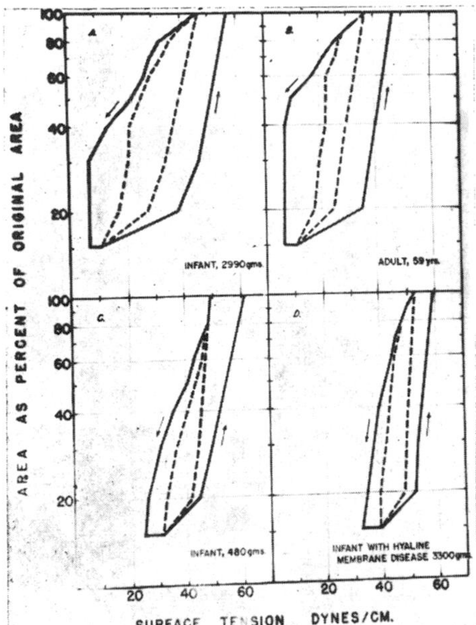

Fig. 2.—Illustrative force-area diagrams. The outer solid line connects the initial values for surface tension obtained when the area was changed. The inner dotted lines connect the values for surface tension after one minute at the given area.

sion of the film. The slope, which is the coefficient of compressibility, is variable, depending on the age of the surface, the number of times cycled and unknown factors. In our experience the least variable values were the lowest and highest tensions recorded. For comparison of the surface behavior of lung extracts from infants of different birth weights, the highest tension reached on extension of the surface, and the lowest tension reached on compression with the means and deviation from the mean are presented in the Table. There is considerable variation in the upper tensions and no pattern is evident. However, a definite pattern appears in the lowest tensions recorded (Fig. 3). The lowest values in the lung extracts of infants under 1,100-1,200 gm. are 20-30 dynes/cm. The lowest tensions in the extracts of heavier infants, older children and adults are under 20 dynes/cm. and usually 5-7 dynes/cm. The only exceptions to this are the lowest tensions measured in the lung extracts of infants dying with hyaline membrane disease. In these, the corresponding figures are all above 20 dynes/cm. and most are above 30 dynes/cm. even though the infants were in the weight group where values below 20 dynes/cm. would be expected. This was true in all nine of the infants with hyaline membrane disease studied. The only infant who did not have the disease whose lung had a surface tension higher than expected was a stillborn infant of a diabetic mother.

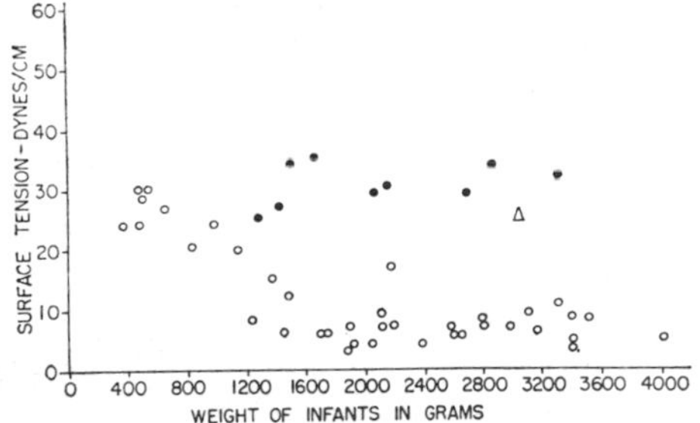

Fig. 3.—Lowest surface tension measured on compression of the surface. Open circles=infants dying from causes other than hyaline membrane disease. Closed circles=infants dying with hyaline membrane disease. Triangle=stillborn infant of a diabetic mother.

The behavior of extracts of lungs of dogs, cats, rabbits, and guinea pigs was much the same as that of human lungs. Washings from the tracheal-bronchial tree had the same surface-tension values as lung extracts. However, other tissues, including plasma, whole blood, gastric juice,

Fig. 4.—The horizontal lines connect the highest and lowest tensions measured in extracts of lungs and other tissues. HMD=hyaline membrane disease; still. IDM=stillborn infant of a diabetic mother.

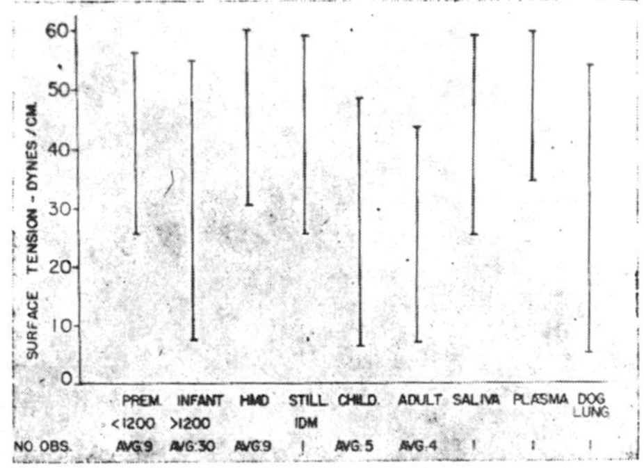

Highest and Lowest Surface Tension of Lung Extracts

Wt., Gm.	Infants Live-born or Stillborn	Highest Tension	Lowest Tension
390	S	49	24.5
470	S	58.2	30.6
480	L	61.5	24.5
500	S	57.5	29
520	L	61	30.5
680	L	56	27
830	L	55	20.8
970	L	59	24.5
1,150	S	49	20
		m=56.2	m=25.7
		± 4.34	± 3.65
1,220	L	52.5	8.6
1,390	L	48	15.2
1,430	L	54	6.6
1,460	L	56	12.2
1,700	L	55	6.1
1,740	L	54	6.1
1,870	L	60	3.6
1,900	S	59	7.3
1,940	S	56	4.9
2,100	S	51.5	9.8
2,125	L	56	7.3
2,180	S	56	17.1
2,180	S	58	7.6
2,390	L	55.5	4.4
2,495	L	61.5	6.8
2,500	L	53	6.1
2,640	L	58	6.1
2,670	L	53.5	6.1
2,800	L	61	8.5
2,800	S	51	7.4
2,990	S	58.2	7.3
3,100	S	61.3	9.8
3,170	S	47	6.1
3,300	S	39.2	11
3,400	L	51	4.9
3,400	L	57.5	8.6
3,400	L	60	3.5
3,515	L	57.5	8.6
4,000	L	52.5	5.4
		m=55	m= 7.6
		± 4.67	± 3.05

	Hyaline Membrane Disease	
Wt., Gm.	Highest Tension	Lowest Tension
1,260	58.8	25.7
1,420	61	27
1,500	60	34.4
1,650	63.5	35.5
2,050	59	29.4
2,150	58	30.5
2,700	62.3	29.5
2,860	59	34.4
3,300	59	32.3
	m=60	m=30.4
	± 1.41	± 3.12

	Children	
Age	Highest Tension	Lowest Tension
9 wk.	54	6.1
3 mo.	51	5.4
8 mo.	51.4	4.9
23 mo.	35.5	7.4
4 yr.	50.6	9.8
	m=48.5	m= 6.7
	± 7.4	± 1.96

	Adults	
Age, Yr.	Highest Tension	Lowest Tension
37	40	9.3
44	41.5	5.4
56	47	7.3
59	46.5	6.8
	m=43.8	m= 7.2
	± 3.53	± 1.61

saliva, synovial fluid, liver, and muscle had surface properties very different from normal lung (Fig. 4).

Comment

The results show that without exception the surface behavior of lung extracts of the nine infants with hyaline membrane disease was different from that of infants dying from other causes and the same as that of infants smaller than 1,200 gm. This suggests that the disease is associated with the absence or delayed appearance of some substance which in the normal subject renders the internal surface capable of attaining a low surface tension when lung volume is decreased.

It is of interest to attempt to relate the results obtained to the pathogenesis of the disease. In all lungs with the first breath, large pressures are necessary to create an air-liquid interface (Table). In this respect the normal lung would not differ from the lung without the surface-active material since surface tension on extension of the surface is similar in both cases. Thereafter, during expiration, the alveolar surface of the normal lung would have diminished tension (Fig. 2), thus reducing the tendency of the air spaces to collapse. On the other hand, in a lung lacking this lining material, surface tension would tend to remain high during expiration; the air spaces would be unstable, and some would collapse. Once a sufficient number had closed, others would remain open inasmuch as the interpleural pressure at end-expiration would be sufficiently negative to prevent further closure. The net mechanical effect would be a lower than normal interpleural pressure, both at end-expiration and, more particularly, at end-inspiration. This is in accord with the measurements of Cook et al. on living infants with the disease in whom the interpleural pressure at end-inspiration can be calculated to be at least -15 cm. H_2O, about a threefold increase over normal.[7]

As a result of an increased mean pressure difference between the thorax and the rest of the body, intrathoracic blood volume would be increased. In atelectatic regions, and for that matter in air-containing regions as well, presumably the pulmonary capillaries would be influenced by the more negative interpleural pressure and would therefore share in the congestion. The evidence presented by Gitlin and Craig[8] that the membranes contain fibrin, derived from the pulmonary circulation as fibrinogen, indicates that transudation occurs in hyaline membrane disease. There is no evidence that the congestion resulting from the increased body to thorax pressure difference would be sufficient to account for this transudation. It is possible that surface forces may produce highly localized distention and leakage of capillaries, although it is probably true that Pattle's estimate of these effects is an oversimplification.[1]

It is of interest that atelectasis, of the type seen in hyaline membrane disease, but without any membrane, has been described.[9,10] Potter suggests that it is an infrequent occurrence seen in infants with a clinical course compatible with the disease.[11] If the primary event is atelectasis with the membrane being formed later, it would be anticipated that some might die before the membrane had developed.

Certain clinical features of hyaline membrane disease could be explained if the disease results from the absence of a surface-active material:

1. The disease has not been described in stillborn infants. The surface forces at an air-fluid interface could not operate before the first breath.

2. The symptoms may begin within the first few minutes after birth, but often do not become severe until several hours later; death or recovery usually ensues in 4 to 72 hours. Although a normal initial expansion of the lungs would be expected, it would take time for the subsequent mechanical difficulties to be evident. If maturation of the lung lining occurred in the first few days of extrauterine life, recovery would be expected.

3. The disease is more common the more premature the infant.[12] Since our data suggest the normal surface behavior usually appears in infants of about 1,100-1,200 gm., its absence from the lungs of certain infants weighing more than this could be an instance of delayed appearance of the normal lung lining material, and more likely the more premature the infant. One could ask if the absence of a specific surface-active material in the lung predisposes to hyaline membrane disease, why do not all infants under 1,100-1,200 gm. (lacking the material) have the disease? The nine such infants thus far studied showed surface tensions similar to those from infants with the disease, but four of the nine were stillborn and two lived only minutes (Fig. 3). In the three who lived more than four hours, long enough to have signs of the disease, the lungs were indeed atelectatic, although there were no membranes. In any case, one cannot expect every very small premature infant to have the disease, without assurance that 1,100-1,200 gm. is a sharp zone of demarcation before which surface-active material never appears.

Among the unexplained features of this disease is the high incidence in infants of diabetic mothers. Whether the resemblance of this group of infants to premature infants is sufficient to assign a similar pathogenesis of the disease remains to be seen.

Finally, the hypothesis presented here that the lack of a normal lining material in the lungs of infants would contribute to the atelectasis seen in hyaline membrane disease does not preclude the possible importance of other factors in the pathogenesis. Immaturity of the lung lining may be associated with immaturity in other respects.[13] A combination of deficiencies or external insults may be required for the complete syndrome. Moreover, other properties or functions of the lung-lining layer deserve investigation.

Summary

Recent observations suggest that a low surface tension in the lining of the lung may permit stability of the alveoli at end-expiration. Lacking such a material, the lung would be predisposed to collapse.

Measurements of the surface tension of lung extracts confirm the presence of a very surface-active substance in lungs of infants over 1,100-1,200 gm. and in children and adults. In lung extracts of very small premature infants and infants dying with hyaline membrane disease the surface tension is higher than expected, suggesting that the surface active material is deficient.

The possible role of this deficiency in the pathogenesis of hyaline membrane disease is discussed.

The authors are particularly indebted to Dr. John Clements, Army Chemical Center, Maryland, for his generous and stimulating advice; also to Dr. Kurt Benirschke and the staff of the Department of Pathology, Boston Lying-In Hospital, and to Dr. John Craig and the staff of the Department of Pathology, Childrens Medical Center, Boston, for permitting us to study human lungs post mortem. Dr. Clement A. Smith reviewed the manuscript.

55 Shattuck St.

REFERENCES

1. Pattle, R. E.: Properties, Function, and Origin of the Alveolar Lining Layer, Proc. Roy. Soc. London, Ser. B 148:217-240, 1958.

2. Pattle, R. E.: Properties, Function, and Origin of the Alveolar Lining Layer, Nature, London 175:1125, 1955.

3. Clements, J. A.: Surface Tension of Lung Extracts, Proc. Soc. Exper. Biol. & Med. 95:170-172, 1957.

4. Brown, E. S.: Lung Area from Surface Tension Effects, Proc. Soc. Exper. Biol. & Med. 95:168-170, 1957.

5. Harkins, W. D.: Physical Chemistry of Surface Films, New York, Reinhold Publishing Corporation, 1952, Chap. 2.

6. Stacy, R. W.; Williams, D. T.; Worden, R. E., and McMorris, R. O.: Essentials of Biological and Medical Physics, New York, McGraw-Hill Book Company, Inc., 1955, Chap. 8.

7. Cook, C. D.; Sutherland, J. M.; Segal, S.; Cherry, R. B.; Mead, J.; McIlroy, M. B., and Smith, C. A.: Studies of Respiratory Physiology in the Newborn Infant: III., J. Clin. Invest. 36:444-448, 1957.

8. Gitlin, D., and Craig, J. M.: The Nature of the Hyaline Membrane in Asphyxia of the Newborn, Pediatrics 17:64, 1956.

9. Gruenwald, P.: Pathologic Aspects of Lung Expansion in Mature and Premature Newborn Infants, Bull. New York Acad. Med. 32:689-692, 1956.

10. Briggs J. N., and Hogg, G.: Perinatal Pulmonary Pathology, Pediatrics 22:41-48, 1958.

11. Potter, E.: Personal communication to the authors.

12. Silverman, W., and Silverman, R.: Letter to the Editor, Lancet 2:588, 1958.

13. Phillips, L. L., and Skrodalis, V.: Fibrinolytic Enzyme System in Maternal and Umbilical-Cord Blood, Pediatrics 22:715-726, 1958.

37

Reprinted from *Physiologist,* 5(1), 12–28 (1962)

SURFACE PHENOMENA IN RELATION TO PULMONARY FUNCTION

John A. Clements

[*Editor's Note:* In the original, material precedes this excerpt.]

It is in this spirit of reaching for the future, of knowledge in flux, of imperfect understanding, that I should like to discuss one step in the development of pulmonary physiology. This step is the recognition that the lungs are "emulsions" of air in tissue and that the bulk properties of such a finely-dispersed system depend to a large extent on the properties of the interface between the two phases. Further, it is the recognition that the presence of materials in either phase that have special affinity for the interfacial region (surfactants), can modify the bulk properties of the system to a very great extent, far out of proportion to their bulk concentrations. Of the several properties that can be so-modified, let us confine our attention to those which can influence bulk elasticity and the distribution of forces in the lungs.

It may be of interest to examine briefly the history of the subject, as it relates to pulmonary function.

It is a remarkable fact that von Neergaard already set forth in 1929 (28) a significant part of what we know now. He stated that 2/3 to 3/4 of the elasticity of the lungs is derived from interfacial forces. He also stated in the summary of his classical paper: "It is possible that the surface tension of the alveoli is decreased below that of other physiological fluids by accumulation of surface-active material, in accordance with Gibbs-Thomsen law." Von Neergaard attempted to extract surfactant from lungs but had slight success, because of the limitations of his methods. It is surprising that his work attracted so little attention. There were sporadic references to it in the German literature of the next two decades. The earliest reference in English that I know of came 25 years later in a paper of Radford (20), although intensive studies of respiratory mechanics had been under way for more than a decade in several academic capitals. The importance of interfacial forces in the initial expansion of the lungs after birth was mentioned by Wilson and Farber (29) in 1933 and by Gruenwald (8) in 1947, but it remained for Mead, Whittenberger, and Radford (14) to clarify the matter in the early 1950's. They essentially repeated von Neergaard's experiments, came to much the same conclusions, and extended them. They showed the dependence of hysteresis in static pulmonary pressure-volume diagrams on surface forces; they emphasized the importance of surface tension in determining alveolar geometry and they made careful measurements of visible airspaces (22). They gave theoretical reasons why the alveolar population should be an unstable one (21). In 1953 Radford also showed how the internal surface area of the lungs could be calculated from pressure-volume diagrams, using an assumed surface tension (5, 20). These investigators apparently thought that pulmonary surface tension is comparatively high, approaching that of serum, although Radford (20) mentioned the possibility that it might be lowered by the presence of intrinsic surfactant.

In 1955 Pattle (15) reported that pulmonary edema foam is very resistant to anti-foam agents and that bubbles expressed from the lung into air-saturated water are stable for long periods. He deduced from these observations that the lungs contain a powerful surfactant, which reduces the surface tension of the alveoli nearly to zero. He concluded tentatively that the material is mucoprotein and lines the alveoli, as had been suggested by Macklin (12).

At Edgewood we had been much intrigued by Radford's method for estimating lung area and had examined his assumptions. Since the calculated area was inversely proportional to the surface tension and since his estimates appeared very low, we reasoned that the value he assumed for pulmonary surface tension might be too high. Brown, Johnson, and I (3) reversed the method of calculation and by assuming how the area of the lungs might change with their volume, worked out values for tension. These traced out a path from serum tension down to very low values, and when Pattle's estimates became available we felt we had nearly achieved a synthesis of Radford's and Pattle's concepts. In addition we felt that the change of surface tension as a function of lung volume was a necessary characteristic for stabilization of the alveolar structure.

How could the surface tension of the airspaces change so much? Was it a plausible physicochemical phenomenon? How might one put the hypothesis to direct test?

As we read the literature of surface physics and chemistry we became convinced that the notion was tenable. Numerous observations had been made on the behavior of monomolecular films of insoluble surface active materials floating on liquids. It had been clearly shown by many workers that such films were sometimes capable of changing the surface tension of aqueous solutions by more than 60 dynes per centimeter when the area of the liquid was changed. Furthermore, the substances that formed these films were ubiquitous biological materials, such as proteins and lipids. The concepts were older than we, and the methods to test their application to the lungs had been hallowed through decades of use by Langmuir, Adam, Harkins, Leathes, Rideal, Schulman, and Danielli. Thus, if our hypothesis was correct, we should be able to extract highly surface active material from the lungs and to measure its activity by standard methods. The result of this test was successful (7), and it launched us on a continuing program of theoretical and practical investigations of pulmonary surface phenomena.

In 1959 Avery and Mead confirmed our findings and applied the same test to the lungs of newborn infants that had died with hyaline membrane disease (1). These infants experienced severe respiratory distress, and at necropsy their lungs were extensively atelectatic and showed deposition of fibrin in the fine airspaces. Although such lungs expand normally with saline, very high pressors are required with air. Extracts of the lungs failed to show high surface activity. These results provided further indirect support of the hypothesis that stability of the alveolar structure requires the presence of surface active material.

In 1960 Bondurant developed a method for the large-scale extraction of surfactant from the lungs (2). This important step made possible unequivocal studies of the chemical composition of the material and greatly extended the vista for investigation of its functional role. It is evident now that the pulmonary surfactant is lipoprotein in nature and contains a large proportion of phospholipids (9, 17). Workers in several laboratories are actively pursuing the physical, chemical, and biological characteristics of the material.

With this hasty chronological review of the subject in mind let us examine the concepts and experimental evidence more closely.

What reasons had von Neergaard and other pioneers of pulmonary physiology to think that surface tension might affect the function of the lungs? The main reasons were the belief that the airspaces are covered with a thin layer of liquid, and the obvious fact that they are small in size. By virtue of its surface tension a liquid surface tends to contract, and if the surface is curved (in the mathematical sense) the pressure must be different on its two sides. The relationship between size, tension, and pressure difference is illustrated in figure 1, which shows a bubble of air in water. If the bubble is small enough, it is nearly

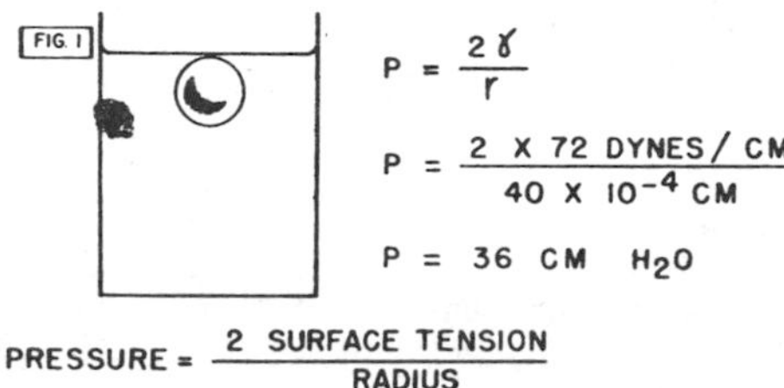

spherical and the pressure of the air exceeds that of the water just outside by twice the surface tension divided by the radius of the bubble. If the bubble is of the average size of the alveoli in an adult dog lung, that is about 40 microns in radius and the surface tension of the water is 72 dynes per centimeter, the air pressure exceeds the water pressure by 36 centimeters of water. Consider a bubble very close to the surface of the water, so that the water pressure is very nearly atmospheric, and the water is saturated with air at atmospheric pressure when the bubble is introduced. Then the air pressure in the bubble is 36 cm H_2O greater than in the atmosphere and the water, and under this gradient air rapidly diffuses out. The bubble contracts and disappears in a few minutes. If the surface tension of the water surrounding the bubble were reduced to zero or nearly zero, the air pressure in it would essentially be atmospheric and the bubble would be stable or would contract very slowly. This is the final behavior of bubbles squeezed from normal lungs into air-saturated water and is the observation that caused Pattle to deduce that their surface tension is nearly zero. We shall return to this phenomenon presently.

If we introduce a tube into the water and deliver air into a bubble at the end of the tube from a microsyringe (figure 2), we find that the same formula governs the relationship between surface tension, curvature, and pressure difference at the air-liquid interface. In addition we can see, as depicted in the graph, that the bubble has a peculiar pressure-volume relationship. As the bubble forms the pressure rises, and reaches a peak when the bubble is hemispherical; as it grows further in volume the pressure declines. For the purpose of our analysis we may call the tube and "airway", the bubble an "alveolus", and the water the wet pulmonary parenchyma. It was this kind of model that von Neergaard (28) and the Harvard group (14) used to explain the effect of surface tension on the lungs.

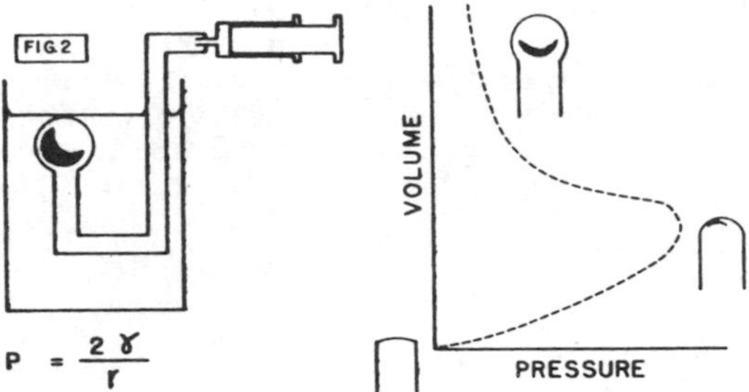

In both instances they put the model to the same test. The surface tension exists because of the contact of the dissimilar materials, gas and watery liquid. They reasoned that if the bubbles were filled with aqueous solution, the surface tension would not exist. Therefore, if surface tension contributed to the elasticity of the lungs the effect would be eliminated by filling them with aqueous liquid.

In figure 3 we see the results of such an experiment (19). The totally collapsed lungs were first filled with saline and emptied and then inflated with air. The loop on the left shows the recoil of the lungs when filled with liquid; that to the right their recoil when filled with air. The

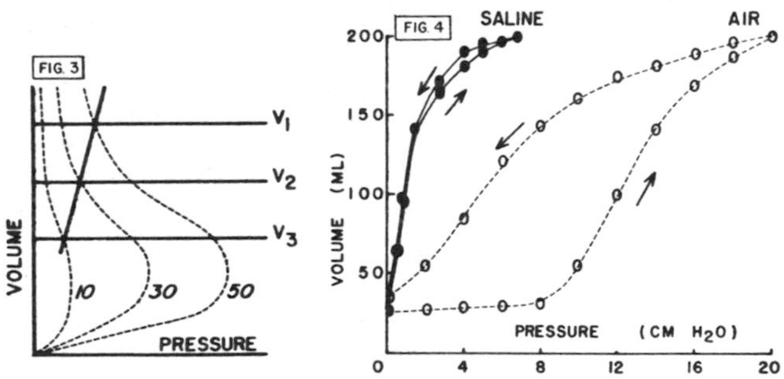

Fig. 3. Effect of changing surface tension on compliance. (Mead: Am. Rev. Resp. Dis. 81:739, 1960).

Fig. 4. Pressure-volume relationship, cat lungs. (Radford: Tissue Elasticity, 1957, p. 185).

same result is obtained if the air is presented first and the saline second. Clearly the force of recoil, measured as pressure on the abscissa, is less with liquid than with gas-filling. The saline pressure-volume loop shows little hystersis and is taken to indicate the true elastic behavior of the pulmonary tissue. The added pressure required for air-filling is attributed to the action of surface tension, and represents about 2/3 of the total.

Let us see if this idea has reasonable consequences. Since we have estimates of the average size of the airspaces and of the pressure due to surface tension at various lung volumes, we can calculate surface tension by the bubble formula. At full volume we get 47 dynes/cm; at mid-volume 9 dynes/cm; and at lower volumes still lower values. We cannot rely on the estimates at small lung volumes because bronchiolar collapse intervenes and the transpulmonary pressure is not a proper measure of the pressure difference across the alveolar "bubbles." However, even at mid-volume, when the airways are manifestly open, the estimate of surface tension is significantly less than that of serum. Thus, one consequence of the idea is that surface tension in the lungs must be much less that that of serum, and as a corrollary to this, that surface active material must be present in the lungs. Another consequence is that the surface tension must change as lung volume changes, and as a corrollary to this, that the surface active material must act as an insoluble film, rather than as the reversibly adsorbed Gibbs film postulated by von Neergaard. A further consequence is that if the surface tension changes so much with volume, the negative slope of the pressure-volume diagram of the "alveolar bubble" is made positive. On this basis we can understand the stability of millions of wet airspaces inflated in parallel.

Figure 4 shows how change in surface tension converts negative to positive compliance (13). Each curve in the family gives the pressure-volume relationship of the bubble at a given, constant, surface tension. If as the volume decreases from V_1 to V_2 to V_3, the tension decreases from 50 to 30 to 10, then the pressure declines rather than rises. An assemblage of bubbles having this positive characteristic is stable, and could be ventilated in parallel. Not so a group of bubbles with negative compliance; in such a system the smaller ones empty into the larger ones, much as an emulsion breaks down by the addition of smaller droplets to larger ones. In the lungs we would call it atelectasis.

At this moment I think you would be quite justified in pointing out that the lungs are obviously more than aggregations of bubbles on tubes: the tissue must at least determine the size and shape of the lungs and the order of airspace size. I admit to having slighted the role of tissue elements. Since it leaves more time for describing the studies of surface tension, I shall continue to neglect the "too, too solid flesh."

We may summarize the consequences of applying the "alveolar bubble" model to pressure-volume data in one statement: the observations can best be accounted for by assuming that the lungs have a moist interior covered with an elastic film of surfactant. This assumption is reasonable only if material exists in the lungs which can form such a film. If one could extract such material, it would be logical to think that it might have been located at the surfaces of the airspaces, especially if it could be washed out the airway without traumatizing the tissue. Several workers have extracted pulmonary surfactant, and I should like to discuss their results now.

Pattle (15) squeezed microscopic bubbles that contained surfactant from cut alveolar tissue. Brown, Johnson, and I (3, 7) made saline extracts in three ways: by touching cut alveolar tissue to saline, by mincing the lung with saline, and by rinsing via the airway with saline. Bondurant (2) prepared artificial pulmonary edema foam that contained large amounts of surfactant.

Pattle's method requires microscopic observation of bubbles in air-saturated water. The other methods require the use of the surface balance, an instrument not so familiar to physiologists as the microscope. Figure 5 shows the essential parts of a surface balance. It consists of a tray filled with liquid; a barrier pushed along the tray to reduce the area of the liquid and compress a surface film if it is present; and a thin, frosted, platinum plate, hanging vertically in the liquid to measure the pull or surface tension of the liquid. The operation can be made automatic,

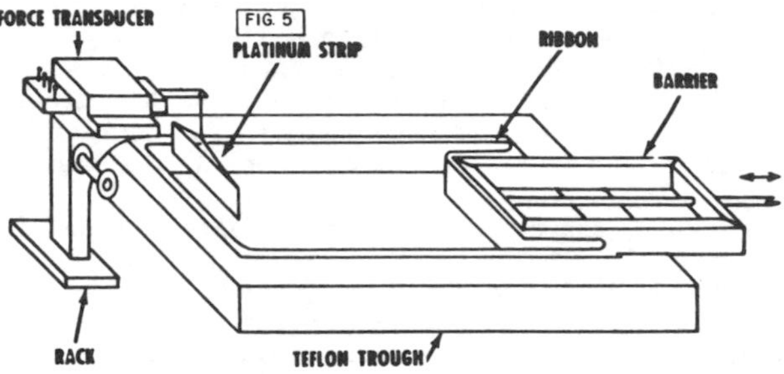

so that area and tension are plotted against each other on an X-Y recorder. When the tray is filled with very clean water, the platinum plate experiences a pull of about 72 dynes per centimeter of its perimeter, and this pull does not change when the barrier is moved. If a tiny amount of a protein or a lipid containing hydrophilic functional groups is dropped on the surface, it spreads out as film and the pull on the platinum plate decreases. If the barrier is now moved, the surface tension falls when the area of the liquid is reduced, and rises when area is increased. When protein is dissolved in the water, it forms a similar surface film by spontaneous adsorption. If a detergent is dissolved in the water, the surface tension falls to about 30 dynes/cm and does not change when the barrier is moved. These relationships between area and surface tension are given diagramatically in figure 6. The thin loop to the right represents clean water with a tension of $\sim$72 dynes/cm; the next curve, blood plasma; the thin loop to the left, 1% Tween 20. The large loop is the type of tension-area diagram found with saline extracts of normal lungs. Similar results have also been obtained with the other methods of extraction. Clearly such lungs contain substances that can bring down surface tension of aqueous solutions to very low values. In addition, the tension varies with the size of the surface. Thus, both assumptions which we made earlier would be borne out if such material came from the alveolar surfaces.

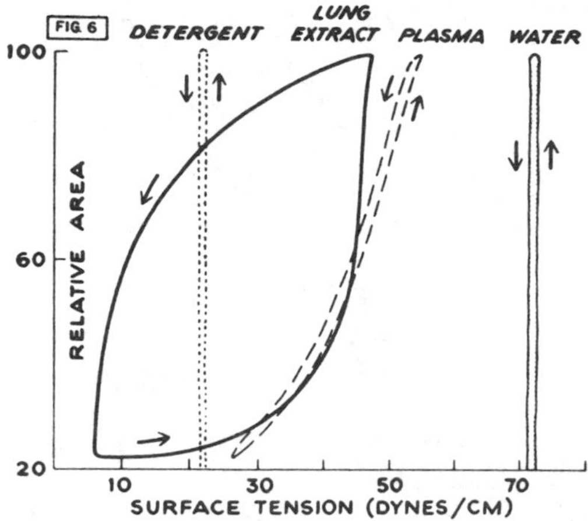

For purposes of comparison figure 7 shows tension-area diagrams recorded on saline extracts of infant lungs. The loop (B) represents a normal lung; the loop (A), one showing congestive atelectasis. Gruenwald, Johnson, Hustead and I have made this determination on 37 neonatal specimens. At autopsy Dr. Gruenwald made pressure-volume measurements on the specimens and calculated an index which expressed numerically how well they remained expanded at physiological pressures, after being fully inflated. Without knowledge of his results we measured the surface tension of saline extracts of the specimens and calculated an index of surface activity for each. The two indices were well correlated (figure 8). Whatever post mortem changes occurred in this material were insufficient to obliterate the correlation.

You recall that Pattle squeezed microscopic bubbles from cut alveolar tissue into air-saturated water and concluded from their stability that their surface tension was nearly zero. We have repeated and confirmed his observations, and are also forced to the conclusion that highly surface active material is present in the alveolar tissue. Since the stable bubbles can be obtained either directly from cut alveolar tissue or indirectly via the airways of undamaged lungs, the surfactant is almost certainly present in a film at the alveolar surfaces. This conclusion is supported by two lines of evidence. First, when a solution of it is placed in the surface balance, the surfactant spontaneously concentrates in the surface. Secondly the electron microscopic studies of Chase (4) show a distinct extracellular film of molecular thickness at the air surfaces of mammalian alveolar membranes.

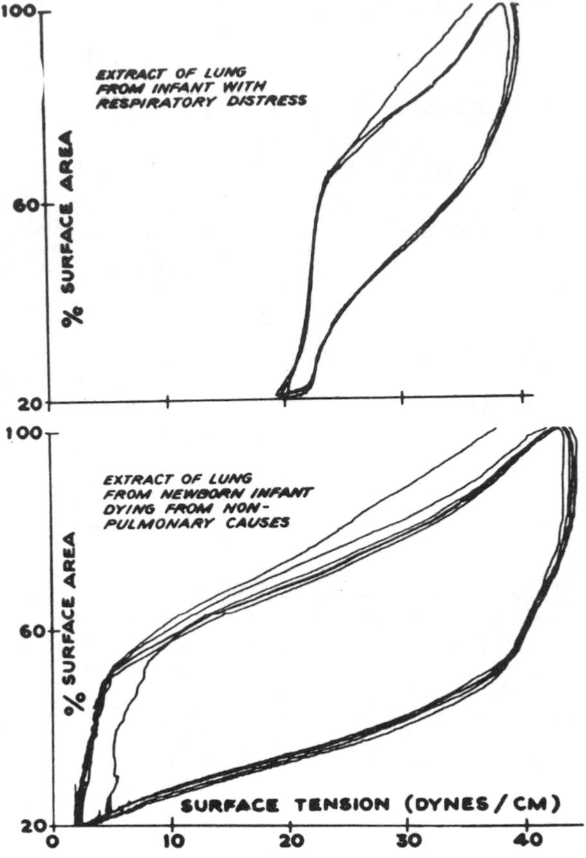

Fig. 7. Respiratory distress in newborn infants.

Let us examine some of Pattle's intriguing data (16). Figure 9 shows a plot of bubble diameter against time. The steep curve to the left indicates how a bubble of air in air-saturated clean water rapidly contracts and disappears from view. The flat curve to the right shows the persistence of an "alveolar bubble" under the same conditions. Using the laws of LaPlace and Fick we have derived an approximate formula (similar to one of Pattle's) which relates the rate of bubble contraction to its surface tension. As the formula in figure 10 indicates, the surface tension is directly proportional to the bubble area and the rate of change of radius, and inversely proportional to the diffusion coefficient and solu-

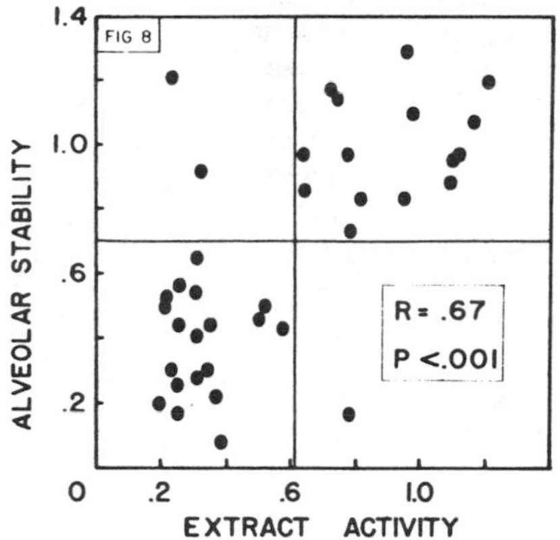

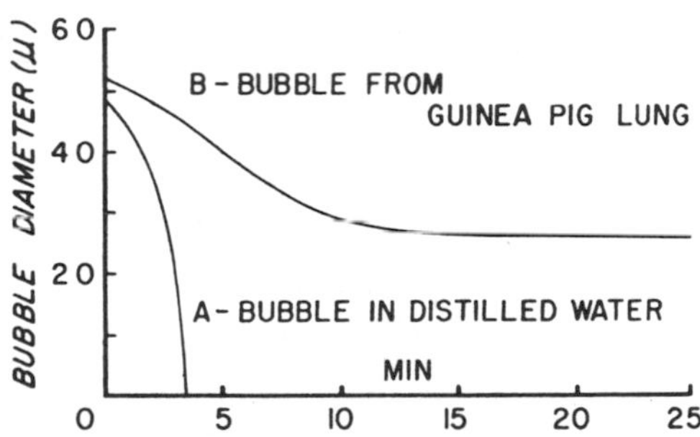

Fig. 9. Contraction of microscopic bubbles in air-saturated water. (Pattle: Proc. Roy. Soc. (London) B 148:223, 1958).

bility of air in water. From Pattle's data (16) we have calculated the relationship between surface area and tension of two "alveolar bubbles". The two curves to the left show that the tension fell from 19 or from 10 dynes/cm to practically zero. The slopes of the curves vary from 0.060 to 0.025 cm/dyne. The third curve is surface balance data on a lung extract; slope varies from 0.025 to 0.099. The curve to the right was calculated from pressure-volume data on a dog lung (3); the slope lies between 0.028 and 0.16. The time interval between points on the curves is about one minute in all cases. When one considers that area-tension slopes for surface films of various biological substances differ by a factor of a million, the six-fold variation shown here does not seem large.

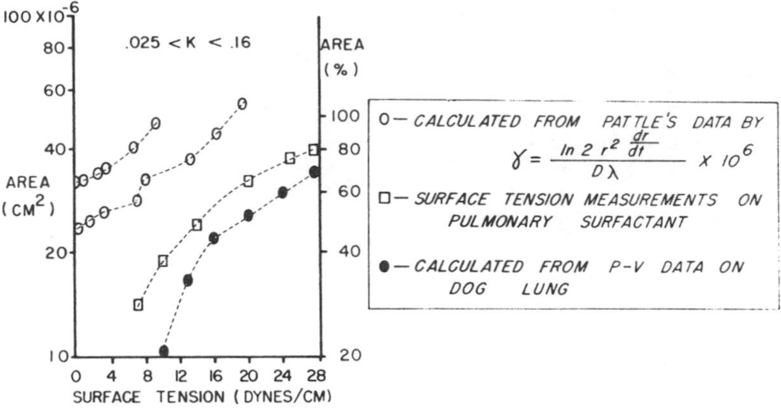

Fig. 10. Tension-area relationship.

Although it has been implied in our previous remarks, we might now make explicit the differential relationship between surface film pressure and surface tension. The effective surface tension of film-covered liquid is the resultant of the contractile strength of the liquid and the force with which the film tends to expand in the surface. Thus, if the water tension is 72 dynes/cm and the film pressure is 60 dynes/cm, the surface tension is 12 dynes/cm. In terms of molecular mechanism there is little difference in this situation between a surface tension of 0.1 and 4 dynes/cm. Although there is a factor of 40 between the tensions, the corresponding film pressures on water are about 68 and 71.9 dynes/cm, a variation of less than 1 part in 20. These considerations make it evident that the change of surface tension that occurs with change of area is really dependent on the elasticity of the surface film; and further that the minimum surface tension that can be achieved in a given system is partly determined by the pressure at which the film collapses. When we say that a material is "highly surface active," we mean that it reduces surface tension to very low values and hence that the surface film it forms is comparatively stable at high pressures. Since the maintenance of moderately low surface tension appears to be important in the lungs, we must therefore be interested in the critical pressure for collapse of films of pulmonary surfactant and the rate at which collapse occurs once initiated. We know from the fundamental studies of Langmuir and Schaefer (10) and others on films of pure substances and on mixtures that these properties depend on molecular size, on the nature, number and arrangement of functional groups in the film molecules, and on the pH and ionic composition of the subjacent liquid. We know that a mixture of two substances can give a film that is more stable than the better component, or less stable, depending upon the nature of the substances. It has also been shown (24) that secondary adsorption of materials from the subphase can unstabilize a surface film, causing it to collapse or desorb from the surface, with a consequent rise in tension; or on the other hand can complex with it, raising the film pressure and lowering surface tension (23). These interactions depend again on the nature of the substances. Studies of this type of phenomena carried out with pulmonary surfactant have been initiated by Tierney and Johnson (26) and have already been helpful in understanding pulmonary responses.

The differential relationship between film pressure and surface tension results in an interesting feedback characteristic in "alveolar bubbles." Let the surface tension be 0.01 dyne/cm, as indicated by Pattle's measurements of the eccentricity of a typical bubble. Then the film pressure is about 71.99 dynes/cm. Let sufficient collapse or desorption of film material occur to lower the film pressure by 0.09 dynes/cm. The surface tension is now 0.1 dyne/cm. The film pressure has diminished about 1 part in 1000 but the surface tension has increased 10-fold. The rate of contraction of the bubble also increases 10-fold, the surface area of the bubble decreases comparatively rapidly, and the remaining film is re-compressed. This occurs because the diffusion of gas from the bubble is increased proportionately 10,000 times as much as film pressure is changed.

Microscopic observation shows this phenomenon to occur periodically, as the surface tension oscillates. If we neglect the oscillation and consider it a slow, steady state of contraction, we can solve the formula shown in figure 10 simultaneously with a general formula relating film pressure, area, and molecular density. The result, given in figure 11, shows that the "steady state" tension is proportional to the size of the bubble and to the rate of loss of film material.

In this situation film pressure, and hence surface tension, are self-determining, and surface area is a dependent variable. We may call it very-low tension state, or the "constant-tension, variable-area," limiting state.

Another limiting state is "constant-area, variable-tension." The lower curve in figure 12 shows the result of compressing an extract of a normal lung in the surface balance to a tension of 4 dynes/cm and holding it at constant area. The tension rises slowly to a higher value, about 36 dynes/cm, as film collapse or desorption occurs. The upper curve gives the result of the same experiment done with an atelectatic newborn lung. The tension rises comparatively rapidly from 28 to about 38 dynes/cm. The rate of change of tension is proportional to the difference between the tension at any time and the final tension. The time constants are about one hour and one minute, respectively. The final tensions are determined by the critical collapse pressures of the films and we shall call them the "critical tensions."

Both the "constant-area" and the "constant-tension" limiting states

$$\gamma_{STEADY} = \frac{\ln 2 \;\; k\,T\,r\,\frac{dn}{dt}_{steady}}{8\,\pi\,D\,\lambda\,\gamma_w} \times 10^6$$

k = *BOLTZMANN CONSTANT*

T = *ABSOLUTE TEMPERATURE*

r = *RADIUS*

D = *DIFFUSION COEFFICIENT OF GAS IN WATER*

λ = *SOLUBILITY OF GAS IN WATER*

γ_w = *SURFACE TENSION OF WATER*

$\frac{dn}{dt}_{steady}$ = *RATE OF FILM COLLAPSE*

Fig. 11. Steady tension $\propto$ radius x rate of film collapse.

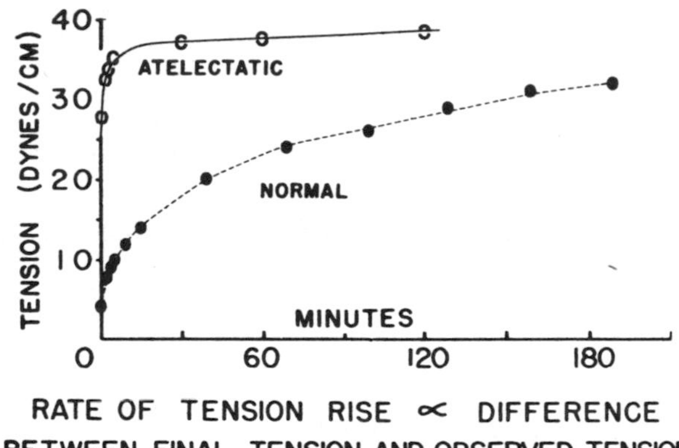

RATE OF TENSION RISE $\propto$ DIFFERENCE BETWEEN FINAL TENSION AND OBSERVED TENSION

$$\frac{d\gamma}{d_t} = K(\gamma_f - \gamma)$$

γ_f = FINAL SURFACE TENSION

K = RATE OF FILM COLLAPSE

Fig. 12

reflect the same property of the surfactant, namely its metastability in the film when compressed above the critical collapse pressure. In the constant-tension state ("alveolar bubbles" in water) the steady tension is nearly zero; in the constant-area state (on the surface balance) about 36 dynes/cm.

Is either of these states apposite to the living lungs? Unfortunately, we cannot come to an irrefutable conclusion by observing the intact organ. It is unlikely that the "very-low-tension state" occurs in normal lungs, because the magnitude of the transpulmonary pressure requires, in addition to tissue recoil, the contribution of significant surface tension. On the other hand, in pathological conditions where transpulmonary pressure is not maintained, the alveolar surfaces might approach the zero-tension state. Indeed, there could be a causal relationship (6).

If the reflexes which regulate lung volume tended to maintain substantially constant alveolar area, the tension might approach 36 dynes/cm. This would be consistent with a transpulmonary pressure of about 10 cm H_2O. However, the maintenance of constant total area would not insure that individual airspaces remained constant, especially in view of their well-known independence of action (21, 22). Since there are very many airspaces, a reasonably small fraction of them could be contracting without significantly changing the average transpulmonary pressure. In terms of a single airspace, this behavior is intermediate between the two limiting states we have been discussing and corresponds to the contraction of a bubble at constant pressure, with rising tension. The relationships between size, tension, and time are complicated but can be approximated by solving simultaneous formulae for alveolar elasticity (including tissue forces), for surface tension versus surface area, and for the rate of film collapse. The resulting expression is given in figure 13 with reasonable values substituted for the variables. At a pressure of 5 cm H_2O the half-life of an average "alveolus" is about equal to the time constant for film collapse, according to the simplified expression at the bottom of the figure. With the time constants from the previous figure, this expression

$$4 \ln \frac{r_i}{r_f} + \frac{2P}{\left(\frac{8E\gamma_{crit}}{r_o} - P^2\right)^{\frac{1}{2}}} \left(\tan^{-1} \frac{\frac{2E}{r_o} r_i - P}{\left(\frac{8E\gamma_{crit}}{r_o} - P^2\right)^{\frac{1}{2}}} - \tan^{-1} \frac{\frac{2E}{r_o} r_f - P}{\left(\frac{8E\gamma_{crit}}{r_o} - P^2\right)^{\frac{1}{2}}} \right) = Kt$$

IF $P = 5$ CM H_2O, $E = 5$ CM H_2O

$r_o = 100\ \mu$, $\gamma_{crit} = 36$

$$t_{50} = \frac{1.06}{K}$$

Fig. 13. Contraction of "alveolus" at constant pressure.

indicates that the alveoli of the normal lung should have half-lives about 60 times as long as those of the lung with hyaline membranes. Needless to say, if the transpulmonary pressure were temporarily raised to expand the airspaces and brought again to low pressure, the individual airspaces would have a new lease on life as their tensions began to rise again from lower values. The frequency of sighs or deep-breaths in the living animal with intact reflexes would be expected to reflect the rate of surface film collapse.

Thus, the time-dependent properties of surface films can endow the lungs with a memory for their volume history. This kind of memory should be limited to about one hour for normal lungs and must be very short for those with hyaline membranes. On this basis we can understand at least qualitatively, the reversible atelectasis and loss of compliance that occur with prolonged shallow breathing at low transpulmonary pressure, and their predilection for dependent regions of the lungs. These calculations of half-life neglect the effect of volume instability on the alveolus. Many airspaces, particularly in lungs with hyaline membranes, collapse or fall to small volumes immediately when transpulmonary pressure is reduced to resting, physiological levels. This action intensifies atelectasis in two ways - by completely removing some units from function, and by shortening the useful lifetime of others.

From quite a different point of view we may expect the tendency for surface tension to rise to have beneficial effects, provided that transpulmonary pressure is maintained at moderate values. The increased pressure gradient required to maintain alveolar volume biases the collapsible portions of the bronchial tree open, and thus acts to homogenize alveolar ventilation. We might speculate that if alveolar surface tension were zero, the tendency to bronchiolar collapse would increase the atelectasis that occurs in the absence of inert gases, especially under circumstances of acceleration and low ambient pressure. Pulmonary function in a space vehicle might be seriously compromised by lack of alveolar surface tension.

I have made a rather long digression to describe microscopic observation of alveolar bubbles and studies of lung extracts with the surface balance, and to develop theoretical notions that might aid the understanding of pulmonary interfacial reactions. If I have dwelt too long on matters of theory it is because some of these concepts also have application to other interfaces in heterogeneous, cellular living things. I do not apologize for the heuristic nature of the argument. I believe, as Henri Poincaré, the great French mathematician and physicist stated, discussing the relations of facts and hypotheses in his "Foundations of Science", that "It is better to foresee even without certainty, than not to foresee at all"(18).

I should like to devote the remaining paragraphs to a discussion of recent advances in the characterization of pulmonary surfactant and related studies of biological reactions of the lungs.

Recently Pattle and Thomas reported (17) that the infrared absorption spectrum of dried pulmonary edema foam is like that of a mixture of 95% lecithin and 5% gelatin. They suggested that the pulmonary surfactant has a similar composition.

In the meantime Klaus, Havel and I had been analyzing the components of dried foam (9) prepared by Bondurant's method (2) from beef lungs. This material is about 70% soluble in 50:50 alcohol-acetone, the remaining material presumptively containing protein. Although the crude powder is highly surface active, neither of these major fractions produces low surface tension in the surface balance. Separation of the lipid fraction on silicic acid columns yields about 74% phospholipids, 8% cholesterol, 10% triglycerides, 8% fatty acids, and essentially no cholesterol esters. At Edgewood, Siakotos (25) separated the lipid fraction by paper chromatography and estimated that the phospholipid fraction is about 40% lecithin and contains several other phosphatides in smaller amounts.

In an elegant experiment Klaus showed that only the phospholipid fraction was capable of giving very low surface tension in the surface balance. This activity disappeared in several hours while the material was in the balance in air. If, however, the measurement was made under nitrogen, the activity remained.

This most important clue may give added insight into the nature of oxygen toxicity not only in the lungs but also in other tissues, where phospholipid-filled membranes are exposed to high partial pressures of oxygen.

The high activity of the crude powder is maintained for several days in air, and it is reasonable to think that it contains substances whose anti-oxidant potential protects the phospholipid fraction. Their presence may be required for preservation of the surfactant film in its normal situation in about 15% oxygen. It is likely that they are the unsaturated lipids of the non-phosphated fractions. Since the combined lipid fraction does not give low surface tensions, the complex most probably is physically stabilized by the presence of protein. Furthermore, the complex surfactant is known to be attacked by trypsin.

The current state of our knowledge indicates that pulmonary surfactant is a complex of at least eight components in fairly definite proportions. These fall into three major categories and a function can be tentatively assigned to each: unsaturated phospholipid to give low tensions; non-phosphated lipid to protect the phospholipids against oxidation; and protein as the skeleton which holds the lipid body together.

The experiments of Tierney and Johnson (26) are of great interest in connection with the properties of the surfactant. They have shown that addition of petroleum ether-soluble lipid from blood, tissue, or even from the strongly active surfactant powder itself can inhibit its activity. The chemically characterized materials thus far known to inhibit the pulmonary surfactant are lipoidal, oxidative, or proteolytic. Tierney and Johnson also found it possible to extract highly surface active material by Bondurant's method from experimentally atelectatic lungs that gave inactive saline extracts. If the surfactant had been destroyed by oxidation or proteolysis, it could not have been extracted by any method. It is possible, therefore, that atelectasis was caused by accumulation of excess free lipid in the alveolar membranes and that the interfering material was rejected in the foam extraction but not in the saline extraction. This concept would fit with the astounding results reported by Tooley, Finley, and Gardner (27). They were studying the mechanism of the respiratory distress that sometimes follows the use of pump-oxygenators on patients undergoing cardiac surgery. By conducting the bypass procedure in experimental animals, they were able to cause the syndrome at will. Both patients and animals died in respiratory failure and at necropsy their lungs were grossly congested and atelectatic. Saline extracts of the lungs were deficient in surface activity.

As the next step in their study Tooley, Finley, and Gardner recirculated donor blood in an extracorporeal circuit and exchange-transfused recipient dogs. If the blood had been pumped 6 hours or longer, the recipients developed congestive atelectasis and died. Saline extracts of their lungs lacked the normal surface activity. In addition these workers found that adding a small quantity of the pumped blood to an active lung extract inhibited it. Normal whole blood had no effect; nor did washed, pumped red cells, hemoglobin, or heparin. Plasma from pumped blood, however, did inhibit an active extract.

These results prove that material is added to the plasma during extracorporeal circulation, which can unstabilize the pulmonary surfactant in extracts and which can produce congestive atelectasis in the living animal. It is tempting to speculate that both effects result from the same interfacial reaction between pulmonary surfactant and free lipid in the plasma. Heparin may play an essential part in the process. Whatever the explanations of these effects may finally prove to be, it is already clear that Tooley, Finley, and Gardner have made an important and exciting contribution to the understanding of pulmonary disease by their demonstration that the lungs can be lethally disturbed by substances liberated in the circulation.

I have restricted this resume of surface phenomena in relation to pulmonary function to mechanical effects and to some chemical and physical properties of interfacial films that may help in explaining such effects. In so doing I have neglected studies of the influence of films on diffusion and electric charge at interfaces. I have said almost nothing about chemical reactions in films and have entirely omitted the interactions of drugs and mediator substances with films, even though these are pertinent to my subject. Studies of such processes are coming into vogue again. It behooves the present-day student to learn the fundamentals of interfacial physics and chemistry well. He will be able to apply them to many fields of biology, as we have already done in a modest and unsophisticated way to pulmonary function. The concepts and methods of surface chemistry and physics which blossomed with such great promise in the '20's and '30's, and which suffered unwonted neglect by biologists in the '40's and '50's may in the '60's and thereafter yield a rich harvest of understanding for physiology.

We follow in the Bowditch tradition. Nathaniel, Henry's father, helped men find their way in the great interface between ocean and sky. Henry performed epochal experiments on excitation and impulse conduction in cells - prime examples of interfacial reactions. Alexander Leathes, professor of physiology at Sheffield, was I believe the first physiologist to use the surface balance and to investigate phospholipid films. He said in his Croonian Lectures (11) before the Royal College of Physicians of London in 1923 that the study of surface films concerns "the very foundations of physiology, though not of physiology alone." And speaking further of surface effects, he said "The role of fats in vital phenomena is a subject on which... much may turn that is important to physiologists and to physicians." Scientists have verified his prediction in part, but his challenge remains.

Acknowledgment

It is a pleasure to acknowledge the stimulation and help of many collaborators and colleagues whose work is the main basis of this lecture.

REFERENCES

1. Avery, M. E., and J. Mead. Am. J. Diseases Children 97:517, 1959.
2. Bondurant, S. J. Clin. Invest. 39:973, 1960.
3. Brown, E. S., R. P. Johnson, and J. A. Clements. J. Appl. Physiol. 14:717, 1959.
4. Chase, W. H. Exptl. Cell Research 18:15, 1959.
5. Chemical Corps Contract DA 18-108 CML 2895, Prog. Rept., 1953.
6. Clements, J. A. Am. Rev. Resp. Diseases 81:741, 1960.
7. Clements, J. A. Proc. Soc. Exptl. Biol. Med. 95:180, 1957.
8. Gruenwald, P. Am. J. Obstet. Gynecol. 53:996, 1947.
9. Klaus, M., J. A. Clements, and R. J. Havel. Program Abstracts, 71st Annual Meeting American Pediatric Soc., May 2-5, 1961, p. 28.
10. Langmuir, I., and V. Schaefer. J. Franklin Inst. 235:119, 1943.
11. Leathes, A. Croonian Lectures, 1923, Lancet 237:851, 1925.
12. Macklin, C. C. Lancet 266:1099, 1954.
13. Mead, J. Am. Rev. Resp. Diseases 81:739, 1960.
14. Mead, J., J. L. Whittenberger, and E. P. Radford, Jr. J. Appl. Physiol. 10:191, 1957.
15. Pattle, R. E. Nature 175:1125, 1955.
16. Pattle, R. E. Proc. Roy. Soc. (London) B 148:217, 1958.
17. Pattle, R. E., and L. C. Thomas Nature 189:844, 1961.
18. Poincare, H. The Foundations of Science, Lancaster, Pa:Science Press, 1946, p. 129.
19. Radford, E. P., Jr. In: Tissue Elasticity. Am. Physiol. Soc. 1957, p. 177.
20. Radford, E. P., Jr. Proc. Soc. Exptl. Biol. Med. 87:58, 1954.
21. Radford, E. P., Jr., N. Lefcoe, and J. Mead. Federation Proc. 13:114, 1954.
22. Radford, E. P., Jr., and M. McLaughlin. Federation Proc. 15:147, 1956.
23. Schulman, J. H., and A. H. Hughes. Biochem. J. 29:1243, 1935.
24. Shanes, A. M., and N. L. Gershfeld. J. Gen. Physiol. 44:345, 1960.
25. Siakotos, A. unpublished observations.
26. Tierney, D. F., and R. P. Johnson. Physiologist 4: 122, 1961.
27. Tooley, W. H., T. N. Finley, and R. Gardner. Physiologist 4:124, 1961.
28. Von Neergaard, K. Z. ges. exptl. Med. 66:373, 1929.
29. Wilson, J. L., and S. Farber. Am. J. Diseases Children 46:590, 1933.

III
PULMONARY CIRCULATION

Papers 38 Through 52

DISCOVERY AND EARLY OBSERVATIONS

38 **IBN NAFĪS**
Excerpts from *Commentary on the Anatomy of the Canon of Avicenna*

39 **SERVETUS**
Excerpt from *Christianismi Restitutio*

40 **HARVEY**
Excerpt from *Movement of the Heart and Blood in Animals*

41 **MALPIGHI**
Excerpt from *Epistle II: About the Lungs*

42 **HOOKE**
An Account of an Experiment Made by M. Hook, of Preserving Animals Alive by Blowing Through Their Lungs with Bellows

43 **LOWER**
Excerpt from *Tractatus de Corde: Item De Motu & Colore Sanguinis et Chyli in cum Transitu*
English translation: *On the Color of the Blood*

PRESSURE AND FLOW

44 **KROGH and LINDHARD**
Excerpts from *Measurements of the Blood Flow Through the Lungs of Man*

45 **LEE and DuBOIS**
Pulmonary Capillary Blood Flow in Man

46 **FORSSMANN**
The Catheterization of the Right Side of the Heart

47 **COURNAND and RANGES**
Catheterization of the Right Auricle in Man

48 **HELLEMS et al.**
Pulmonary "Capillary" Pressure in Man

49 VON EULER and LILJESTRAND
Excerpts from *Observations on the Pulmonary Arterial Blood Pressure in the Cat*

50 BALL et al.
Excerpts from *Regional Pulmonary Function Studied with Xenon*[133]

NONRESPIRATORY FUNCTIONS

51 COLIN
Excerpt from *On Absorption in Airways*

52 GADDUM et al.
5-Hydroxytryptamine. Pharmacological Action and Destruction in Perfused Lungs

EDITOR'S COMMENTS

DISCOVERY AND EARLY OBSERVATIONS

The discovery and rediscovery of pulmonary circulation extended over more than 400 years. Ibn Nafīs, a Damascus physician living in the thirteenth century, was the first to question Galen's view that blood "sweated" from the right to the left ventricle through invisible pores in the interventricular septum (Paper 38). Ibn Nafīs described in unequivocal terms the motion of blood through the lungs; however, his account was unknown to the Western world until 1922.

The next discovery, by Michael Servetus, appeared in a religious tract, "Christianismi Restitutio," in 1553 (Paper 39). Servetus, a Spanish theologian, apparently intrigued with the statement in Genesis that God breathed the divine spirit, the breath of life, into the nostrils of man, performed anatomical studies on the lungs and concluded that the communication between the right and left heart is "not through the middle wall of the heart . . . but by a very ingenious arrangement the subtle blood is urged forward by a long course through the lungs." Because earlier he had challenged religious dogma ("Errors of the Trinity") and continued to challenge Calvin, Servetus was burned at the stake in 1553.

Although not the first to describe the pulmonary circulation,

Harvey (Paper 40) was the first to gain acceptance for his studies. He first presented his observations in a lecture in 1616 and then in *De Motu Cordis* in 1628. Today, 12 years would be a very long lag between a momentous discovery and its publication, but Harvey had no reason to be concerned that another might publish before him. Few had the courage to court Servetus's fate, and Harvey carefully worded his own classic account in a way that would convince sceptics that his observations were correct and at the same time avoid charges of perilous innovation. He succeeded. William Cruikshank, writing in 1790, said:

> When Harvey discovered the circulation of the blood, his opponents first attempted to prove that he was wrong; but finding their ground untenable, they then asserted that it was known long before; Servetus, Colombo and Cesalpinus, all knew it: and when they were informed, that if these gentlemen did know anything of the matter, the world at large were totally ignorant of the fact, and likely to have continued so, except for Harvey, they once more shifted their ground, and said the discovery was of no use.

The course that blood takes from the right to the left ventricle is commonplace knowledge today, but Harvey had no microscope and it took imagination and courage to insist that blood could flow where there were no visible openings. And Harvey, in 1628, knew nothing of oxygen and hemoglobin (that soaked up oxygen) and had to concern himself with how air in the lungs influenced blood when there were never any visible gas bubbles in blood.

Malpighi (Paper 41), a celebrated microscopist of Bologna, completed the circle for Harvey by finding pulmonary capillaries in the frog. "Harvey made the existence of capillaries a logical necessity; Malpighi made it a histological certainty."

Robert Hooke (Paper 42) and Richard Lower (Paper 43), also without knowledge of oxygen and hemoglobin, joined forces in the 1660s to prove that the change in color of venous blood occurs in the lungs because of some interaction with air. Lower used Hooke's continuously inflated lung preparation to show that the color change occurs in air-distended lungs even when the thorax is open and the dog is dead. Hooke used the preparation to prove that the movements of the lung were not essential either for pulmonary blood flow or for life. Note that in his last sentence (his page 540), Hooke says "I shall shortly further try, whether suffering the blood to circulate through a vessel, so as it may be openly exposed to the fresh air, will not suffice for the life of the animal." This promissory note is probably the first recorded allusion to extracorporeal circulation and oxygenation.

PRESSURE AND FLOW

The modern era of measuring pulmonary blood flow started with Krogh and Lindhard, who in 1912 measured pulmonary uptake of nitrous oxide in man (Paper 44). Modified by many investigators between 1912 and 1945, gas uptake methods fell into disuse with the advent of cardiac catheterization and use of the Fick equation. But 10 years later, Lee and DuBois (Paper 45) ingeniously made use of the body plethysmograph to measure pulmonary capillary blood flow on a beat-by-beat basis; this was the first continuous "noninvasive" method to measure pulmonary capillary blood flow (approximately equal, in normal subjects and in many patients, to cardiac output).

Forssmann (Paper 46), Cournand (Paper 47), and Richards won the Nobel prize in physiology or medicine in 1956 for revolutionizing the quantitative study of the whole cardiovascular system and of its separate components by cardiovascular catheterization in man. Forssmann's original goal had been to develop a safe method for giving intracardiac drugs in an emergency (to avoid blind puncture through the chest and myocardial wall), and Cournand and Richards's goal initially had been to obtain mixed venous blood, essential to their physiological study of how air and blood are distributed to alveoli throughout the lung. A few years later, Hellems, Haynes, and Dexter devised a method for estimating left atrial and "pulmonary capillary" pressure in man, another important technical advance needed to study pulmonary circulation (Paper 48).

Regulation of pulmonary circulation was largely ignored until von Euler and Liljestrand's 1946 study (Paper 49). There seemed to be no reason for overall vasoconstriction or for redistribution of total flow within the lungs, although both were obviously useful and had been widely studied in the systemic circulation. Von Euler and Liljestrand found that hypoxia, probably by local action, constricted pulmonary arterioles; their work opened the door to physiological and pharmacological studies of this circulation in the fetus, newborn, and adult.

Another technical advance of great importance was the use of radioactive gases that could be inhaled into the lungs or, dissolved in saline, injected intravenously; their concentration in various regions of the lungs could then be detected by counters applied to the chest wall. The ^{133}xenon technique, as used by Ball and associates (Paper 50), has led to a number of modified techniques now widely employed in diagnostic clinics and physiological laboratories.

NONRESPIRATORY FUNCTIONS

The lungs and pulmonary circulation have important functions other than that of exchanging gases. The arteriolar and capillary beds act as a filter to protect the systemic circulation from emboli; the pulmonary vessels act as a reservoir (in series with the left atrium) for the left ventricle; reflexes from the upper and lower airways protect against some toxic materials in inspired air; the low pulmonary capillary blood pressure provides an elegant mechanism to speed absorption into the blood of fluid in alveoli; and the lung has metabolic functions that trap and inactivate substances in the venous blood or that synthesize materials needed locally or systemically.

Two papers are included to emphasize functions of the pulmonary circulation that are not concerned with gas exchange. The first, Paper 51, is by Colin, who in 1873 reported the very rapid disappearance of large quantities of fluid introduced into the trachea of large animals and who also noted the very rapid appearance in blood (and then in the urine) of some inhaled materials; his experiments called attention to the absorptive capacity of the lungs for fluid and salts and the potential dangers of rapid absorption of poisons into blood flowing through the pulmonary capillary bed.

The second, Paper 52, by Gaddum and associates, opened the exciting new field of the metabolic functions of the lungs when they found that the pulmonary vascular bed takes up 5-OH-tryptamine coming to it in mixed venous blood. Since then, other investigators have found that endothelial cells lining pulmonary capillaries inactivate some materials and convert others from inactive to active substances. Use of the light microscope had strengthened the belief that the alveolar capillary walls were fantastically thin membranes designed for rapid exchange of gases, but use of the electron microscope clearly showed the presence of a variety of cells in the lungs morphologically capable of handling special metabolic functions other than maintaining the integrity of membranes for gas exchange.

38

Reprinted from *Ann. Surg.*, **104**(1), 3, 5, 7 (1936)

A FORGOTTEN CHAPTER IN THE HISTORY OF THE CIRCULATION OF THE BLOOD

Sami I. Haddad, M.D., and Amin A. Khairallah, M.D.

[*Editor's Note:* Pages 287–289 contain translated excerpts from "Commentary on the Anatomy of the Canon of Avicenna," by Ibn Nafīs, dean of the Mansoury Hospital in Cairo, Egypt, in the thirteenth century.]

In the manuscript in our possession —Commentary on the Anatomy of the Canon of Avicenna—Ibn Nafīs clearly and repeatedly describes the pulmonary circulation. The following are literal translations of some of the passages in which he describes it. ". . . Our purpose now is to set forth what we have been able to find of the discussions of the Sheikh, the Rais, Abi Ali al-Husein Ibn Abdallah Ibn Sina, on anatomy in his Canon, and that by collecting what he wrote in the first book of the Canon and the third book of the same, and so arrange properly all that he wrote on anatomy. What has deterred us from engaging in dissection is the authority of the law and our inherent compassion. So we see fit to depend, for the description of the internal organs, on the words of those who have preceded us—of those engaging in dissection—especially the honorable Galen, as his books are the best books that have come down to us on this subject. . . . We have relied chiefly . . . on his sayings, except in a few details which we thought might be mistakes of copyists or the fact that his description had not been given after a thorough observation. In describing the use of these organs we have depended on true observation and honest study, regardless of whether or not these fit the theories of those who have preceded us. . . . We see fit, before starting the discussion of anatomy, to write a preface that will help us to understand this science. The preface contains five discussions. The first is on the difference that animals show regarding their organs. . . ."

In describing the pulmonary vessels and their structure Ibn Nafīs disagrees with Galen and his predecessors as to the cause of the difference in structure between these vessels and the vessels in the other parts of the body. ". . . And we say, and God is the All-Knowing, whereas, one of the functions of the heart is the creation of the spirit from very thin blood strongly miscible with air, and air, so it is necessary to make, in the heart, very thin blood to make possible the creation of the spirit from that mixture. The place where the spirit is created is in the left cavity of the two cavities of the heart. Therefore, it is necessary, in the heart of man and his like—of those who have lungs—

to have another cavity where the blood is thinned to become fit for mixing with the air. For if the air is mixed with the blood while it is still thick, it would not make a homogeneous mixture. This cavity (where the blood is thinned) is the right cavity of the two cavities of the heart. If the blood is thinned in this cavity it must of necessity pass to the left cavity where the spirit is created. *But between these two cavities there is no passage as that part of the heart is closed and has no apparent openings as some believed and no non-apparent opening fit for the passage of this blood as Galen believed.* The pores of the heart there are obliterated and its body is thick, and there is no doubt that the blood, when thinned, *passes in the vena arteriosa to the lung to permeate its substance and mingle with the air, its thinned part purified; and then passes in the arteria venosa to reach the left cavity of the two cavities of the heart; having mixed with the air and* become fit for the creation of the spirit. What is left of this mixture, less attenuated, the lung uses for its own nourishment. This is the reason why the vena arteriosa is made of thick walls and of two coats, so that what passes through its pores be very thin, and the arteria venosa thin and of one coat."

In describing the anatomy of the lung Ibn Nafīs states: "The lung is composed of parts one of which is the bronchi, the second the branches of the arteria venosa and the third the branches of the vena arteriosa, and all of these are connected by loose porous flesh. . . . *The need of the lung for the vena arteriosa is to transport to it the blood that has been thinned and warmed in the heart, so that what seeps through the pores of the branches of this vessel into the alveoli of the lung may mix with what there is of air therein and combine with it, the resultant composite becoming fit to be spirit when this mixing takes place in the left cavity of the heart. The mixture is carried to the left cavity by the arteria venosa.* What is left of that blood in the inside of the branches of the vena arteriosa and passes through its apertures to the body of the lung, would be thicker than the blood that seeps through and more watery, and fit for the nourishment of the lung. This vena arteriosa while it brings to the lung its nourishment, also brings the blood that is very thin and that is fit to become animal spirit when mixed with the air. The use of arteria venosa is to transmit this air that is mixed with the thinned blood to the left cavity of the two cavities of the heart to become spirit. Another use is for the passage of what is left in this cavity of that mixture which was not fit for the creation of the spirit and of what is left in it of air that is overheated and useless. Both of these must come out of the cavity to make space for what comes afterwards of air alone or of air mixed with greatly thinned blood. So this vessel carries back these things to the lung to be discharged with the returning breath (expiration)."

[*Editor's Note:* Material has been omitted at this point.]

"*Therefore, for the nourishment of the spirit that is in the heart, it is necessary for the blood to become attenuated in the heart and its consistency very much thinned, then pass to the lung and mix with what there is of air there and be cooked in it until it is tempered and become fit for the nourishment of the spirit, and afterwards pass to the spirit that is in the heart and mix with it and nourish it. . . .*

[*Editor's Note:* Material has been omitted at this point.]

" the heart has only two ventricles, one filled with blood on the right side and the other filled with the spirit on the left side, *and between these two there is absolutely no opening for if there were, the blood would pass to the place of the spirit and spoil its essence. Also dissection gives the lie to what they said, as the septum between these two cavities is much thicker than elsewhere, lest some blood or spirit pass through and get lost.* . . . Again, his (Avicenna's) statement that the blood that is in the right side is to nourish the heart is not true at all, for the nourishment to the heart is from the blood that goes through the vessels that permeate the body of the heart. . . . *The benefit of this blood (that is in the right cavity) when it is thinned and attenuated is to go up to the lung, mix with what is in the lung of air, then pass through the arteria venosa to the left cavity of the two cavities of the heart and of that mixture is created the animal spirit.*"

[*Editor's Note:* Material has been omitted at this point.]

39

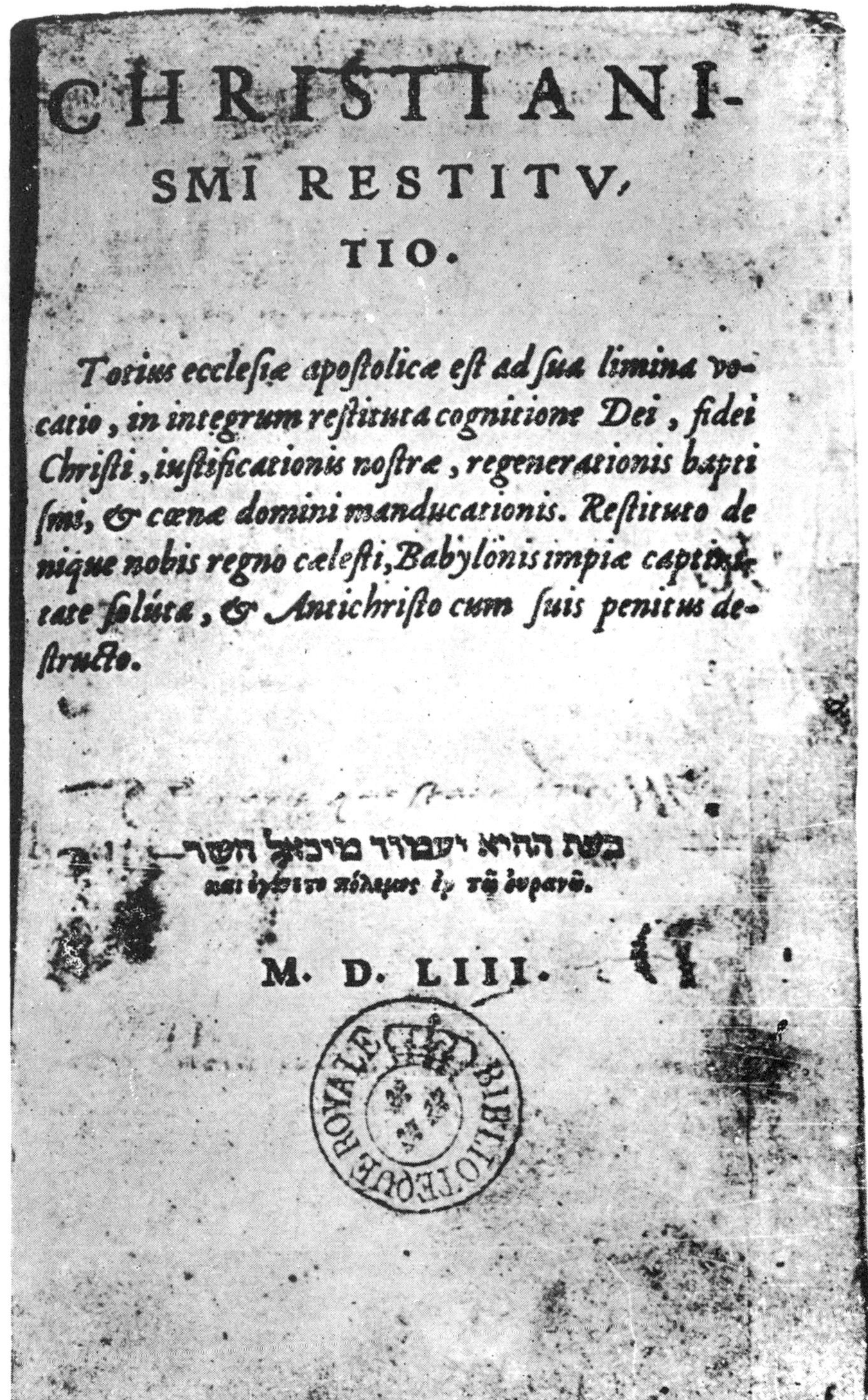

CHRISTIANI-
SMI RESTITV-
TIO.

Totius ecclesiæ apostolicæ est ad sua limina vocatio, in integrum restituta cognitione Dei, fidei Christi, iustificationis nostræ, regenerationis baptismi, & cœnæ domini manducationis. Restituto denique nobis regno cælesti, Babylonis impiæ captiuitate solúta, & Antichristo cum suis penitus destructo.

בעת ההיא יעמוד מיכאל השר
καὶ ἐγένετο πόλεμος ἐν τῷ οὐρανῷ.

M. D. LIII.

Reprinted from *Michael Servetus, A Translation of His Geographical, Medical and Astrological Writings with Introductions and Notes,* C. D. O'Malley, trans., American Philosophical Society, Philadelphia, 1953, pp. 204–205

[*Editor's Note:* In the original, material precedes this excerpt.]

In this matter there must first be understood the substantial generation of the vital spirit which is composed of a very subtle blood nourished by the inspired air. The vital spirit has its origin in the left ventricle of the heart, and the lungs assist greatly in its generation. It is a rarefied spirit, elaborated by the force of heat, reddish-yellow (*flavo*) and of fiery potency, so that it is a kind of clear vapor from very pure blood, containing in itself the substance of water, air and fire. It is generated in the lungs from a mixture of inspired air with elaborated, subtle blood which the right ventricle of the heart communicates to the left. However, this communication is made not through the middle wall of the heart, as is commonly believed, but by a very ingenious arrangement the subtle blood is urged forward by a long course through the lungs; it is elaborated by the lungs, becomes reddish-yellow and is poured from the pulmonary artery into the pulmonary vein. Then in the pulmonary vein it is mixed with inspired air and through expiration it is cleansed of its sooty vapors. Thus finally the whole mixture, suitably prepared for the production of the vital spirit, is drawn onward from the left ventricle of the heart by diastole.

That the communication and elaboration are accomplished in this way through the lungs we are taught by the different conjunctions and the communication of the pulmonary artery with the pulmonary vein in the lungs. The notable size of the pulmonary artery confirms this; that is, it was not made of such sort or of such size, nor does it emit so great a force of pure blood from the heart itself into the lungs merely for their nourishment; nor would the heart be of such service to the lungs, since at an earlier stage, in the embryo, the lungs, as Galen teaches, are nourished from elsewhere because those little membranes or valvules of the heart are not opened until the time of birth. Therefore that the blood is poured from the heart into the lungs at the very time of birth, and so copiously, is for another purpose. Likewise, not merely air, but air mixed with blood, is sent from the lungs to the heart through the pulmonary vein; therefore the mixture occurs in the lungs. That reddish-yellow color is given to the spirituous blood by the lungs; it is not from the heart.

[*Editor's Note:* Material has been omitted at this point.]

40

EXERCITATIO

ANATOMICA DE MOTU CORDIS ET SAN-GUINIS IN ANIMALI-BUS,

GUILIELMI HARVEI ANGLI,

Medici Regii, & Professoris Anatomiæ in Col-legio Medicorum Londinensi.

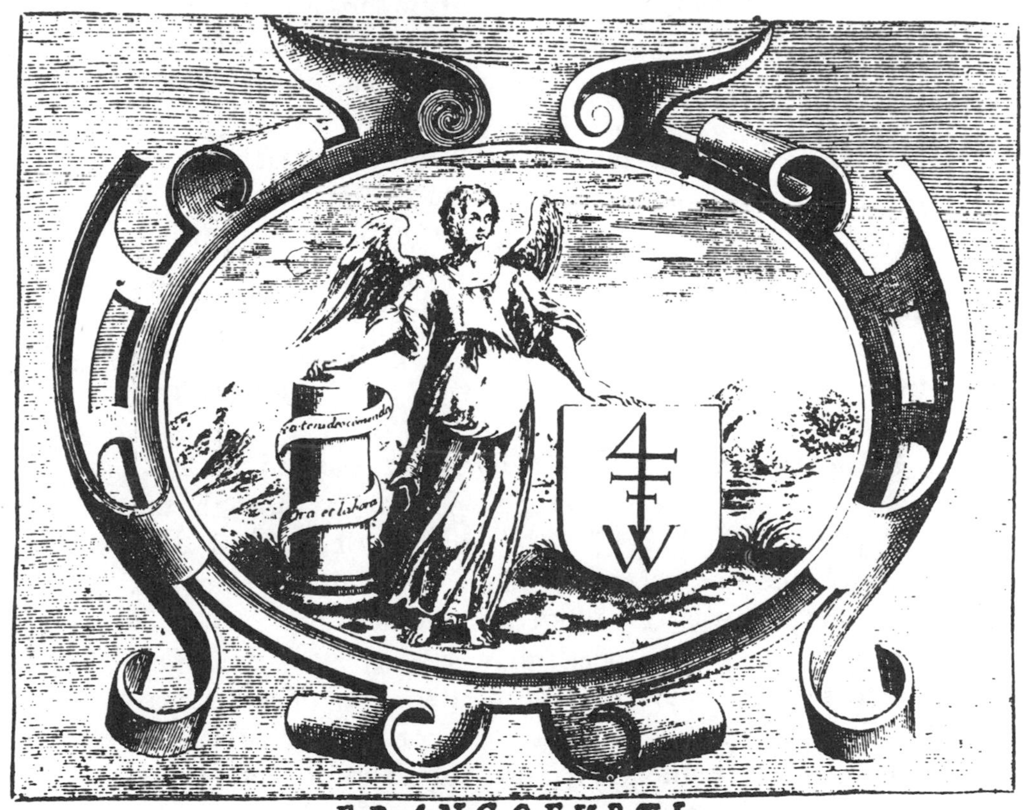

FRANCOFURTI,

Sumptibus GUILIELMI FITZERI.

ANNO M. DC. XXVIII.

Reprinted from *Movement of the Heart and Blood in Animals, An Anatomical Essay by William Harvey, 1628,* Kenneth Franklin, trans. Blackwell Scientific Publications Ltd., Oxford, 1957, pp. 51–56, 87

CHAPTER SEVEN

The blood permeates from the right ventricle of the heart through the parenchyma of the lungs into the vein-like artery and the left ventricle

WE may agree that this can happen and that there is nothing to prevent it from happening when we think how water, permeating through the earth's substance, gives rise to streams and springs; or observe how sweats pass through the skin, or urine through the parenchyma of the kidneys. It is to be noted in those who use the waters of Spa, or the so-called waters of 'our Lady' in the Paduan countryside, or other waters of a mineral or sulphurous character, or in people who just measure their drink in gallons, that one to two hours suffice for them to pass it all out through the bladder as urine. The digestion of such a quantity must take a little while; and it must flow on through the liver (which all agree produces each day a double flow of juice from the food ingested), the veins, the parenchyma of the kidneys, and the ureters into the bladder.

Whom then do I hear denying that blood, indeed, the whole mass of the blood, permeates through the substance of the lungs just as the juice of the food does through the liver, saying that such cannot happen, and must be regarded as altogether incredible? Such folk (in the words of the poet) allow readily that something can take place when they wish it so, but deny its possibility completely when they do not wish it so. They fear to assert it when it is necessary, and do not fear so when it is unnecessary.

The parenchyma of the liver is denser by far, and that

of the kidneys likewise. That of the lungs is of much finer texture, and spongy by comparison with the kidneys and the liver. In the liver there is no inthrust, no driving force; in the lung, the blood is pushed in by the pulsation of the right ventricle of the heart, and by this inthrust the vessels and porosities of the lungs must be distended. Moreover,* in breathing the lungs rise and fall, movement that necessitates the opening and closing respectively of the porosities and vessels; as happens in sponges, and in all parts having a spongy-make-up, when they constrict and subsequently dilate. The liver, on the other hand, remains quiescent and has not been seen to dilate and constrict in this way.

Lastly, everyone agrees that the whole of the juice of the ingesta can pass through the liver into the vena cava in man as in the ox or in very large animals, and people have had to admit exactly this if nutriment is somehow to get through the liver to the veins for the purpose of nutrition and no other way is available. Why, in these circumstances, should they not have equal faith in the same proofs of the passage of blood through the lungs in these post-natal subjects, and assert and believe as did the very skilful and learned anatomist, Colombo, from the size and structure of the vessels of the lungs, and from the fact that the vein-like artery and likewise the ventricle are always full of blood which must have come to them through the veins and by no other path than an intrapulmonary one? He was, and we are, convinced of the truth of this by what has already been stated, by what has been seen in inspection of living animals, and by other proofs.

Since, however, there are some who defer only to duly adduced authorities, let these men know that this truth can be established from Galen's own words.

* *Galenus, De usu partium.*

Indeed, not only can blood pass from the artery-like vein into the vein-like artery and thence into the left ventricle of the heart and afterwards into the arteries, but this happens because of the continuous pulsations of the heart, and of the movement of the lungs in breathing.

There are in the opening into the artery-like vein three sigmoid or crescentic valves which completely prevent blood discharged into the artery-like vein from returning into the heart. That is known to all; indeed, Galen* explains the need and function of these valves in the following words. *Throughout*, he says, *there is a mutual intercommunication and opening up of arterio-venous connections, and they exchange blood and spirit through certain invisible and quite narrow passages. Had the entry into the artery-like vein likewise remained patent all the while, and had Nature not found a means of shutting it at need and of re-opening it, the blood could never (in the contracted state of the thorax) have been transferred into the arteries through invisible narrow connections. However, neither indrawing nor expulsion are completely simple processes. For, on the one hand, that which is light is more easily drawn in than that which is heavier when the means of access are dilated, and more easily expressed when they are contracted. On the other hand, a wide passage is more conducive than a narrow one to swift indrawing and subsequent expulsion. When the thorax contracts, the vein-like arteries in the lung, pushed and pressed in upon from all sides, express indeed their contained spirit, but also take up through those delicate connections that have been mentioned a certain portion of the blood. This could certainly never have happened had the blood been able to move back towards the heart through a large opening, such as that of the artery-like vein. As it is, with the return through the large opening shut off, it distils off a small amount into the arteries through*

* *Galen. de usu part., lib.* vi, *cap.* 10.

the small openings that have been mentioned. And in a closely following chapter he says: *The more the thorax contracts increasingly strongly in squeezing out the blood, the more the membranes (i.e. the sigmoid valves) occlude with ever greater precision the opening itself, and permit of no backflow.* Just before this in the same Chapter Ten he says: *Without the valves, a triple inconvenience would ensue. The blood itself would keep travelling over this long course to no purpose, flowing forwards it is true in the diastoles of the lung and refilling all the veins within the organ, but in its systoles, like a sea-tide patterned on Euripus, continually reversing the movement to all parts, which would in no way suit the blood. In itself this may appear of little moment, but the fact that meanwhile it upsets the object of respiration itself can certainly not be regarded as trifling,* and so forth. And a little later he adds: *And still a third inconvenience would have ensued, and that by no means an insignificant one, for the blood would have gone backwards in the acts of expiration, had not our Creator devised that outgrowth of membranes.* This leads on to his conclusion in the Eleventh Chapter. *The common purpose of them all* (i.e. of the valves) *is to prevent things from moving backwards again. But each kind has its own special purpose. In the cases of those which direct things out of the heart it is to prevent backflow into that organ; in the cases of those which direct things into the heart, it is to prevent any outflow from it. For Nature did not wish the heart to be tired by unnecessary work, such as on occasion distributing to a part from which it has been preferable to receive, or frequently withdrawing from another part which should have been receiving. As there are altogether four openings, two in each ventricle, one of each pair leads in and the other out.* And a little later he adds: *Further, since there is one vessel, consisting of a single coat, inserted into the heart, and another, consisting of two coats, extending away from it, a place common to both*

(Galen had in mind the right ventricle, but the present writer finds the left ventricle equally indicated) *had to be prepared to serve as a kind of pool to which both belong, but into which blood is carried by one vessel and from which it is dispatched by the other.*

The proof which Galen adduces for the passage of blood from the vena cava through the right ventricle and into the lungs can more rightly be used, if only the names are changed, for the passage of blood from the veins through the heart into the arteries, and I should like so to use it. Thus extracts from the writings of Galen, the revered Sire of Physicians, clearly show that blood passes from the artery-like vein through the lungs and into the small branches of the vein-like artery because of the pulsation of the heart and the movement of the lungs and thorax. They show, further, that the heart is constantly receiving and discharging blood, with the ventricles acting as pools, and that for this reason, of the four kinds of valve present, two subserve entry and two exit of blood. This ensures that the blood does not follow Euripus and become unduly disturbed, moving hither and thither or even backwards to the spot which it should have left, and flowing away from the part to which it should have been directed. In this way the heart would become tired by useless work, and the respiration of the lungs would be impeded.* Finally, there is support for our claim that blood is continuously and unceasingly passing through the porosities of the lungs from the right to the left ventricle, from the vena cava into the aorta. For, as blood is continuously discharged from the right ventricle into the lungs through the artery-like vein, and is likewise continuously drawn from the lungs into the left ventricle (as is clear from what

* See the Commentary of the learned Hofmann on Galen, *De usu partium*, lib. 6. I saw this book after writing these passages.

has been said, and from the position of the valves), it must continuously make the complete circuit.

In like manner, as blood is always continuously entering the right ventricle of the heart, and continuously emerging from the left one (as reason and sense alike show it to be), it cannot do other than pass right through from the vena cava into the aorta.

Thus that which dissection establishes as occurring through very wide passages in the majority of animals, and certainly in all animals before they are fully developed, is equally well established as occurring (according to Galen's statements and to what I have said above) in these fully developed animals through the invisible porosities of their lungs and the minute connections of the lung vessels. From which it is clear that one ventricle of the heart (namely, the left one) would suffice to distribute the blood through the body and to withdraw it from the vena cava (which indeed is the way it happens in all lungless creatures). When, however, Nature wished the blood to be filtered through lungs, she was forced to make the extra provision of a right ventricle so that its pulsation would drive the blood through these very lungs from the vena cava to the region of the left ventricle. Thus one has to regard the right ventricle as having been made for the sake of the lungs and the transfer of blood, and not merely for nutrition. It is altogether incongruous to suppose that the lungs need for their nourishment so large a supply of food, so pulsatorily delivered, and also so much purer and more spirituous (as being supplied direct from the ventricles of the heart). For they cannot need such more than does the extremely pure substance of the brain, or the very fine and ineffable fabric of the eyes, or the flesh of the heart itself (which is more directly nourished through the coronary artery).

[*Editor's Note:* Material has been omitted at this point.]

CHAPTER FOURTEEN

Conclusion of my description of the circuit of the blood

MAY I now be permitted to summarize my view about the circuit of the blood, and to make it generally known!

Since calculations and visual demonstrations have confirmed all my suppositions, to wit, that the blood is passed through the lungs and the heart by the pulsation of the ventricles, is forcibly ejected to all parts of the body, therein steals into the veins and the porosities of the flesh, flows back everywhere through those very veins from the circumference to the centre, from small veins into larger ones, and thence comes at last into the vena cava and to the auricle of the heart; all this, too, in such amount and with so large a flux and reflux—from the heart out to the periphery, and back from the periphery to the heart—that it cannot be supplied from the ingesta, and is also in much greater bulk than would suffice for nutrition.

I am obliged to conclude that in animals the blood is driven round a circuit with an unceasing, circular sort of movement, that this is an activity or function of the heart which it carries out by virtue of its pulsation, and that in sum it constitutes the sole reason for that heart's pulsatile movement.

41

Reprinted from *De Pulmonibus* by Marcellus Malpighi (1661), James Young, trans., *Proc. R. Soc. Med.*, **23**, 7–11 (1929–1930)

EPISTLE II: ABOUT THE LUNGS

Marcellus Malpighi

[*Editor's Note:* In the original, material precedes this excerpt.]

There is this difficulty and obscurity to be met with in natural things, that there seems to be something in them that is not to be determined altogether by our senses. And so, steadfastly working with very great labour, we may contemplate Nature showing herself in her beginnings, as it were in a volume elaborated through mysteries. And when we try to unravel the obscure things in the viscera of animals, at length by our efforts, and only with great weariness, we conclude that the truth of our observations is made out. We borrow illumination, as if by degrees, from dissection, sometimes of insects, sometimes of perfect animals. For Nature is accustomed to rehearse with certain large, perhaps baser, and all classes of wild (animals), and to place in the imperfect the rudiments of the perfect animals.

And now, most famous man, I will handle the matter more closely. There were two things which, in my epistle about observation on the lungs, I left as doubtful and to be investigated with more exact study.

(1) The first was what may be the network described therein, where certain bladders and sinuses are bound together in a certain way in the lungs.

(2) The other was whether the vessels of the lungs are connected by mutual anastomosis, or gape into the common substance of the lungs and sinuses.

The solution of these problems may prepare the way for greater things and will place the operations of nature more clearly before the eyes. For the unloosing of these knots I have destroyed almost the whole race of frogs, which does not happen in that savage Batrachomyomachia of Homer. For in the anatomy of frogs, which, by favour of my very excellent colleague D. Carolo Fracassato, I had set on foot in order to become more certain about the membranous substance of the lungs, it happened to me to see such things that not undeservedly I can better make use of that (saying) of Homer for the present matter—

"I see with my eyes a work trusty and great."

For in this (frog anatomy) owing to the simplicity of the structure, and the almost complete transparency of the vessels which admits the eye into the interior, things are more clearly shown so that they will bring the light to other more obscure matters.

In the frog, therefore, the abdomen being laid open lengthwise, the lungs, adhering on each side to the heart, come forth. They are not slack as in other animals, but remain tense for the animal's requirements. They are nothing more than a membranous bladder, which at first sight seems to be spattered with very small spots, arranged in order after the fashion of the skin of the dogfish—

commonly called Sagrino. In form and surface protuberances it resembles the cone of a pine: but internally and externally a certain texture of vessels diversely prolonged is connected together, which, by the pulse, by contrary movement, and the insertion of the vein, are pulmonary arteries. In the concave and interior part of this (bladder) it almost fades into an empty space devoted to the reception of air, but it is not everywhere smooth but is interrupted by the occurrence of alveoli. These are produced by membranous walls raised to a little height. They are not all of this shape, but when the walls are produced out in length and width and connected together, the bays (sinuses) are formed almost into hexagons; and bent at the corners of the sinuses the membrane is extended a little as an infundibulum is constituted; and thus the lungs of the smaller frogs are fashioned. But in those which are larger, the walls are raised higher, and from the middle of the enclosed floor three come out very visibly increasing. The partitions in the smaller frogs are almost unobservable, but those in the bigger ones are bound into three other sinuses as they divide the greater sinus very much. The area, or the floor of the sinuses, admits the vessels spoken of above, and the artery itself sometimes ends inconspicuously, fork-like in the middle, but further on is spread out at the greater passage and sometimes manifestly produces another branch, but the vein glides down the inner slopes of the walls and is mingled with these, and, the branches having been sent down through the walls, at length runs into the area.

Observation by means of the microscope will reveal more wonderful things than those viewed in regard to mere structure and connection: for while the heart is still beating the contrary (i.e., in opposite directions in the different vessels) movement of the blood is observed in the vessels,—though with difficulty,—so that the circulation of the blood is clearly exposed. This is more clearly recognized in the mesentery and in the other greater veins contained in the abdomen.

Thus by this impulse the blood is driven in very small (streams) through the arteries like a flood into the several cells, one or other branch clearly passing through or ending there. Thus the blood, much divided, puts off its red colour, and, carried round in a winding way, is poured out on all sides till at length it may reach the walls, the angles, and the absorbing branches of the veins.

The power of the eye could not be extended further in the opened living animal, hence I had believed that this body of the blood breaks into the empty space, and is collected again by a gaping vessel and by the structure of the walls. The tortuous and diffused motion of the blood in divers directions, and its union at a determinate place offered a handle to this. But the dried lung of the frog made my belief dubious. This lung had, by chance, preserved the redness of the blood in (what afterwards proved to be) the smallest vessels, where by means of a more perfect lens, no more there met the eye the points forming the skin called Sagrino, but vessels mingled annularly. And, so great is the divarication of these vessels as they go out, here from a vein, there from an artery, that order is no longer preserved, but a network appears made up of the prolongations of both vessels. This network occupies not only the whole floor, but extends also to the walls, and is attached to the outgoing vessel, as I could see with greater difficulty but more abundantly in the oblong lung of a tortoise, which is similarly membranous and transparent. Here it was clear to sense that the blood flows away through the tortuous vessels, that it is not poured into spaces but always works through tubules, and is dispersed by the multiplex winding of the vessels. Nor is it a new practice of Nature to join together the extremities of vessels, since the same holds in the intestines and other parts; nay, what seems more wonderful, she joins the upper and the lower ends of veins to one another by visible anastomosis, as the most learned Fallopius has very well observed.

But in order that you may more easily get hold of what I have said, and follow it with your own sight, tie with a thread, just where it joins the heart, the projecting swollen lung of an opened frog while it is bathed on every side with abundant blood. This, when dried, will preserve the vessels turgid with blood. You will see this very well if you examine it by the microscope of one lens against the horizontal sun. Or you may institute another method of seeing these things. Place the lung on a crystal plate illuminated below through a tube by a lighted candle. To it bring a microscope of two lenses, and thus the vessels distributed in a ring-like fashion will be disclosed to you. By the same arrangement of the instruments and light, you will observe the movement of the blood through the vessels in question. You will yourself be able to contrive it by different degrees of light, which escape description by the pen. About the movement of the blood, however, one thing shows itself, worthy of your speculation. The auricle and the heart being ligatured, and thus deprived of motion and the impulse which might be derived from the heart into the connected vessels, the blood is still moved by the veins toward the heart so that it distends the vessels by its effort and copious flow. This lasts several hours. At the end, however, especially if it is exposed to the solar rays, it is agitated, not by the same continued motion, but, as if impelled by changing impulses, it advances and recedes fluctuating along the same way. This takes place when the heart and auricle are removed from the body.

From these things, therefore, as to the first problems to be solved, from analogy and the simplicity which Nature uses in all her operations, it can be inferred that that network which formerly I believed to be nervous in nature, mingled in the bladders and sinuses, is (really) a vessel carrying the body of blood thither or carrying it away. Also that, although in the lungs of perfect animals the vessels seem sometimes to gape and end in the midst of the network of rings, nevertheless, it is likely that, as in the cells of frogs and tortoises, that vessel is prolonged further into very small vessels in the form of a network, and these escape the senses on account of their exquisite smallness.

Also from these things can be solved with the greatest probability the question of the mutual union and anastomosis of the vessels. For if Nature turns the blood about in vessels, and combines the ends of the vessels in a network, it is likely that in other cases an anastomosis joins them ; this is clearly recognized in the bladder of frogs swollen with urine, in which the above described motion of the blood is observed through the transparent vessels joined together by anastomosis, and not that those vessels have received that connection and course which the veins or fibres mark out in the leaves of nearly all trees.

To what purpose all these things may be made, beyond those which I dealt with in the last letter concerning the pulmonary mixing of the blood, you yourself seemed to recognize readily, nor is the opinion to be lessened by your very famous device, because by your kindness you have entrusted me with elaborate letters in which you philosophised subtly by observing the strange portents of Nature in vegetables, when we wonder that apples hang from trunks not their own, and that by grafting of plants the processes have produced bastards in happy association with legitimates. We see that one and the same tree has assumed diverse fashions in its branches,—while here the hanging fruits please the taste by a grateful acidity, there they fulfil every desire by their nectar-like sweetness, and you furnish credibility to the truth at which you wondered when in Rome, that the vine and the jasmine had come forth from the bole of the Massilian apple. He who cultivated the gardens with a light inserted fork made these clever things with bigger branches, and he taught the unreluctant trees the bringing forth of divers things. About this matter Virgil in the Georgics fitly sang :—

"They ingraft the sprout from the alien tree
And teach it to grow from the moist inner bark."

You lay bare the secret of this wonderful result by your philosophising method, for we might consider the acid juice of the Massilian apple sweetens to the nature of pure wine as far as the particles of that juice may run through the small openings of the trunk proper, but not in the same way can they come up into the continued tubules of the vine. Here, stirred by their own motion, and torn away beyond their usual order by the impulse of those following after, and broken up, they must conform themselves to the superinduced form of the passage, and put on the new nature by which the vine or the jasmine is brought forth. Nature pursues a like mode of operation in the lungs, for the turbid blood returns from the ambit of the body, widowed elsewhere of particles, to which a new humour from the subclavian vein is added to be perfected by the further action of Nature. This happens in order that it may be arranged and prepared into the nature of particles of flesh, bone, nerve, etc., while it enters the myriad vessels of the lungs. It is conducted into divers very small threads. Thus a new form, situation, and motion is prepared for the particles of the blood, from which flesh, bone, and spirits may be formed. The trustworthiness of your saying is increased by the like structure of the seminal vessels as if a certain nutrition of the living animal were also its regeneration.

I have put these few little observations into a letter that I might increase the things found out about the lungs. If I have set in motion all the point of my observations I have owed the addition to the frog. You will bring out the truth and dignity of these matters by your authority and contrivance. Meantime, apply yourself happily to philosophy, and may you go on to render me altogether happy by increasing a little my very unimportant thoughts of your writings "De Animalium Motu."

Farewell! Bologna, 1661.

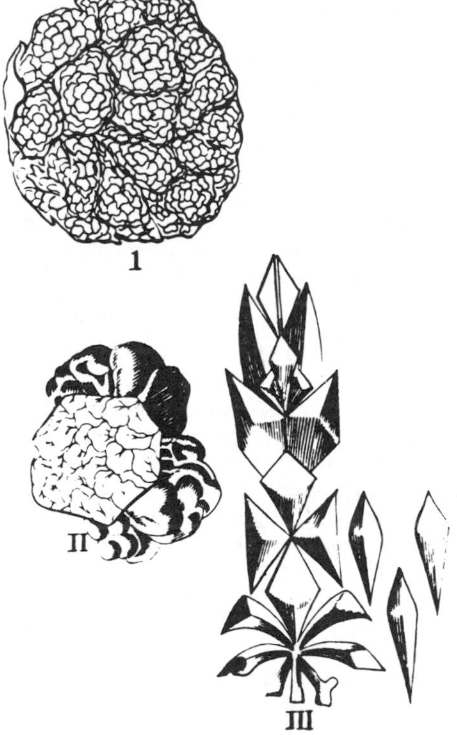

Tabula I.

FIG. I.—Outermost piece of dried lung showing the rete.

FIG. II.—Interior vesicles and sinuses sketched with portion of the interstitium in the upper part. The beginning and complete prolongation could not be exhibited to the eye by the picture.

FIG. III.—Adaptation over the trachea and the pulmonary vessels which also, parted from their usual site, are shown for easier understanding.

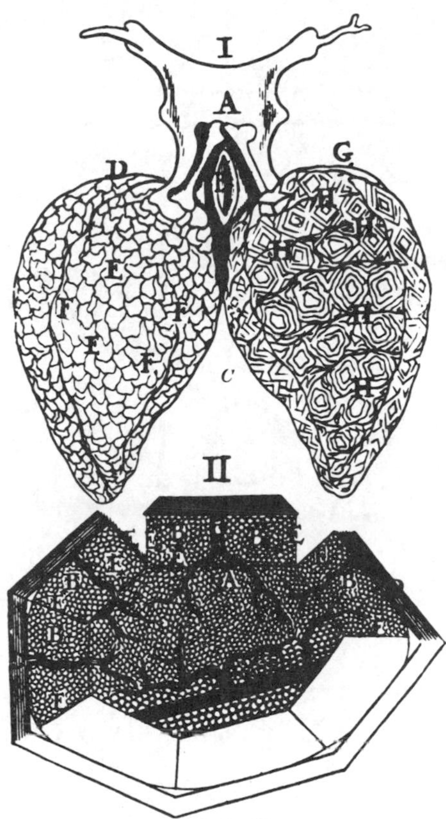

Tabula II.

FIG. I.—Showing lungs of frogs with trachea attached. (*A*) Larynx, which is semi-cartilaginous. (*B*) Rima, which is accurately closed and opened at the animal's need. Air being enclosed it keeps the lungs expanded. (*C*) Site of the heart. (*D*) External part of the lung. (*E*) Prolonged rete of the cells. (*F*) Prolongation of the pulmonary artery. (*G*) Concave part of the lung divided through the middle. (*H*) Prolongation of the pulmonary vein running through the apices.

FIG. II.—Containing the most simple cell without the intermediate walls (magnified). (*A*) Interior floor of the cell. (*B*) Parietes separated and bent. (*C*) Trunk of pulmonary artery with attached branches, as if ending in a network. (*D*) Trunk of pulmonary vein wandering with its branches over the slopes of the walls. (*E*) Vessel in the bottom and corners of the walls with the ramifications of the rete continued.

PHILOSOPHICAL

Tranſactions:

GIVING SOME

ACCOMPT

OF THE

Preſent Undertakings, Studies, and Labours

OF THE

INGENIOUS

IN MANY

CONSIDERABLE PARTS

OF THE

WORLD.

VOL. II.

For *Anno* 1667.

In the *SAVOY*.

Printed by *T. N.* for *John Martyn* at the Bell, a little without *Temple-Bar*, Printer to the *Royal Society*.

Reprinted from *Philos. Trans.*, **2**, 539–540 (1667)

AN ACCOUNT OF AN EXPERIMENT MADE BY M. HOOK, OF PRESERVING ANIMALS ALIVE BY BLOWING THROUGH THEIR LUNGS WITH BELLOWS

Robert Hooke

This Noble Experiment came not to the Publisher's *hands, till all the preceding Particulars were already sent to the Press, and almost all Printed off, (for which cause also it could not be mentioned among the* Contents:) *And it might have been reserved for the next opportunity, had not the considerableness thereof been a motive to hasten its Publication. It shall be here annexed in the Ingenious* Author *his own words, as he presented it to the* Royal Society, Octob. 24. 1667. *the Experiment it self having been* both *repeated (after a former successful trial of it, made by the same hand a good while agoe)* and *improved the week before, at their* publick Assembly. *The Relation it self followes*;

I Did heretofore give this *Illustrious Society* an account of an Experiment I formerly tryed of keeping a Dog alive after his *Thorax* was all display'd by the cutting away of the *Ribbs* and *Diaphragme*; and after the *Pericardium* of the Heart also was taken off. But divers persons seeming to doubt of the certainty of the Experiment (by reason that some Tryals of this matter, made by some other hands, failed of success) I caus'd at the last Meeting the same Experiment to be shewn in the presence of this *Noble Company*, and that with the same success, as it had been made by me at first; the Dog being kept alive by the Reciprocal blowing up of his Lungs with *Bellowes*, and they suffered to subside, for the space of an hour or more, after his *Thorax* had been so display'd, and his *Aspera arteria* cut off just below the *Epiglottis*, and bound on upon the nose of the Bellows.

And because some Eminent Physitians had affirm'd, that the *Motion of the Lungs* was necessary to Life upon the account of promoting the Circulation of the Blood, and that it was conceiv'd, the Animal would immediately be suffocated as soon as the Lungs should cease to be moved, I did (the better to fortifie my own *Hypothesis* of this matter, and to be the better able to judge of several others) make the following additional Experiment; *viz.*

The Dog having been kept alive, (as I have now mentioned) for above an houre, in which time the Tryal had been often repeated, in suffering the Dog to fall into *Convulsive* motions by ceasing to blow the Bellows, and permitting the Lungs to subside and lye still, and of suddenly reviving him again by renewing the blast, and consequently the motion of the Lungs: This, I say, having been done, and the Judicious Spectators fully satisfied of the reallity of the former Experiment; I caused another pair of Bellowes to be immediately joyn'd to the first, by a contrivance, I had prepar'd, and pricking all the outer-coat of the Lungs with the slender point of a very sharp pen-knife, this second pair

pair of Bellows was mov'd very quick, whereby the first pair was alwayes kept full and alwayes blowing into the Lungs; by which means the Lungs also were alwayes kept very full, and without any motion; there being a continual blast of Air forc'd into the Lungs by the first pair of Bellows, supplying it as fast, as it could find its way quite through the Coat of the Lungs by the small holes pricked in it, as was said before. This being continued for a pretty while, the Dog, as I exspected, lay still, as before, his eyes being all the time very quick, and his Heart beating very regularly: But, upon ceasing this blast, and suffering the Lungs to fall and lye still, the Dogg would immediately fall into Dying convulsive fits; but be as soon reviv'd again by the renewing the fulness of his Lungs with the constant blast of fresh Air.

Towards the latter end of this Experiment a piece of the Lungs was cut quite off; where 'twas observable, that the Blood did freely circulate, and pass thorow the Lungs, not only when the Lungs were kept thus constantly extended, but also when they were suffer'd to subside and lye still. Which seem to be Arguments, that as the *bare* Motion of the Lungs *without fresh Air* contributes nothing to the life of the Animal, he being found to survive as well, when they were not mov'd, as when they were; so it was not the subsiding or movelesness of the Lungs, that was the immediate cause of Death, or the stopping the Circulation of the Blood through the Lungs, but the *want* of a sufficient *supply of fresh Air.*

I shall shortly further try, whether the suffering the Blood to circulate through a vessel, so as it may be openly exposed to the fresh Air, will not suffice for the life of an Animal; and make some other Experiments, which, I hope, will throughly discover the *Genuine use of Respiration*; and afterwards consider of what benefit this may be to Mankinde.

FINIS.

43

Reprinted from *Tractatus de Corde: Item de Motu & Colore Sanguinis et Chyli in cum Transitu,* Elzevir edition, 1669, p. 176; translation by K. J. Franklin, reproduced from *Early Science in Oxford,* Vol. 9, R. T. Gunther, Clarendon Press, Oxford, 1932

TRACTATUS DE CORDE: ITEM DE MOTU & COLORE SANGUINIS ET CHYLI IN CUM TRANSITU

Richard Lower

Quocirca cum ita ſe res habeat, proximo in loco videndum eſt, cui tandem ſanguis acceptum refert quod colore tam rutilo & purpureo penitus imbuatur: Atque hoc pulmonibus totum tribuendum eſt, ſiquidem expertus ſum ſanguinem, qui totus venoſi inſtar atro colore pulmones intrat, arterioſum omnino & floridum ex illis redire; ſi enim abſciſſa anteriore parte pectoris & folle in aſperam arteriam immiſſo pulmonibus continenter inſufflatis, &, quo liber per eos aëri tranſitus fiat, acu ſimul undique perforatis, vena pneumonica prope auriculam ſiniſtram pertundatur, ſanguis totus purpureus & floridus in admo-

ON THE COLOUR OF THE BLOOD

This being so, we must next see to what the blood is indebted for this deep red colouration. This must be attributed entirely to the lungs, as I have found that the blood which enters the lungs completely venous and dark in colour, returns from them quite arterial and bright. For if the anterior part of the chest is cut away and the lungs are continuously insufflated by a pair of bellows inserted into the trachea, and they are also pricked with a needle in various places to allow free passage of air from them, then, on the pulmonary vein being cut near the left auricle, the blood will flow out into a suitably placed receptacle completely bright red in color . . . .

44

Reprinted from *Skand. Arch. Physiol.*, **27**, 100–105, 106–109, 118–121, 124–125 (1912)

Measurements of the Blood Flow through the Lungs of Man.[1]

By

August Krogh and **J. Lindhard.**

(From the Laboratory of Zoophysiology, University of Copenhagen.)

In a series of experiments shortly to be published, undertaken to study the regulation of the respiratory functions during heavy muscular work, we found that a very marked rise in oxygen absorption took place immediately after the beginning of such work on a stationary bicycle ergometer. We have recorded in one instance an increase in oxygen absorption from the resting value of 230 ccm per minute to 1340 during the period from 6 to 19 seconds after the work had begun, whereupon a slower rise took place until the level corresponding to the work (about 2500 ccm) had been reached in about 1·5 minutes. As it seemed to us extremely unlikely that any considerable alteration in the oxygen content of the venous blood, reaching the lungs, should take place in so short a time as 6—19 seconds, and as there did not appear to be the slightest reason to believé that any (hypothetical) consumption of oxygen in the lungs themselves should suddenly become more intense, we were forced to the conclusion that the flow of blood through the lungs must be almost instantly increased in about the same proportion as the absorption of O_2, since this absorption must, when all other things are equal, be proportional to the supply of venous blood.[2]

[1] Der Redaktion am 1. Februar 1912 zugegangen.

[2] Krogh, The Mechanism of Gas Exchange. *Skand. Arch. Physiol.* 1910. Bd. XXIII. p. 267. **We want to emphasize that we base the conclusion on the initial rise of the O_2 absorption and on that alone. As soon as the blood from the working muscles actually reaches the lungs, the conditions regarding O_2 content and possibly oxidable substances may be altered to such a degree that it would be rash to draw definite inferences from the O_2 absorption to the supply of venous blood.**

This result did not in the least agree with our expectations[1] while it supported definitely the views of Zuntz and Hagemann, Plesch, Bornstein[2] and others as to the blood flow during work, and we thought it desirable therefore to concentrate our attention upon this most important problem and endeavour to obtain direct and absolute measurements of the blood flow through the lungs during rest as well as during work. For this purpose we intended to apply the ingenious principle introduced in 1910 by Bornstein.[3]

Briefly stated Bornsteins principle amounts to this: To produce a definite tension difference between the blood and the alveolar air with regard to a certain neutral gas (e. g. nitrogen) and to measure the quantity of the gas liberated or absorbed during a certain time. On the assumption that the blood leaving the lungs is in tension equilibrium with the alveolar air, the quantity of blood which must have passed during the time can be calculated from these data.

Bornstein washed out his lungs rapidly with oxygen and thereupon breathed through a cartridge with potash into a bag filled with oxygen. The total volumes of air in the apparatus and the lungs and the nitrogen percentages were determined before the experiment and after a definite period. If this period were short enough to prevent the blood from coming in contact with the gas in the lungs more than once, the N_2-tension in the blood reaching the lungs could be taken as 80 % and an absolute value could be obtained for the blood flow. Bornstein, however, made experiments of longer duration and attempted only to obtain by a somewhat complicated calculation relative values for the minute volume, taking the flow during complete rest as his starting point. It is obvious, however, that if his figures are used for calculation of the absolute flow of blood, minimum values must be obtained, since the N_2-tension of the blood must be steadily decreasing. If we calculate in this manner we find from his experiments of 1·5 minutes duration a minute volume of 6 liter, and from the 3 minutes experiments a minute volume of 5 liter, Bornstein finds that during work the flow is increased up to ten times, giving the impossible minute volume of 60 liter.

[1] Our expectations were based upon current notions regarding the blood flow and especially upon the argumentation given by Bohr, *Skand. Arch. Physiol.* 1909. Bd. XXII. p. 228—234.

[2] Zuntz u. Hagemann, *Stoffwechsel d. Pferdes.* Berlin 1899. Plesch, *Hämodynamische Studien.* Berlin 1909. Bornstein, Pflügers *Archiv.* 1910. Bd. CXXXII. p. 312.

[3] Eine Methode zur vergleichenden Messung des Herzschlagvolumens beim Menschen. Pflügers *Archiv.* 1910. Bd. CXXXII. p. 307—318.

We could not therefore accept Bornstein's work as conclusive, but we hoped by suitable modifications of his method to find the errors and to obtain reliable results. We made at first some trials with nitrogen but found the difficulties very great, chiefly because the differences in N_2-percentage were too small compared with the analytical accuracy obtainable. This is due to the fact that the solubility of nitrogen in blood is very small, the absorption coefficient not exceeding 0·015. We therefore resolved to try a more soluble gas and selected nitrous oxide, which possesses according to the determinations of Siebeck[1] the absorption coefficient of 0·43 at 37° without entering into chemical combination with any substance in the blood. We knew from the determinations of diffusion constants for the lungs of man[2] that the diffusion would be in all cases so rapid that the blood leaving the lungs would be practically completely saturated at the tension of N_2O obtaining in the alveoli, and the narcotic properties of the gas could do no harm when low concentrations only were employed. We succeeded after a few trials in working out suitable experimental and analytical methods for this gas. When our methods were completed and a number of experiments made, Zuntz, Müller and Markoff published a preliminary paper[3] on the same subject. They have also, and before us, employed nitrous oxide, but in other respects their method is very different from ours and, in the form published, not very reliable. The four determinations recorded differ rather widely, and when we calculate the O_2 absorption from the analytical data given, we find that in two cases oxygen appears to have been eliminated from the body during the experiments (Versuch III 88 ccm, Versuch II 130 ccm) while in a third so much has apparently been absorbed that it amounts to 252 ccm per liter blood (Versuch IV). According to a communication by letter from prof. Zuntz the discrepancies are probably due to incomplete mixture of the gases in the spirometer employed.

Methodics.

The details of the method employed by us are as follows.

1. We prepare a suitable gas mixture generally containing 10—25% N_2O and 20—25% O_2.

2. A small recording spirometer is filled with about 4·5 liter of

[1] *Skand. Arch. Physiol.* 1909. Bd. XXI. p. 368.
[2] A. and M. Krogh, *Skand. Arch. Physiol.* 1910. Bd. XXIII. p. 247.
[3] *Zeitschr. f. Balneologie.* 1911. Bd. IV. No. 14—15.

this mixture. The spirometer (fig. 1) is constructed on the principle of the aeroplethysmograph. The movable part is made of very thin aluminium and turns on knife edges. The water surface has been made as small as possible. A screw (*1*) is provided to mix the gases thoroughly. The apparatus has been very carefully calibrated and a special scale made to measure the curves recorded.[1] By means of

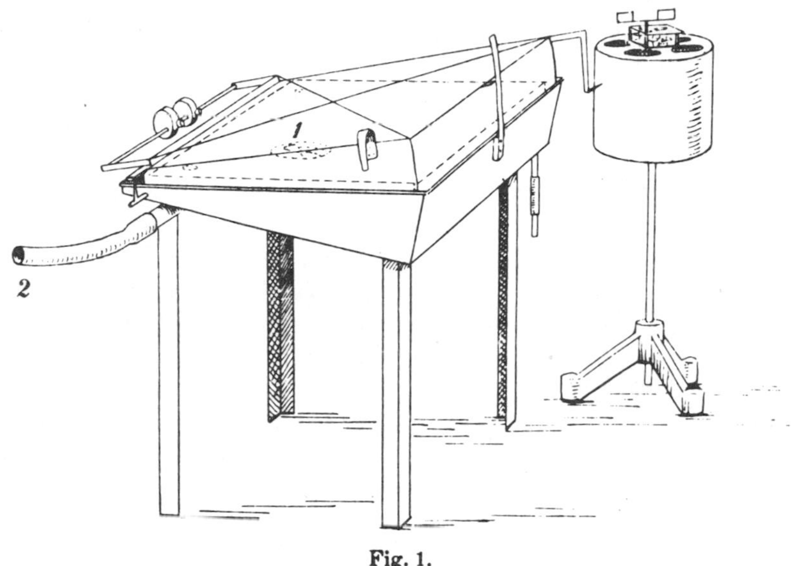

Fig. 1.

flexible rubber tubing, 20 ^{mm} wide (*2*), the spirometer is connected with a brass three way tap (fig. 2, *1*) of the same bore bearing a mouthpiece. As shown on figure 2 the subject breathing through the mouthpiece (*2*) may be connected through the tap either with the valves (*3*) and through them with a respiration apparatus, by which the respiratory exchange can be measured in brief periods, or with the recording spirometer. A very narrow (0·5 ^{mm}) lead tube (*4*) connects the mouthpiece with two sampling vessels of 20 ^{ccm} capacity each (*5*). If a sample is drawn at the close of a deep expiration it will consist of unmixed alveolar air.

3. The subject is seated in a chair or on the bicycle ergometer. The tap with mouthpiece etc. is suspended before him at such a height that his position is easy. For experiments on the blood flow

[1] The apparatus is made by the Laboratory Workshop. Ny Vestergade 11 Copenhagen, and can be provided at a price of 75 Kr. (£ 4/4).

during rest we have found it essential that he shall sit still for at least 15 minutes before the determination is made. A respiration experiment of 1—2 minutes duration is performed immediately before the blood flow experiment.

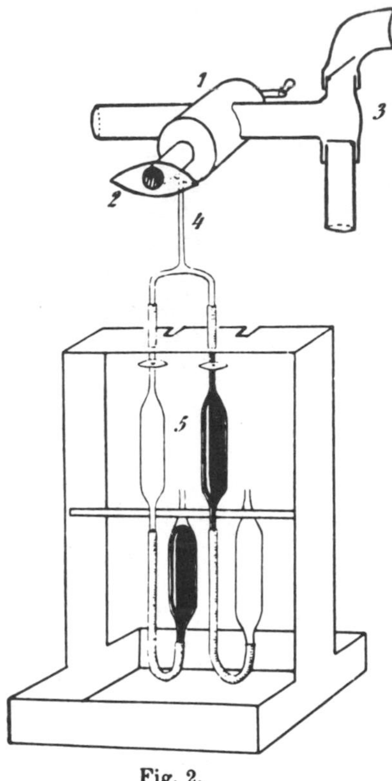

Fig. 2.

4. The recording drum is put in motion. The subject makes an expiration of the greatest possible depth. The tap is turned and he makes a deep inspiration from the spirometer. The tap is closed and the breath held for a few (generally 5—15) seconds. This is called the *introductory period.*

5. The tap is again opened to the spirometer and a sharp expiration of at least 1 liter is made. The tap is closed and a sample of air is drawn, representing the composition of the alveolar air at the beginning of the experimental period.

6. The breath is held during the experiment proper which lasts a suitable number of seconds (6—25). The tap is then opened a second time for a large sharp expiration and the final sample of alveolar air drawn. The curve produced during an experiment is

26./10. A. K. No. 3. N_2O.

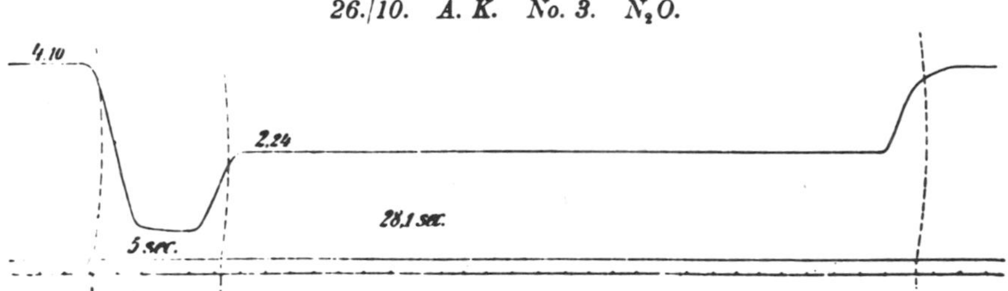

Fig. 3. ($^1/_3$ actual size.)

shown in fig. 3. The volume of air enclosed in the lungs during the experiment is represented by the vertical distance between the first and third horizontal portion of the curve + the residual air of the subject.[1] The duration of the experiment is represented by the horizontal distance between the lines showing the moments of sampling. These lines are drawn so as to intersect the expirations at a vertical distance from their tops equal to the dead space of the subject and the mouthpiece.

7. The analyses of the gas mixtures are performed in a Haldane apparatus with a burette holding 10 ^{ccm} and divided from 6·5 to 10 in 1/100 parts of a ccm. This apparatus has been used extensively before by both of us. The analysis of the nitrous oxide has necessitated only two slight modifications. For the absorption of CO_2 60 % KOH is employed instead of the usual 10 % in order to minimize the absorption of the readily soluble N_2O. The combustion pipette fig. 4 (*1*) is provided with a three way tap (2), one tube of which is permanently connected with a small hydrogen generator. The hydrogen

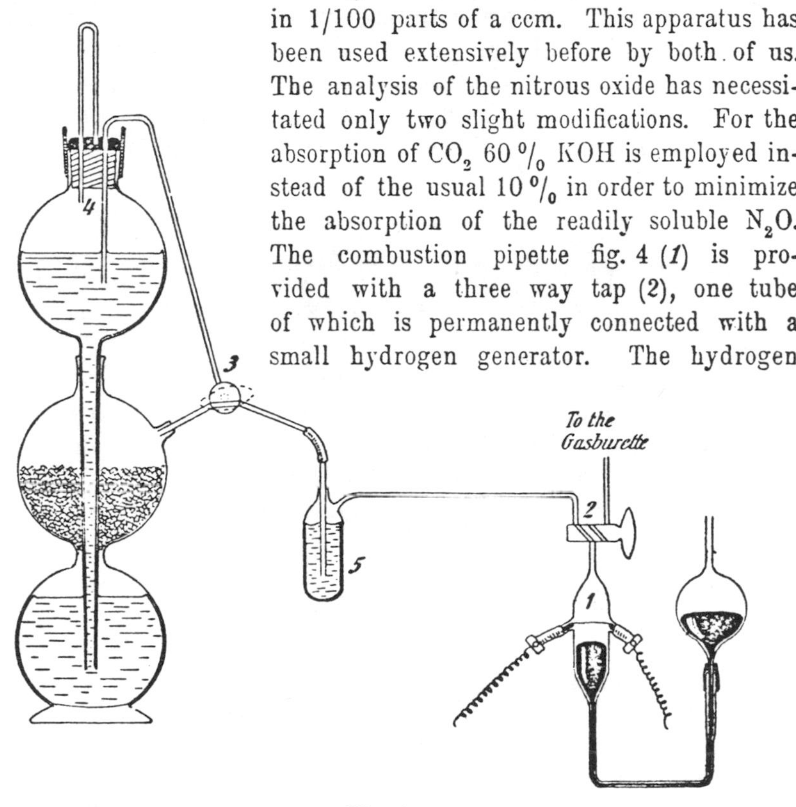

Fig. 4.

is evolved in a Kipp apparatus from pure zink and sulphuric acid.

[*Editor's Note:* Material has been omitted at this point.]

The analyses gave:

	Sample I	Sample II
CO_2	4·15 %	6·17 %
O_2	17·18	12·72
N_2O . . .	12·04	9·90
N_2	66·63	71·21

It is apparent that the nitrogen percentage has risen during the experiment. This is due partly to a slight liberation of nitrogen from the blood which can be calculated approximately as follows, taking the quantity of blood passing as 3 liter, the absorption coefficient for N_2 as 0·015 and the mean tension difference between the blood and the air in the lungs during the experiment as $79 - 69\,\% = 10\,\%$

$$3000 \times 0{\cdot}015 \times \frac{10}{100} = 4{\cdot}5^{\text{ccm}}$$

or 0·13 % of the 3·3 liter air present. This rise is so slight that it may be left out of account, and it has been so left in all our determinations.

Apart from this, the rise in nitrogen percentage is brought about by a contraction of the volume of air enclosed in the lungs due to absorption of oxygen and nitrous oxide and only partly counterbalanced by elimination of carbon dioxide. Taking the quantity of nitrogen as unaltered, the final volume is calculated from the initial

$$\frac{66{\cdot}63}{71{\cdot}21} \times 3{\cdot}26 = 3{\cdot}05$$

that is a contraction of 210 ^{ccm} (3260—3050) in 28 seconds or 7·3 per second.

A similar contraction takes place during the introductory period. This cannot be directly measured but is estimated from that found in the experimental period. We take it as about 6 ^{ccm} per second. This contraction + the volume of the first sample of alveolar air must be deduced as above from the initial volume of air in the lungs.

We calculate the quantities of nitrous oxide and oxygen present in the lungs at the beginning and at the end of the experimental period

$$N_2O\ \text{I} = 3{\cdot}26 \times \frac{12{\cdot}04}{100} = 0{\cdot}3925\ \text{l.} \quad O_2\ \text{I} = 3{\cdot}26 \times \frac{17{\cdot}18}{100} = 0{\cdot}560\ \text{l.}$$

$$N_2O\ \text{II} = 3{\cdot}05 \times \frac{9{\cdot}90}{100} = 0{\cdot}302\ \text{l.} \quad O_2\ \text{II} = 3{\cdot}05 \times \frac{12{\cdot}72}{100} = 0{\cdot}3875\ \text{l.}$$

N_2O absorbed 0·0905 l. O_2 absorbed 0·1725 l.

From the determinations of Siebeck, quoted above, we have the absorption coefficient for N_2O in blood at 37° = 0'43. The mean percentage of N_2O in the lungs during the experiment can without serious error be taken as

$$\frac{12\cdot04 + 9\cdot90}{2} = 10\cdot97\,\%.$$

The volume of blood necessary to absorb 0·0905 ccm N_2O must therefore be

$$\frac{0\cdot0905 \times 100}{0\cdot43 \times 10\cdot97} = 1\cdot92\,l,$$

which must have passed the lungs during the 28'1 seconds of the experiment. The volume passing during one minute therefore amounts to

$$1\cdot92\,\frac{60}{28\cdot1} = 4\cdot10\,l.$$

This figure requires correction, because the 0·0905 liter should be reduced from 740'4 mm and 15'7° to 760 mm and 0°, while the mean tension 10'97 % should be multiplied by (740·4 — 47): 760 to give the tension expressed in per cents of an atmosphere. We have found, however, that at ordinary temperatures and pressures these two corrections counterbalance each other almost exactly, leaving only a correction of 99/100 by which the result must be multiplied.

In practice we never reduce the volume enclosed in the lungs, but instead of that we reduce the percentages in the second sample of alveolar air to what they would have been, had the volume kept unaltered.

We have

	Sample I	Sample II	II corrected	Difference I—II corr.	Mean $\frac{I + II}{2}$
CO_2 %	4·15	6·17	5·78		
O_2	17·18	12·72	11·91	5·27	
N_2O	12·04	9·90	9·27	2·77	10·97
N_2	66·63	71·21	(66·63)		

and the whole calculation of the minute volume in put as follows

$$\frac{3\cdot26 \times 2\cdot77 \times 100 \times 60 \times 99}{0\cdot43 \times 100 \times 10\cdot97 \times 28\cdot1 \times 100} = 4\cdot05\,l.$$

and worked out by means of the slide rule. The accuracy really obtainable is not large enough to warrant any more elaborate calculation or correction.

The quantity of oxygen absorbed per minute during the experiment is calculated in like manner from the analyses

$$\frac{3\cdot 26 \times 5\cdot 27 \times 60}{100 \times 28\cdot 1} = 0\cdot 3661$$

and reduced to 760 ^{mm} and 0° = 332 ^{ccm}.

[*Editor's Note:* Material has been omitted at this point.]

The blood flow during rest. Our experiments have mostly been made on subjects sitting on a bicycle with the feet resting on special supports arranged for that purpose. The position is fairly easy, but is not of course comparable to complete rest in a chair or on a bed. In our first determinations we let the subject sit still for a few minutes only before a determination, but we found later that it was essential for getting constant results that the subject should keep quiet for not less than 15 minutes and better for 1/2 hour before any determinations were made.

We find that, when the blood flow measurements are repeated several times, while the subject remains at rest in a constant position, the results are remarkably constant when reduced to the normal absorption of oxygen, though they may show a small but steady decrease or increase.

Instances are exp. 24—26, 30—32, and 34—36 on the subject A. K. showing the reduced minute volumes:

3·3, 3·05, 2·75 mean 3·03
4·7, 4·25, 5·0 mean 4·65
4·6, 4·55, 4·15 mean 4·43

and 38—41 on M. K. giving

4·0, 4·15, 4·5, 4·6 mean 4·3

The variation found within each of these series hardly go beyond the possible experimental errors, but we believe nevertheless that most of them are real.

On separate days very distinct differences manifest themselves ranging from 2·8 liter per minute as the lowest figure recorded for each of the three adult subjects to 5·7 liter in the case of J. L., 5·0 in the case of A. K. and 4·6 in the case of M. K.

We do not of course lay any special stress on the limits observed. They may possibly be considerably widened by further extension of the observations.

The utilization of the oxygen carrying capacity of the blood has varied in our experiments between 0·28 and 0·60, and if we assume that no oxygen has been used for metabolic processes within the lungs the venous blood must have been from 60 to 40% saturated with oxygen.

The blood flow during muscular work. Our determinations were made on a stationary bicycle ergometer which allowed a direct weighing of the work done. The work is given in the tables in kilogrammeter per minute.

To make determinations during heavy work is very difficult, because the breath can be held only for very few seconds, but with moderate work of 400—600 kg-m per minute the determinations do not present any serious difficulties, though the experiments must be brief. We have used introductory periods of about 5 seconds and experiments of 5 to 7 seconds duration. The residual air is augmented during work and must be specially determined while a similar amount of work is being done as that employed in the experiment. In spite of this precaution the accuracy is no doubt diminished. It is essential that some oxygen should be added to the air in the recording spirometer in order to obtain values for the O_2 absorption comparable to those obtained during the preceding respiration experiment. This precaution has been omitted in exp. 19 where the O_2 percentage in the alveoli has fallen to 9% which is so low that the saturation of the blood leaving the lungs must have been incomplete.

No.	Subject	Work kg-m per m	Observed		Resp. exp. O_2 absorbed ccm per m	Reduced Blood flow l. per m	Coeff. of utilizat.	Pulse per m	Output of heart per beat
			O_2 absorbed ccm per m	Blood flow l. per m					
3	J. L.	Rest	—	3·7					
4	—	heavy W.	—	19·1					
18	J. L.	Rest	386	3·4	320	2·8	0·60		
19	—	458	1600	11·6	1350	9·8	0·73		
20	—	1 m after W.	374	4·45	—	—	0·44		
27	A. K.	Rest	382	4·7	240	2·95	0·46	(70)	(42)
28	—	446	1745	21·2	1320	16·0	0·47		
29	—	524	1537	17·2	1570	17·6	0·51	152	116

Our experiments afford a very striking confirmation of the views of Zuntz[1] on the circulation during muscular work. We find that the minute volume can rise from about 3 liter during rest to 18 or even to 21 liter during a work representing only one half of the maximum attainable by man.

The experiments 19 and 28 show very different reactions on the part of the two subjects to practically identical amounts of muscular work. J. L. performs the work with a minute volume of 9·8 liter and a coefficient of utilization of the oxygen of 0·73, while in A. K. the minute volume goes up to 16 liter and the coefficient of utilization is about the same as during rest, 0·47. There can be no doubt that the former reaction, by which the work thrown on the heart is very moderate, is the more economical of the two. The subjective sensations of the individuals bear this out. J. L. felt the work as being very easy and had no unpleasant sensations whatever, while A. K. felt very much done at the time when exp. 28 was made. On continuing the work, however, these symptoms disappeared, the amount of work performed rose, and in the second experiment (29) the coefficient of utilization has risen slightly (0·51). Still, however, the utilization is no better than it can be during rest, and the circulation is performed in an uneconomical way. It is extremely probable that the differences noted depend upon the very different degrees of muscular training of the two subjects.

We have reason to believe that the maximum output of the average human heart is not much higher than the 21·6 liter observed in one of our experiments. The pulse rate has not been observed in this case, but, to judge from countings made in similar conditions, it must have been something between 160 and 180, say 170, which would give an output per beat of 127 ^{ccm}. Hiffelsheim[2] has made some determinations of the capacity of the human ventricles. He found on three male adults capacities of 168, 143 and 158 ^{ccm} (mean 156 ^{ccm}) for the left ventricle, while the right ventricles were found to be a little larger. The differences between the two ventricles were no doubt due to the method (filling with wax), and the figures even for the left ventricles are probably higher than the real capacities of the hearts when living. The maximum output per beat must always be somewhat less than the maximum capacity, because the systole, especially

[1] Zuntz u. Hagemann, Stoffwechsel des Pferdes. *Landwirtschaftl. Jahrbücher.* 1897.

[2] *Journ. de l'anat. et de physiol.* 1864. T. I. p. 469.

of the left ventricle, will never completely obliterate the internal space, while the relaxation, especially with a rapid pulse rate, may also fall short of completeness. The maximum output per beat of an average human heart (capacity 156 ccm) cannot therefore be higher than about 140 ccm from each ventricle. The maximum pulse rate is perhaps 180, and even this can probably be maintained for short periods only and is beyond the limit of economical working. An output of 140 ccm with a pulse of 180 would give a minute volume of 25 liter. If we assume an oxygen capacity of 200 ccm per liter and a coefficient of utilization of 0·75 (the highest value observed by us being 0·73) we get an oxygen absorption of 3750 ccm per minute while the highest actually recorded is about 3200 ccm.[1]

Our results point to the conclusion that the circulation will in all cases be able to carry the necessary amount of oxygen to the tissues. They lend no support to the theory, that respiratory processes of considerable magnitude take place in the lungs themselves, but they cannot of course say anything against the possibility of such processes.

The most important fact brought out by our experiments is the very great variability in the output of the heart ranging from 2·8 liter during rest to 21·6 liter per minute during muscular work. The output per beat has varied during rest between 39 ccm (exp. 26) and 103 ccm (exp. 32, during the determination). The higher of these figures falls very little short of the largest output recorded (116 ccm) or assumed (127 ccm) during work. From all what is known about the behaviour of the heart we are forced to conclude that the volume of the heart in systole, when the subject is at rest and with a slow pulse, is practically a constant quantity. It is absolutely impossible that the heart should normally be filled to the limit of its capacity during diastole, but should discharge in some cases only one third, more often one half and sometimes the whole of its contents.

[1] In a paper on the Significance of the Pulse Rate in *Transact. Oxford Jun. Scientific Soc.* 1909. p. 351—365 Miss Buchanan points out the very interesting fact that people who are capable of very great muscular exertion (rowers in the University Boat Race) often have a very slow pulse. She mentions a case with a pulse of 45 per minute during rest and with a very prolonged systole (0·36 sec). This she takes as an indication of a very large heart. During training the length of the systole increased still further to 0·42 sec. It is probable that the output of such a heart during work may rise considerably above 25 l. per minute.

[*Editor's Note:* Material has been omitted at this point.]

The great variations in output cannot therefore be due to anything but variations in diastolic volume or, in other words, to variations in the filling of the heart during diastole. The conclusion that ***the supply of venous blood must be variable within very wide limits and must during rest almost always be inadequate to fill the ventricles*** appears to us to be inevitable.

A more elaborate discussion of the significance of this fact and of the mechanisms by which the venous supply is regulated will be given in two subsequent papers. Here we shall only attempt to estimate the limits between which the output of the average human heart may vary during rest. The upper limit is obviously determined by the capacity of the heart. When the venous supply is adequate the heart will be filled completely during each diastole, and the systolic discharge may reach the maximum assumed for work viz. 140 ^{ccm}. A pulse rate of 70 will then produce a minute volume of 9·8 liter. If the O_2 metabolism is taken as 250 ^{ccm} the oxygen absorbed per liter is only 26 ^{ccm}.

The lower limit for the circulation is determined by the oxygen supply, which must not fall below 200 ^{ccm} (1 Calorie) per minute. The limit of utilization observed during rest is 113 ^{ccm} per liter blood (0·60) necessitating a minute volume of 1·8 liter or, with a pulse rate of 70, an output per beat of 26 ^{ccm}.

Further series of determinations of the blood flow through the lungs in man by our methods are in progress. They comprise:

1. The extension of the investigation to a larger number of individuals and a study of the influence of a number of factors such as body position, meals, light baths etc. on the blood flow during rest.
2. A further study of the blood flow in several stages of moderate and severe muscular work.

Summary.

1. Methods are described by which it is possible to measure with considerable accuracy the blood flow through the lungs (the minute volume) in man. The methods can with slight modifications be applied also to animals.

2. The blood flow during rest is shown to vary between very wide limits (from 2·8—8·7 liter per minute) depending on the variable supply of venous blood to the right heart. When a series of consecutive determinations are made a remarkable constancy is, however, generally observed.

3. During muscular work the rapidity of the circulation is greatly increased. The maximum observed is 21·6 liter per minute. The systolic discharge may become very nearly maximal in spite of a greatly increased pulse rate.

4. The utilization of the O_2 *carrying capacity of the blood, i. e. the quantity of oxygen absorbed by 1 liter blood during its passage through the lungs divided by its total oxygen capacity, has been found varying between 0·28 and 0·60 during rest, but has reached 0·73 during muscular work. Athletic training appears to influence the circulation during work in the direction of a better utilization of the oxygen and consequently a less rapid flow of blood and a more economical working of the heart.*

Reprinted from *J. Clin. Invest.*, **34**(9), 1380–1390 (1955)

PULMONARY CAPILLARY BLOOD FLOW IN MAN [1,2]

By G. de J. Lee [3] and A. B. DuBois

(*From the Department of Physiology and Pharmacology, Graduate School of Medicine, University of Pennsylvania, Philadelphia, Pa.*)

(Submitted for publication March 2, 1955; accepted May 11, 1955)

Although it is obvious that the blood flow through the pulmonary artery is pulsatile, it is not so certain that it remains so within the pulmonary capillaries. On the contrary, the direct Fick method for measuring cardiac output expresses mean flow per unit time, and calculation of pulmonary arteriolar resistance tacitly assumes the existence of a non-pulsatile blood flow. Furthermore, it is not known whether the rate of gas diffusion from alveolus to capillary varies with the phase of the cardiac cycle.

The present communication describes a method for measuring instantaneous blood flow in the pulmonary capillary bed in man. A continuous recording of pressure within an airtight body plethysmograph is made before and after the inhalation of nitrous oxide. As the gas is absorbed by the blood entering the lung capillaries, the pressure within the body plethysmograph falls. This fall in pressure is proportional to the pulmonary capillary blood flow, and was found to vary according to the phase of the cardiac cycle.

METHOD

An airtight body plethysmograph of approximately 600 liters capacity, previously constructed for the measurement of alveolar pressure (1) was used (Figure 1).

The differential pressure between the plethysmograph chamber and an adjacent "compensatory" chamber was measured, using a Lilly capacitance manometer, Brush D.C. amplifier and recorder. This arrangement eliminated artefacts produced by extraneous sounds in the laboratory, alterations in room temperature and changes in ambient barometric pressure. The sensitivity of the recording system was .04 cm. H_2O per cm. deflection, and the response time was satisfactory up to a rate of 35 cycles per second. The pressure between the plethysmograph and compensatory chamber could be equalized by a valve, and the plethysmograph could be vented to the exterior by a solenoid operated valve in the wall of the chamber.

The subjects, who had been active in the laboratory, were permitted to sit for 5 to 15 minutes before entering the plethysmograph. During the test, they were required to breathe in a special way, and to turn valves; they were by no means basal. The subject sat in the closed plethysmograph with two 5-liter bags and two sampling tubes. His electrocardiograph (lead CF.4) was recorded simultaneously with the plethysmograph pressure, using a second Brush D.C. amplifier operating the remaining pen of the Brush recorder. Two minutes were allowed for temperature equilibration to occur, but in spite of this, some slight rise in pressure within the plethysmograph continued owing to continued heating of the contained air by the subject's body. To measure this and also R.Q. effects during the subsequent breath-holding procedures a control record was first obtained. The subject twice exhaled almost to his residual capacity and then took a deep inspiration. After the second inspiration, he exhaled to resting lung volume and held his breath with the glottis open for a few seconds while simultaneous records of plethysmograph pressure and ECG were obtained. In addition to the pressure changes

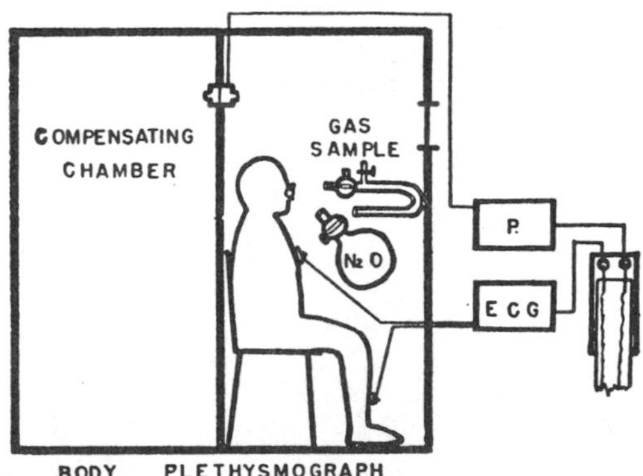

Fig. 1. Diagram of Body Plethysmograph, Manometer, and Electrocardiograph Recording System

For pictorial clarity, valves between the plethysmograph, compensating chamber, and the exterior are not shown.

[1] These studies were aided in part by a contract between the Office of Naval Research, Department of the Navy, and the University of Pennsylvania, Graduate School of Medicine, NR 112-323.

[2] Presented in preliminary form at the Fall Meetings of the American Physiological Society, 1954. DuBois, A. B., and Lee, G. de J., (Am. J. Physiol., In press).

[3] Holding a Travelling Fellowship from St. Thomas's Hospital, London. Present address: St. Thomas's Hospital, London, England.

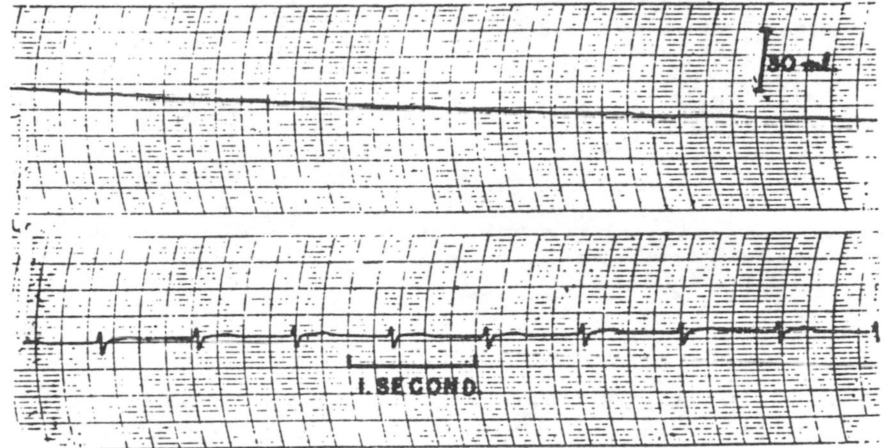

FIG. 2. CONTROL RECORD DURING BREATHHOLDING AFTER AIR INHALATION

Plethysmograph pressure record (inverted) above, calibrated as a volume change. ECG shown below.

occurring from heating and R.Q. effects, small variations in pressure were seen to occur in association with the heart beat (Figure 2).

After a short period of normal breathing, the subject again exhaled almost to his residual volume and then took a deep inspiration from a 5-liter bag containing 100 per cent oxygen. This was done to raise the alveolar oxygen content so that when nitrous oxide was subsequently breathed, the resultant alveolar gas mixture would contain approximately the normal concentration of oxygen. Next, the subject again fully exhaled and took a maximal inspiration of 100 per cent nitrous oxide from a second 5-liter bag. He then exhaled through a Haldane gas sampling tube to resting lung volume and held his breath with the glottis open. The plethysmograph pressure fell in a characteristic fashion as the nitrous oxide was absorbed by the blood entering the lung capillaries (Figure 3). After 5 to 10 seconds breathholding the subject exhaled maximally through a second Haldane gas sampling tube.

The two expiratory samples were taken for subsequent analysis for nitrous oxide in a mass spectrometer. From these samples, the mean alveolar gas concentration during each cardiac cycle was calculated. The subject usually began to feel slightly 'intoxicated' some 15 to 20 seconds after inhaling the gas; this sensation disappeared rapidly after inhaling several breaths of air from the plethysmograph; it was more marked if oxygen was not inspired prior to the nitrous oxide inspiration.

The calculation of mean alveolar gas concentration from expired air samples assumes satisfactory distribution of the inspired gases within the lungs. All the subjects studied were healthy young adults. Under such circumstances it has been shown that the alveolar plateau recorded by a rapid gas analyzer can be extrapolated backward to the dead space (2, 3) and forward to the residual volume (4, 5). Since the mean concentration of alveolar gas is the mean of the integral of the product of concentration and volume over the entire range of lung volume, it is reasonable to assume that the mean alveolar concentration is represented as a point located at approximately mid expired volume on the alveolar plateau in a normal subject.

Expiration into a rapid gas analyzer showed that after a single breath of nitrous oxide, the alveolar gas concentration was approximately 58 per cent N_2O. However, if the breath was held at resting volume for varying intervals of time before exhaling into the analyzer, the alveolar concentration fell progressively at approximately 0.5 per cent N_2O per second. After exercise, the rate of decline was considerably faster (0.7 to 1.8 per cent N_2O per second).

The change in pressure in the plethysmograph was converted to volume change by calibrating with a small volume of air alternately injected and withdrawn, using a 30 ml. syringe or a diaphragm type pump. The calibrating volume under ambient conditions at 26° to 28° C., and 40 to 50 per cent saturated (unpublished measurements by Botelho) was converted to BTPS by an appropriate factor, assuming a barometric pressure of 760 mm. Hg. It produced a deflection of approximately 12 mm. on the record.

Having completed the procedure under resting conditions, the whole procedure was repeated after half a minute of knee-bending exercises in the plethysmograph.

Calculation of blood flow

The solubility of nitrous oxide (S_{N_2O}) in whole blood is 47 vol. per 100 ml. blood per atmosphere at BTPS (6). Since the volume of N_2O (V_{N_2O}) which dissolves in the blood is proportional to the alveolar fraction of N_2O

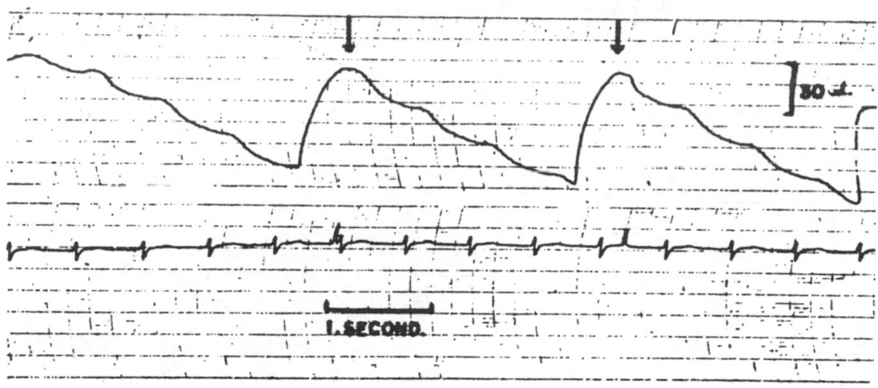

FIG. 3. RECORD OBTAINED DURING BREATHHOLDING AFTER N_2O INHALATION

Plethysmograph pressure record above, calibrated as a volume change. ECG shown below. Plethysmograph vented at arrows.

($F_{A_{N_2O}}$), it is necessary to calculate the latter from the samples which have been analyzed, as the fraction of dry gas (F_{N_2O}), by the formula: $F_{A_{N_2O}} = F_{N_2O} \cdot \frac{B-47}{760}$, where the symbols are standard (7).

The volume of gas absorbed in a given time (t) is also proportional to the quantity of blood (Q) equilibrated with the gas at that time. Combining terms

$$V_{N_2O} = S_{N_2O} \cdot F_{A_{N_2O}} \cdot Q.$$

Rearranging and differentiating with respect to time

$$Q = \frac{\dot{V}_{N_2O}}{S_{N_2O} \cdot F_{A_{N_2O}}},$$

where Q = cardiac output

$\dot{V}_{N_2O}$ = rate of absorption } of nitrous oxide

S_{N_2O} = solubility in whole blood } of nitrous oxide

all terms being expressed in liters per minute at BTPS.

Two separate methods for measuring the rate of gas absorption ($\dot{V}$) were employed:

(a) Four consecutive cardiac cycles were measured for pressure deflection at 0.04 second intervals, commencing in time with each R-wave of the ECG. The pressure changes during corresponding intervals of time in each cycle were then averaged to obtain a succession of mean values of $\dot{V}$ and so eliminate effects of random noise artefact.

The same was done for the control period, and the control values were subtracted from those obtained during the N_2O period in order to eliminate the recurrent variations produced by mechanical gas compression with the heart beat, temperature, and R.Q. changes already mentioned.

(b) The output from the capacitance manometer amplifier recording the plethysmograph pressure (V) was led through a 'differentiating' circuit consisting of a capacitance (C) and resistance (R); the voltage across the resistance was measured by a Brush DC amplifier and recorder. The values of C and R were selected to give a time constant of 0.06 second. The output was approximately proportional to the rate of change of pressure in the plethysmograph and hence proportional to the rate of blood flow (Figure 4).

It was considered that part of the pressure drop in the plethysmograph during nitrous oxide uptake might possibly be due to uptake in the lung tissues themselves, rather than by the blood. This possibility was therefore tested, using the trachea, heart and lungs of dogs, obtained immediately following the termination of other experiments in which the lungs had not been involved. These isolated lungs contained blood that was not flowing. The preparation was placed in a plethysmograph of approximately 25 liters capacity and inflation experiments were made which were identical with the procedure carried out by our subjects in the body plethysmograph. After the first second following inflation of the dog's lungs with 100 per cent nitrous oxide, only minor changes in plethysmograph pressure occurred:

Dog 1: 0.09 ml. per sec. N_2O uptake. Weight of lungs: 176 gm.

Dog 2: 0.13 ml. per sec. N_2O uptake. Weight of lungs: 155 gm.

Dog 3: 0.02 ml. per sec. N_2O uptake. Weight of lungs: 174 gm. (Average: 0.08 ml. per sec. N_2O uptake.)

Assuming that human lungs are approximately four times as heavy as those of the dog, then approximately 0.3 ml. N_2O per sec. would be taken up, due to delayed equilibration. However, the uptake due to blood flow is approximately 30 ml. N_2O per sec., so that the factor of delayed lung tissue equilibration is negligible in the present study on man.

Although N_2O is an inert gas chemically, it seemed possible that it might be evoking a local vasodilator effect upon the lung vessels. This could have led to the production of a pulsatile blood flow within the lung capillaries not necessarily present in the normal state. To test this possibility, the pressures obtained via a catheter

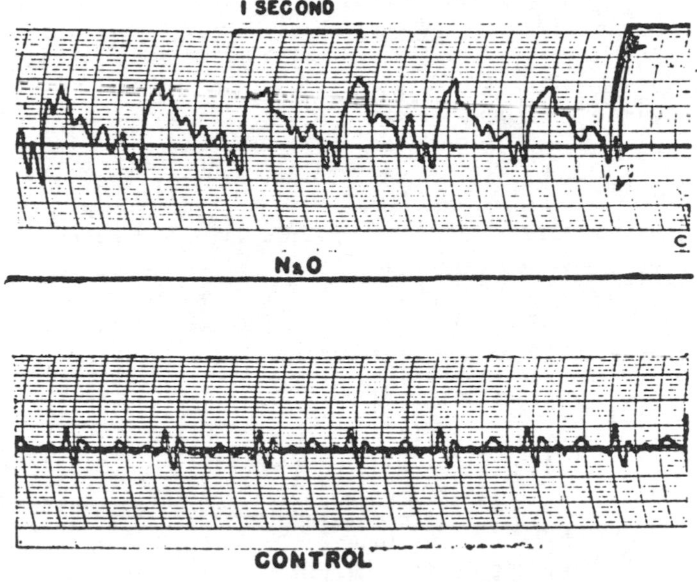

FIG. 4A. G. L. AT RESTING LUNG VOLUME
Control record, on air, is below, and gas absorption record, on N_2O is above.

wedged in the pulmonary vein of three open-chested dogs under light Nembutal® anesthesia were studied. The animals alternately breathed room air and 50 per cent N_2O in oxygen. No alteration in the pressure pulsations was obtained when the N_2O mixture was breathed. This suggested that no change in the physical state of the vessels had occurred.

RESULTS

Instantaneous pulmonary capillary blood flow measurements with simultaneous electrocardiograph records were obtained from five healthy young male subjects sitting at rest following laboratory activity and again immediately after moderate exercise. The results are shown graphically in Figures 5 and 6, where instantaneous flow rates expressed in liters per minute are shown in relation to the electrocardiographic events. In all instances the rate of pulmonary capillary blood flow is seen to vary markedly, being slowest shortly after the QRS complex of the ECG and most

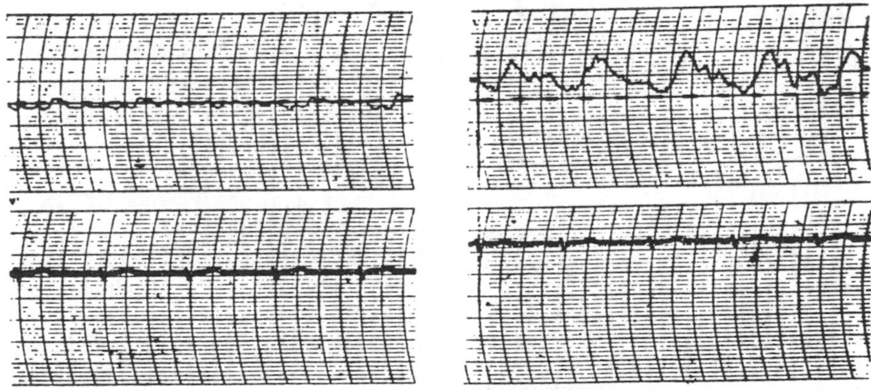

FIG. 4B. DuB IN EXPIRATORY POSITION, GLOTTIS OPEN
Control record, upper left, with ECG beneath. N_2O record, upper right, with ECG below.

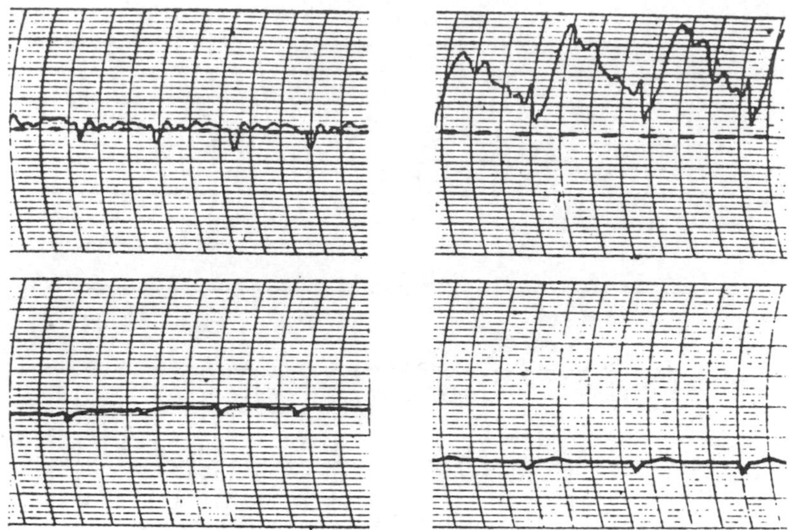

FIG. 4C. DuB AFTER EXERCISE

Control record, upper left, with ECG underneath. N_2O record, upper right, with ECG below.

FIG. 4. "DIFFERENTIATED" PLETHYSMOGRAPH PRESSURE RECORDS

rapid subsequent to onset of the T wave. The closed circles in Figure 5 represent instantaneous flow rate measurements at each 0.04 second following the R wave (zero time) obtained from four consecutive heart cycles (see section on *Calculation of blood flow*). The solid line represents the average instantaneous flow rate of the four cycles. The dashed horizontal line represents the mean flow rate or mean cardiac output. In Figure 6, for the sake of pictorial clarity, only the line representing the average instantaneous flow rates of four cardiac cycles have been shown.

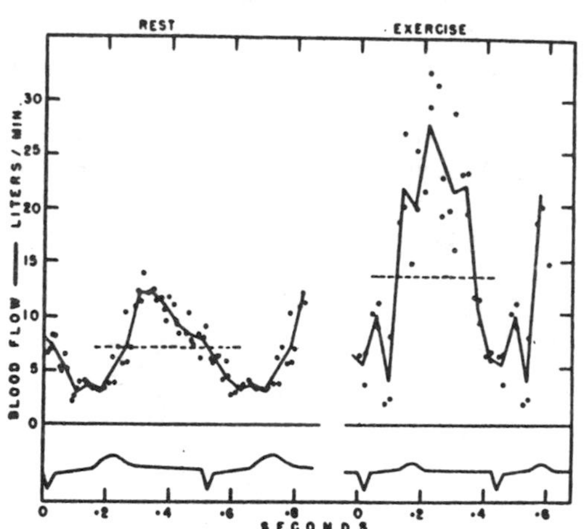

FIG. 5. INSTANTANEOUS PULMONARY CAPILLARY BLOOD FLOW RATES AT REST AND AFTER EXERCISE OBTAINED FROM ONE SUBJECT

Zero time arbitrarily taken as the R wave of the ECG, shown below each flow curve. Closed circles represent instantaneous flow rates at every 0.04 sec. from four consecutive heart cycles. Solid line represents the average instantaneous flow rate obtained from those points. Dashed line represents mean cardiac output per minute.

Sharp transient changes in flow rate occur in the regions at highest and lowest flow rate, as are shown in Figures 5 and 6. Table I shows the maximal and minimal instantaneous flow rates that were obtained in each subject at rest and after exercise. The figures are approximate and have been obtained by visual inspection of Figures 5 and 6.

In all five subjects, both at rest and after exercise, the instantaneous pulmonary capillary blood flow rates were found to be pulsatile. They varied between 40 and 70 ml. per sec. (2.4 and 4.2 L. per min.) during the period of minimal flow, and 203 and 426 ml. per sec. (12.2 and 25.6 L. per min.) at maximal flow during rest. Following exercise, the minimal pulmonary capillary blood flow rates varied between 40 and 128 ml. per sec. (2.4 and 7.7 L. per min.) and the maximal flow rates varied

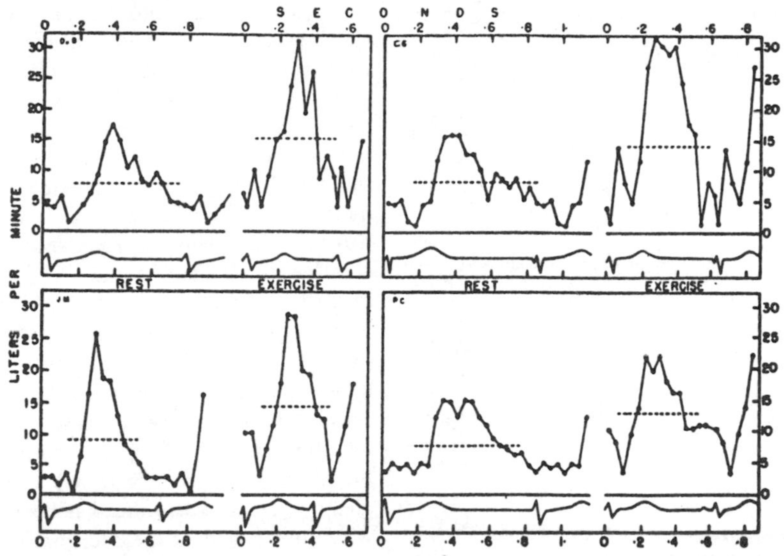

FIG. 6. THE AVERAGE INSTANTANEOUS PULMONARY CAPILLARY FLOW RATE CURVES OBTAINED FROM FOUR CONSECUTIVE CARDIAC CYCLES OF FOUR HEALTHY SUBJECTS AT REST, AND AFTER EXERCISE

Zero time is arbitrarily taken as the R wave of the ECG, shown below each flow curve. The dashed line represents mean cardiac output per minute.

between 370 and 530 ml. per sec. (22.2 and 31.8 L. per min.).

In one individual (subject M) although the mean cardiac output per minute rose after exercise, the instantaneous flow rates per beat remained virtually unaltered. The rise in cardiac output was accomplished in this instance by change in cardiac frequency alone. In the other four subjects, both changes in cardiac frequency and increases in instantaneous pulmonary capillary blood flow rates (stroke output) were responsible for the rise in cardiac output. The ratio of maximal to minimal flow rates in the five subjects varied between 3.6 and 10.7 at rest, and 3.1 and 12.0 after exercise.

Stroke volume measurements can be made from the instantaneous flow curves (Figures 5 and 6), since the area of each curve represents pulmonary capillary blood flow per cardiac cycle. Hence, knowing the pulse rate, or from measurement of the mean slope of the plethysmograph pressure curve during N_2O breathing (Figure 3), the mean cardiac output per minute can be obtained (Figure 7 and Table II).

The mean cardiac output in our resting, nonbasal subjects, was 7.9 L. per min. S.E. ± .26

TABLE I

The maximal and minimal instantaneous pulmonary capillary blood flow rates compared with the mean cardiac output estimations in each of five healthy male subjects before and after moderate exercise

	Rest						Exercise						Rest	Exercise
	Cardiac frequency *pulse/min.*	Minimum		Maximum		Maximum/Minimum	Cardiac frequency *pulse/min.*	Minimum		Maximum		Maximum/Minimum	Mean cardiac output *L./min.*	
Subject		*ml./sec.*	*L./min.*	*ml./sec.*	*L./min.*			*ml./sec.*	*L./min.*	*ml./sec.*	*L./min.*			
C.	72	70	4.2	252	15.1	3.6	97	120	7.2	370	22.2	3.1	7.8	13.1
DuB.	79	43	2.6	290	17.4	6.7	121	128	7.7	526	31.6	4.1	7.8	15.4
G.	72	56	3.4	265	15.9	4.7	97	80	4.8	530	31.8	6.6	8.2	14.2
M.	96	40	2.4	426	25.6	10.7	156	40	2.4	480	28.8	12.0	8.7	14.2
L.	118	55	3.3	203	12.2	3.7	141	88	5.3	466	28.0	5.3	7.1	13.8

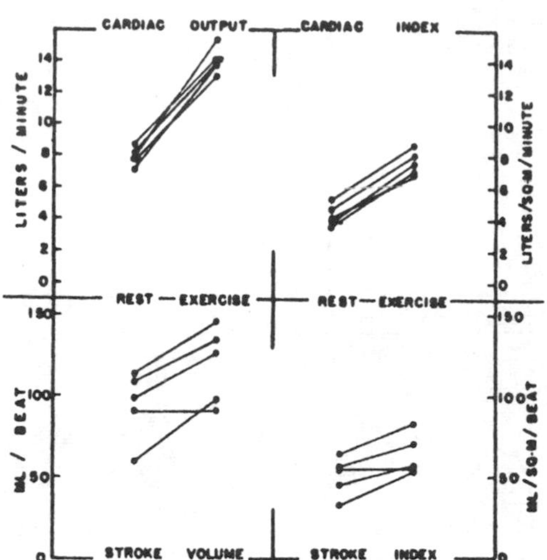

FIG. 7. MEAN CARDIAC OUTPUT AND STROKE VOLUME RESULTS OBTAINED FROM FIVE HEALTHY MALE SUBJECTS BEFORE AND AFTER EXERCISE

(4.3 L. per sq. meter per min.: S.E. ± .32); and after exercise 14.1 L. per min. S.E. ± .37 (7.6 L. per sq. meter per min.: S.E. ± .39).

No simultaneous estimates of cardiac output by other methods were carried out. However, the mean cardiac output by the direct Fick method or by the Hamilton dye injection technique on resting subjects appears to be less than the mean value on these subjects who were actively participating in the procedure.

DISCUSSION

The method here described for measuring pulmonary capillary blood flow incorporate some features of Krogh and Lindhard's single breath technique for measuring pulmonary blood flow in man, using nitrous oxide (8). It differs by using a differential manometric respirometer which allows instantaneous changes in gas uptake to be measured. It suffers from some of the disadvantages that previous indirect Fick methods for cardiac output measurement have had, whether using nitrous oxide, ethyl iodide, acetylene or carbon dioxide. These limitations result from re-circulation of blood during the gas breathing period, alterations of blood flow with each phase of respiration, and the necessity for obtaining a mean alveolar gas sample, which is only possible in subjects with reasonably uniform gas distribution in the lungs. However, accuracy of the alveolar gas sample is not so critical by this method. It also has the disadvantage, compared with the direct Fick method, that the subject must enter a closed chamber, and must be trained in the breathing procedure. Further, no associated data such as pressure measurements, or blood gas samples from various sites in the circulation, can be obtained as with catheter techniques. However it has the advantage of being the only method at present available for instantaneous blood flow in the pulmonary capillaries. Contrasted with it, the dye or isotope dilution methods for measuring cardiac output record the mean flow rate occurring over a period of several heart beats. The present technique allows instantaneous pulmonary capillary blood flow measurements to be made, and also makes possible measurement of the stroke volume of individual right ventricular contractions in man.

TABLE II

Cardiac output and stroke volume data obtained from five healthy male subjects at rest and after moderate exercise

	Rest					Exercise				
Subject	Cardiac frequency *pulses per min.*	Cardiac output *L./min.*	Cardiac index *L./sq. m./min.*	Stroke volume *ml./beat*	Stroke volume index *ml./sq. m./beat*	Cardiac frequency *pulses per min.*	Cardiac output *L./min.*	Cardiac index *L./sq. m./min.*	Stroke volume *ml./beat*	Stroke volume index *ml./sq. m./beat*
C.	72	7.8	4.1	109	57	97	13.1	6.9	135	71
DuB.	79	7.8	3.5	99	45	121	15.4	7.0	127	58
G.	72	8.2	4.7	114	65	97	14.2	8.1	146	84
M.	96	8.7	5.3	91	56	156	14.2	8.7	91	56
L.	118	7.1	3.9	60	33	141	13.8	7.5	98	54
Mean	87	7.9	4.3	95	51	122	14.1	7.6	119	65
S.D.		.59	.71	13.2	12.4		.83	.87	5.0	3.6
S.E.		.26	.32	5.9	5.5		.37	.39	2.2	1.6

Two qualifications need to be made when interpreting flow data indicated by nitrous oxide uptake in the lungs. Firstly, since nitrous oxide diffuses with approximately the same speed as carbon dioxide, the equilibration between alveolar N_2O and blood entering the pulmonary capillaries is theoretically complete long before the equilibration for oxygen, probably within the first 1/20th of the capillary length (6). The method therefore measures the rate of blood flow at the arteriolar end of the pulmonary capillary only, and gives no information about the blood flow at the venous end of the system. The second qualification concerns pulmonary ventilation-perfusion relationships. A region of lung receiving no ventilation, or presenting an impervious diffusion barrier, will absorb no N_2O despite the presence of blood flow through that area. Such blood must be considered to be passing through a 'physiological shunt' and is not measured by the method.

The instantaneous pulmonary capillary blood flow curves obtained from the nitrous oxide uptake studies do not show a constant flow rate but are pulsatile, having the form and degree shown in the graphs of our five subjects (Figures 5 and 6). The blood flow tends to increase in pulsatility with exercise. Differential pressures between the pulmonary artery and "capillary" curves in man suggested the likelihood of pulsatile capillary flow (9).

Although the amplitude of pulsatility varied among the different subjects and under different physiological conditions, there were certain features to the curves that were consistent and reproducible. The pulmonary blood flow reached its slowest rate approximately 0.1 second after electrical systole and then rapidly accelerated during the period of the T wave, to reach a peak blood flow approximately twice the mean blood flow. The rate of flow then diminished to reach a minimum rate, which was usually less than half the mean flow rate and approximately a fifth of peak flow rate. The instantaneous flow records show that these events do not occur in a smooth or sinusoidal wave form, but with abrupt angulations. Following peak flow there was usually a notch or sharp angulation in the curve; similarly, during the period of minimum flow there were sharp transient changes in the instantaneous flow rate. These sharp changes may be due to artefacts resulting from mechanical compression by the heart of the gases within the lungs (10). On the other hand, since they appear so consistently it seems possible that they may represent real alterations in flow rate associated with the notch in the pulmonary arterial pressure record at the time of pulmonary valve closure in the first instance (11), and with left atrial systole in the second instance. These events would produce transient changes in pressure gradient across the capillary and hence affect capillary flow rates at these instants.

Since many calculations which use pulmonary blood flow as one of their parameters tacitly assume that the pulmonary capillary flow rate is constant, it is interesting to review these and consider whether errors may be introduced by the assumption of a steady flow. The following sections of the discussion are speculative rather than experimental.

Gas exchange

The concepts of ventilation and perfusion, and the ratio $\dot{V}/\dot{Q}$ presume a steady ventilation and steady blood flow for convenience of calculation. Calculation of the variation of alveolar gas tensions during the respiratory cycle (12) shows that under normal conditions and during the steady state it is satisfactory to assume a steady ventilation. The exceptions to this are that the alveolar gas concentrations during a single respiratory cycle and during sudden changes in ventilatory rate do not fluctuate along the same line as the $\dot{V}/\dot{Q}$ ratio. A superficial examination of the effects of pulsatile blood flow will reveal much the same state of affairs. Exchange of oxygen and carbon dioxide between the capillary blood and alveolar gas should mostly take place during the rapid phase of blood flow (systole) and very little during the slow phase (diastole). This intermittent exchange would result in a halting type of progression round the loop describing fluctuations of P_{O_2} and P_{CO_2} on the O_2–CO_2 diagram during a single respiratory cycle (12). Since the respiratory loop itself causes little effect on the $\dot{V}/\dot{Q}$ ratio, intermittent progression round the loop should have little additional effect. In other words, under most circumstances it is satisfactory to assume a constant pulmonary blood flow as far as the $\dot{V}/\dot{Q}$ ratio is concerned. Again, the exception occurs when rapid changes in alveolar gas concentration are measured. Under such circumstances, instead of a smooth and continuous change in gas concentration as previously supposed, one would expect to find changes occurring in an intermittent fashion. It is of interest that such an intermittency of concentration change has already been noted by Bartels, Severinghaus, Forster, Briscoe, and Bates from continuous analysis of the expired air for O_2, CO_2, and N_2, using a rapid gas analyzer (13).

Analysis of the alveolar-arterial oxygen gradient is based on the $\dot{V}/\dot{Q}$ ratios discussed above. With the presence of a pulsatile capillary blood flow it is possible to conceive of a situation where an A-a gradient, not present in a steady system, could exist. This would exist where the diffusing capacity for oxygen were such that the systolic spurts of blood flow would pass through the capillaries too rapidly to become saturated and where the diastolic pauses could not make up for the systolic rush. Here saturation would be reached at the mean flow rate, and not improved by a slow diastolic flow rate. Such a situation would require that various elements of the stroke output stay in the capillary system unequal lengths of time. This has not been determined experimentally as far as we know.

Hemodynamics

There is no theoretical reason to challenge the direct Fick method for cardiac output measurement during the steady state on the grounds of pulsatile blood flow, but it is interesting to note that the mean blood flow actually exists during only two brief instants of the cardiac cycle during the rise and fall of the instantaneous flow curve. To test the method further, simultaneous direct Fick and plethysmograph measurements of cardiac output need to be made. In the present investigation, the phase of respiration at which the breath was held was seen to influence the stroke volume, which was greatest during inspiration and least during the expiratory phase. In preliminary experiments, the Valsalva maneuver was studied and was found to be associated with a marked increase in stroke volume during the period of the hypertensive overshoot. This is not in agreement with the findings of others who reported a fall in cardiac output during the overshoot period, using the dye technique (14). The stroke volume events associated with the Valsalva maneuver are a gross example of the unsteady state. Calculations were made from constantly timed blood samples, with the result that a disproportionately large concentration of dye was collected during the overshoot period when the stroke volume was large. With the plethysmograph method, nitrous oxide uptake is entirely dependent on flow. The importance of obtaining constant volume samples rather than constant time samples in any modification of the Fick principle for cardiac output measurement is thus well demonstrated in situations where the unsteady state exists (15, 16).

The combination of the elasticity of the arteries and the resistance of the arterioles is capable of converting the pulsatile output of the left ventricle into a constant capillary blood flow in the systemic vascular system. However, the findings here reported regarding pulmonary capillary flow indicate that, although the elasticity of the pulmonary arteries maintains a certain diastolic capillary flow, the combination of this elasticity and the pulmonary arteriolar resistance is not sufficient to induce a constant capillary blood flow. With techniques now available it should be possible, from simultaneous pressure flow data, to separate the factors of elasticity, resistance, and inertia in the pulmonary arterial system. In the absence of such information, it seems likely that the ratio of mean pressure to mean flow commonly used to express "pulmonary arteriolar resistance" will include components of elasticity and inertia. We believe that it would be more logical to calculate the "pulmonary impedance" until the elasticity and inertia factors are computable.

In a pulsatile system it is difficult to conceive of a single value for pulmonary capillary blood volume during all phases of the blood flow, unless the pulmonary capillary inflow exactly matches outflow in time and degree. If this were the case, the oxygen diffusing capacity would tend to decrease with exercise (pulsatile variation of the A-a gradient), the reverse in fact being the case. It would seem more likely that in such a system the pulmonary capillary volume would be capable of increasing to accommodate sharp increases in flow, with the result that the transit time through the alveolar capillary would remain approximately constant. Exercise would then be associated with an increase in oxygen diffusing capacity, as has been shown to be the case (17–19). The change in pulmonary capillary volume could occur by passive dilatation of already patent vessels as flow increased. Alternatively, the capillary volume could increase by the opening up of previously closed capillaries as flow rate increased and the pressure within the vessels exceeded a certain critical value. Regulation of pulmonary capillary volume by such a critical opening mechanism is an attractive hypothesis (20, 21). Maintenance of a constant pulmonary artery pressure in the face of large and rapid flow changes would become explicable on a physical basis, and the apparent lack of neurogenic control of pulmonary vascular tone would become less perplexing. In addition, opening of fresh vessels at high flow rates would allow both capillary transit time and the diameter of each open capillary to remain constant, with the result that conditions of gas diffusion would remain optimal at all flow rates. Microscopic observation showed opening or closing of lung capillaries in the anesthetized cat (22) and also various types of blood flow, sometimes pulsatile, sometimes steady.

In summary, conditions of pulsatile flow may be expected to produce certain hemodynamic and gas exchange effects which would be absent if the pulmonary capillary blood flow were constant as has sometimes previously been assumed.

SUMMARY

1. A method is described for measuring instantaneous pulmonary capillary blood flow in man.

The subject sat in a body plethysmograph and the plethysmograph pressure was continuously recorded during breathholding after inspiration of nitrous oxide. The plethysmograph pressure fell as the gas was absorbed by the blood entering the pulmonary capillaries. The rate of uptake of nitrous oxide so measured was proportional to the pulmonary capillary blood flow.

2. Observations were made on five healthy male subjects before and after moderate exercise. Pulmonary capillary blood flow was not steady but pulsatile.

Following electrical systole, there was a rapid acceleration of flow to a rate about twice the mean cardiac output, followed by a more gradual decline to low rates of flow. The cycle was repeated with each heart beat.

3. The possible effects on gas exchange and upon the hemodynamics of the pulmonary circulation are discussed.

ACKNOWLEDGMENTS

We wish to thank Dr. Robert E. Forster for help and advice in using the mass spectrometer for nitrous oxide analysis; also Dr. Julius H. Comroe, Jr., and Dr. Stella Y. Botelho who designed and built the plethysmograph; and Dr. Carl C. Gruhzit for help during the animal experiments.

REFERENCES

1. DuBois, A. B., Botelho, S. Y., and Comroe, J. H., Jr., Resistance to airflow through the tracheobronchial tree as measured by means of a body plethysmograph. J. Clin. Invest., 1954, **33**, 929.
2. Fowler, W. S., Lung function studies. II. The respiratory dead space. Am. J. Physiol., 1948, **154**, 405.
3. Fowler, W. S., and Forster, R. E., II. A method for producing uniform distribution of inspired gas. Federation Proc., 1952, **11**, 48.
4. Lilly, J. C., Mixing of gases within respiratory system with a new type nitrogen meter. Am. J. Physiol., 1950, **161**, 342.
5. Lanphier, E. H., Determination of residual volume and residual volume/total capacity ratio by single breath technics. J. Applied Physiol., 1953, **5**, 361.
6. Kety, S. S., The theory and applications of the exchange of inert gas at the lungs and tissues. Pharm. Rev., 1951, **3**, 1.
7. Pappenheimer, J., *et al.*, Standardization of definitions and symbols in respiratory physiology. Federation Proc., 1950, **9**, 602.
8. Krogh, A., and Lindhard, J., Measurements of the blood flow through the lungs of man. Skandinav. Arch. f. Physiol., 1912, **27**, 100.
9. Cournand, A., Some aspects of the pulmonary circulation in normal man and in chronic cardiopulmonary diseases. The fourth Walter Wile Hamburger Memorial Lecture, Institute of Medicine, Chicago. Circulation, 1950, **2**, 641.
10. Blair, H. A., and Wedd, A. M., The action of cardiac ejection on venous return. Am. J. Physiol., 1946, **145**, 528.
11. Bloomfield, R. A., Lauson, H. D., Cournand, A., Breed, E. S., and Richards, D. W., Jr., Recording of right heart pressures in normal subjects and in patients with chronic pulmonary disease and various types of cardio-circulatory disease. J. Clin. Invest., 1946, **25**, 639.

12. DuBois, A. B., Alveolar CO_2 and O_2 during breath holding, expiration, and inspiration. J. Applied Physiol., 1952, **5**, 1.
13. Bartels, J., Severinghaus, J. W., Forster, R. E., Briscoe, W. A., and Bates, D. V., The respiratory dead space measured by single breath analysis of oxygen, carbon dioxide, nitrogen or helium. J. Clin. Invest., 1954, **33**, 41.
14. McIntosh, H. D., Burnum, J. F., Hickam, J. B., and Warren, J. V., Circulatory changes produced by the Valsalva maneuver in normal subjects, patients with mitral stenosis, and autonomic nervous system alterations. Circulation, 1954, **9**, 511.
15. Visscher, M. B., and Johnson, J. A., The Fick principle: Analysis of potential errors in its conventional application. J. Applied Physiol., 1953, **5**, 635.
16. Stow, R. W., Systematic errors in flow determinations by the Fick method. Minnesota Med., 1954, **37**, 30.
17. Krogh, M., The diffusion of gases through the lungs of man. J. Physiol., 1915, **49**, 271.
18. Lilienthal, J. L., Jr., Riley, R. L., Proemmel, D. D., and Franke, R. E., An experimental analysis in man of the oxygen pressure gradient from alveolar air to arterial blood during rest and exercise at sea level and at altitude. Am. J. Physiol., 1946, **147**, 199.
19. Riley, R. L., Shepard, R. H., Cohn, J. E., Carroll, D. G., and Armstrong, B. W., Maximal diffusing capacity of the lungs. J. Applied Physiol., 1954, **6**, 573.
20. Burton, A. C., On the physical equilibrium of small blood vessels. Am. J. Physiol., 1951, **164**, 319.
21. Nichol, J., Girling, F., Jerrard, W., Claxton, E. B., and Burton, A. C., Fundamental instability of the small blood vessels and critical closing pressures in vascular beds. Am. J. Physiol., 1951, **164**, 330.
22. Wearn, J. T., Ernstene, A. C., Bromer, A. W., Barr, J. S., German, W. J., and Zschiesche, L. J., Normal behavior of pulmonary blood vessels with observations on intermittence of flow of blood in arterioles and capillaries. Am. J. Physiol., 1934, **109**, 236.

46

THE CATHETERIZATION OF THE RIGHT SIDE OF THE HEART

Werner Forssmann

This article was translated by Stanley A. Hartman from "Die Sondierung des rechten Herzens," Klin. Wochenschr., ***8**(45), 2085–2087 (1929)*

In sudden emergencies threatening the patient with cessation of heart activity, that is, in conditions of acute collapse, heart ailments, or even anesthetic accidents or cases of poisoning, quick local medical treatment must be undertaken. Often the only way to save the patient is to attempt an intracardiac injection, which is occasionally successful. Nonetheless, intracardiac injection remains a dangerous procedure; in numerous cases it has led, upon puncture of the heart wall, to injury of the coronary blood vessels and their branches, bleeding into the pericardium, and death by cardiac tamponade. Likewise, injury of the pleura can cause a fatal pneumothorax. Incidents of this sort make it necessary to delay intracardiac injections until the last moment, resulting in loss of valuable time for application of medicine at the heart itself. These experiences compelled me to look for a new way, a less dangerous way, to penetrate into the heart, and I tried the *catheterization of the right side of the heart from the venous system.*

The anatomy of the venous system is such that the heart can be reached from all points in the vessels, except, naturally, from points in the portal venous system. Since the catheter is going in the direction of blood flow, there are no obstacles to overcome, and since the valves are already set against backflow the catheter slides over without resistance. A wrong turn at the branching points of the vessels is also impossible, since they always form an acute angle, with the apex pointing in the direction of blood flow.

I tested these considerations in experiments with cadavers. Through a vein picked at random, I probed from a point near the elbow joint and, working toward the heart with no resistance, reached the right ventricle with a feather-light gliding. It was here that the catheter met its first resistance. The position of the catheter was investigated by performing an autopsy. In the process we slid upward through the vena cephalica or the vena brachialis, in which the presence of the catheter could be felt, came through Mohrenheim's fossa under the collar bone into the vena subclavia and from there, via the innominate vein and the superior vena cava, into the right side of the heart. It appears advisable to choose the path from the left arm, since, because of the arrangement of the convergence of large veins, the left innominate vein is longer and empties into the superior vena cava at a less acute angle.

After the successful experiments on the cadaver, I undertook the first tests on a living person, using myself as the subject of the experiment. First, as a preliminary test, I had a colleague, who kindly made himself available for this purpose, puncture my right elbow vein with a large-bore needle. Then, as in the tests with the cadaver, I slid a well-oiled ureteral catheter of four Charrieres thickness through the cannula and into the vein. The catheter slid in for 35 cm with playful ease. Since my colleague considered it too dangerous to continue, we stopped the test, after which I felt completely well. A week later I undertook a further test by myself. In my left elbow vein I made a venesection using local anesthesia (since doing a venous puncture with a large-bore needle on one's own body is technically very difficult) and slid the entire catheter 65 cm into my body without resistance. This distance seemed to me to be the distance from my left elbow to my heart, based on external body measurements. While sliding the catheter in, I had a feeling of slight warmth on my vein wall, similar to the feeling when calcium chloride is injected intravenously. When moving backward, the catheter would jam on the upper rear wall of the subclavian vein, and I sensed an especially intense warmth behind the clavicle near the insertion of the sternocleidomastoid muscle; at the same time, probably from irritation of rami of the vagus nerve, I had a dry cough. I examined the position of the catheter in an x-ray photograph, and I myself observed the forward sliding of the catheter in a mirror held in front of the radioscopy screen by the nurse.

In Figure 1 we see the shadow of the contrasting catheter running up as far as the right armpit (long-range photo). Figure 2 is a photograph of the second test: the catheter lies, extending up from the left arm, on the chest wall, disappears behind the clavicle and makes a downward bend at the same height as the junction with the left jugular vein, lays itself on the right edge of the vessel shadow and stays there, partially covered by the shadow of the spinal column, until it ends in the right atrium. The catheter was not long enough for further probing.

Aside from the sensations described (I paid particular attention to phenomena of irritation of the conduction system of the heart), I felt nothing. In our establishment it is a fairly long way from the operating room to the x-ray room, and even walking this distance with the catheter in my heart did not cause any discomfort. Insertion and extraction of the catheter were entirely painless, causing only the sensations described. Later I felt nothing detrimental aside from a slight inflammation at the site of the venesection, which probably resulted from faulty sterilization during my self-operation. I believe that the playfully easy movement of the well-oiled probe rules out any damage to the vein wall and thus any danger of clotting or thrombosis formation.

Of course, from wartime and postwar literature there are known cases of foreign objects being lodged in the heart for months with no disturbance. Likewise, Volkmann described a patient in whom an aspirating needle stayed in the right ventricle for 15 minutes, causing no damage.

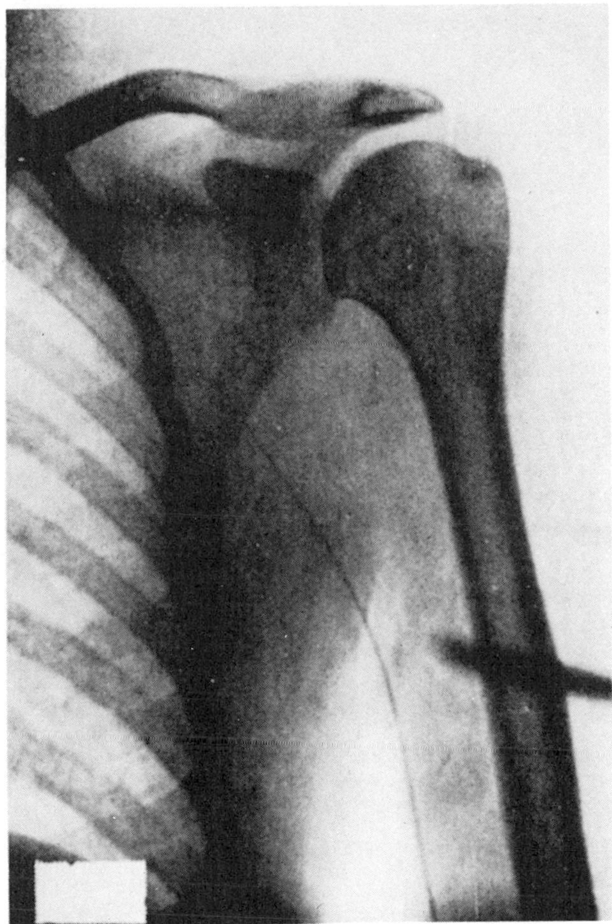

Figure 1 The catheter is inserted in the right cephalic vein to the height of the armpit. (Reproduced from *Klin. Wochenschr.*, **8**(45), 2085–2087 (1929); copyright © 1929 by Springer-Verlag, Berlin.)

Also, measurements of blood pressure were undertaken in animals in 1861 by Chauveau and Marey, who introduced measuring instruments into the heart from the jugular vein and the common carotid artery. All these observations prove the safety of such incursions into the heart. Of course, caution is urged in cases where either a tendency toward thrombosis or thrombosis itself is evident.

I had the first opportunity for a clinical application in a patient who had purulent peritonitis as a complication to a spreading inflammation of the appendix.

The patient was in extraordinarily bad condition and seemed to have a general circulatory disturbance—a small, soft, frequently varying pulse, blue patches on the limbs, labored shallow breathing, and blurring of consciousness. At 9:30 a venesection was made on the right arm and a

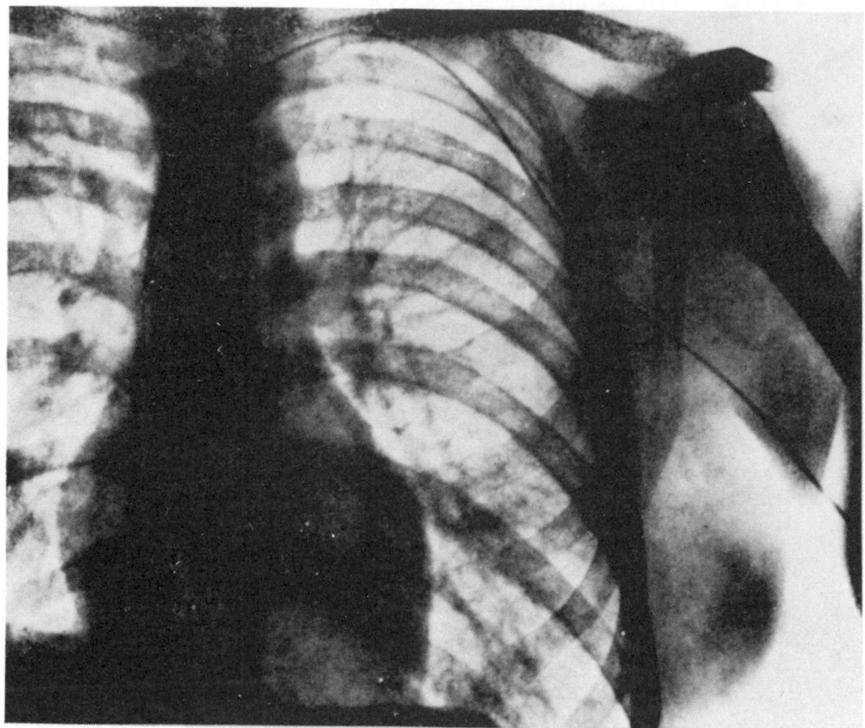

Figure 2 The catheter extends from the left cephalic vein downward into the right atrium. (Reproduced from *Klin. Wochenschr.*, **8**(45), 2085–2087 (1929); copyright © 1929 by Springer-Verlag, Berlin.)

catheter was inserted. A resistance met at about 30 cm was easily overcome by lifting the arm slightly, and the catheter was inserted to 60 cm. Following this, 1 liter of glucose with 0.002 Suprarenin hydrochloride and 0.001 strophanthin was infused continuously over 1 hour; visible improvement became apparent within minutes. The pulse became slow and strong, and breathing and consciousness normal. After the infusion, 0.25 ml of citrate solution was injected and the stylet was introduced. At 12:30 the patient's condition had deteriorated markedly, and I repeated the infusion without strophanthin. After slight fleeting improvements, death occurred at 3:10. Cardiac activity outlasted breathing by 6 minutes. I let the catheter remain, and at autopsy found it extending as intended from the vena cephalica to the right atrium; from there it went 2 cm more into the inferior vena cava. No change in the lining of the vessels was apparent and there was no thrombus formation, only some postmortem clotting in the vessel, just as in the other arm.

The findings show that not even the continuous presence of the catheter for 6½ hours in a weakened patient causes pathological changes in the blood vessels and heart. It is noteworthy that, in contrast to the cadaver experiment, the catheter did not enter the right ventricle but was in the inferior vena cava. This contradiction is explained by the fact that, in the cadaver, the blood vessels were collapsed and the catheter took the large opening into the chamber, whereas in the living person the wide open inferior vena cava, extending in the same direction as the superior vena cava, was the easier way. Experience must yet teach us the proper distance of the path from the elbow to the heart so that the heart will not be overshot.

I recommend that the method that I worked out be further tested, with puncture in favorable circumstances, with venesection in serious cases. In addition, I might also remark that it certainly is not obligatory to enter the vessels in the arm, and that any other part of the body can be used in deference to the individual anatomical circumstances. My method seems to me especially advantageous because it avoids the dangerous path through the chest wall and heart muscles and along with that the feared pericardial shock, and because it proceeds to the heart along a natural path. It is also especially suited in cases where time is short, since the catheter can be inserted in 3–4 seconds. It is also useful because, as my tests prove, it can be carried out in patients with poor circulation as well as in those with good heart function. Naturally, when the circulation is slow, a central infustion is significantly faster and much more effective than a peripheral infusion that must first be transported centrally. Along with the possibility of sampling blood with a syringe, there is also the possibility of relieving the right side of the heart, of having a central bloodletting. Concerning the various therapeutic indications, I refer the reader to the excellent comprehensive work of Henschen on resuscitation of the heart. I would only like to point out expressly that it is important not to waste extremely valuable time of as much as 10–15 minutes for resuscitation in cases of an anesthetic accident or death by shock.

I furthermore consider the method useful for performing slow intravenous injections, as for example during the administration of contrast media for studying the gall bladder and renal pelvis, or even for infusions. The catheter can be inserted for short distances, 20–30 cm (see Figure 1), and the injection may then be carried out as slowly as desired without fear of losing the vein.

For this purpose a sterile ureteral catheter is kept on supply, in sterile olive oil, along with attachable cannulas. Therefore, I suggest a nourishing oil and not a neutral lubricant such as liquid paraffin, so that any very small fat embolism of pulmonary capillaries can be immediately saponified and eliminated by the fat-splitting enzymes of the blood. That the stylet must also be well oiled to be handled easily goes without saying.

In conclusion I would like to mention that the method that I used opens up countless vistas of new possibilities for studies of metabolism and cardiac activity, which I am already pursuing.

BIBLIOGRAPHY

L. Aschoff, *Pathologische Anatomie,* 1923.
Esch, *Münch. med. Wschr.,* **1916**:786.
Henschen, Die Wiederbelebung des Herzens durch peri- und intrakardiale Injection, durch Herzaderlass und Herzinfusion. *Schweizer med. Wschr.,* **1**:261–270 (1920).
Landois-Rosemann, *Lehrbuch der Physiologie des Menschen,* 1923.
E. Vogt, *Verh. dtsch. Ges. Chir.,* **45**:26.
Volkmann, *Med. Klin.,* **1917,** No. 52, 1357.

47

Reprinted from *Proc. Soc. Exp. Biol. Med.*, **46**(3), 462–466 (1941)

CATHETERIZATION OF THE RIGHT AURICLE IN MAN

Andre Cournand and Hilmert A. Ranges*

From the Departments of Medicine, College of Physicians and Surgeons, Columbia University, and of New York University College of Medicine, and the Third Medical Division (N.Y.U.), Bellevue Hospital, New York City.

Forssmann[1] first used catheterization of the right heart on himself, after exposure of a vein of the arm by a surgeon. Numerous other investigators since have used right heart catheterization for visualization of the right chamber of the heart and pulmonary vascular trees by means of contrast substance.[2–7] The introduction of the Robb and Steinberg method,[8] however, renders this method unnecessary for the latter purpose. Collection of right heart blood by catheterization of the right auricle for determining cardiac output in man[9] is mentioned by Grollman,[10] who discredits it because of the possible

*Supported by a grant from the Commonwealth Fund.

1 Forssmann, W., *Klin. Wchschr.*, 1929, **8**, 2085.

2 Forssmann, W., *Muench. Med. Wchschr.*, 1931, **78**, 489.

3 Egas Moniz, Lopo de Carvalho, and Almeida Lima, *Presse med.*, 1931, **39**, 996.

4 Heuser, C., *Rev. Asoc. med. argent.*, 1932, **46**, 1119.

5 Conte, E., and Costa, A., *Radiology*, 1933, **21**, 461.

6 Ravina, A., *Progres med.*, November 3, 1934, p. 1701.

7 Ameuille, P., Ronneaux, G., Hinault, V., DeGrez, and Lemoine, J. M., *Bull. et mem. Soc. med. d. hop. de Paris*, 1936, **60**, 720.

8 Robb, G. P., and Steinberg, I., *J. Clin. Invest.*, 1938, **17**, 507.

9 Klein, O., *Muench. Med. Wchschr.*, 1930, **77**, 1311.

10 Grollman, A., *The Cardiac Output of Man in Health and Disease*, Monograph, Williams and Wilkins Co., Baltimore, 1932.

dangers and numerous misleading factors associated with it. In animal experimentation it is widely used and its innocuity established.

Because it is apparently the soundest method for obtaining mixed venous blood for respiratory gas determinations, and because of the numerous problems of hemodynamics it might help solve, a method of right heart catheterization was developed which attempts to overcome objections to former methods. The principal objections included the possibility of venous thrombi and thrombophlebitis that might be associated with introduction of a foreign body in the blood stream, the formation of thrombi within the catheter, and the psychic effects accompanying the procedure with possible alterations in the cardiac output.

The following equipment was used in our method: a specially made 10 gauge Lindeman type of needle; a 3-way stopcock with a Luer lock, tightly fitting adapter; a No. 8 French flexible radiopaque ureteral catheter with 2 holes, one at the rounded tip and another about 1 cm from the tip. The catheter is silk with a smooth varnish finish. A saline reservoir with rubber tubing and clamp for controlling the rate of flow was also used.

Under the strictest asepsis a nick is made in the skin over the median basilic vein of either the right or left arm after a preliminary infiltration with 2% novocain. After applying a tourniquet and fixing the distal portion of the vein with the fingers, the special needle is introduced. The catheter is next introduced into the vein through the needle. The end of the catheter is connected to the saline reservoir by a screw adapter, and a constant flow of saline at the rate of 15 drops per minute allowed to flow through the catheter throughout the procedure. When the catheter has been inserted about 12 cm into the vein, the needle is removed. This is done to prevent the possibility of cutting or shaving the catheter when it is withdrawn or pulled back in manipulation. The further passage of the catheter is done on a horizontal fluoroscopic table, using the fluoroscope in guiding the catheter to the desired position.

Occasionally resistance in passing the catheter may be encountered in the axillary region or at the level of the first rib. This can usually be overcome by drawing the catheter back slightly and placing the arm at a lower level than the table and rotating it inwardly. Several possible false routes may be encountered. It is conceivable that the flexible catheter might find its way into one of the jugular veins, but we have not encountered this. The catheter has on 2 occasions passed into the innominate vein of the opposite side, and occurrence immediately recognized under the fluoroscope. In either case the

TABLE I.

Influence of Right Auricle Catheterization and Arterial Blood Puncture upon Various Respiratory and Circulatory Measurements in 8 Successive Experiments.

Subject	Date	Time	Ventil. 1/min	Rate per min	Gas exchange CO_2 cc/min	Gas exchange O_2 cc/min	R.Q.	Pulse per min	Venous pressure, mm	C.I.* 1/min sq.m.B.S.	S.V.* cc Beat	Observations
G.B.	10/25/40	Before	9.14	21	201	261	.77	89	132			Catheter in position 15′.
Malignant		During	9.38	22	201	275	.73	88	132†			
hypertension,	31	Before	14.57	29				93		2.29	35.5	,, ,, ,, 20′.
heart failure		During	16.42	26	221	272	.81	95		2.50	37.9	
P.T.	11/27	Before	12.67	19	223	316	.71	115		3.11	42.2	,, ,, ,, 50′.
Carcinoma		During	11.63	18	194	282	.69	114	80†	2.71	36.2	Intra-auricular pressure = 10 mm change between inspiration and expiration
liver (?)												
F.L.	12/20	Before	8.08	21	158	201	.79	79	34	2.92	61.3	Catheter in position 30′.
Carcinoma		During 1	7.78	22	168	214	.79					15′ interval between Exp. 1 and 2
stomach		,, 2	8.46	22	168	216	.79	66	34	2.72	68.3	
	27	Before	7.44	19	157	200	.79	72				Catheter in position 40′.
		During 1	8.69	22	191	236	.81	66				15′ between Exp. 1 and 2.
		,, 2	9.14	25	189	237	.80	66				
	31	Before	8.32	22	167	218	.77	80		3.13	65.0	Catheter in position 25′.
		During	8.95	19	192	225	.85	68		2.80	68.4	
G.T.	1/14/41	Before	7.92	15	174	191	.91	88		2.66	45.8	Catheter in position 50′.
Carcinoma		During 1	8.72	21	178	205	.87	86				20′ between Exp. 1 and 2.
stomach		,, 2	8.07	20	158	193	.82	80		2.46	46.6	
	21	Before	6.54	16	156	208	.75	81				Catheter in position 60′.
		During 1	7.36	19	175	225	.78	80	30†	2.17	40.6	
		,, 2	7.50	19	168	221	.76	88	30†	2.29	40.8	20′ between Exp. 1 and 2.

*Stroke volume and cardiac index calculated from ballistocardiogram tracings (wave area formula) and cross-section area of the aorta (Bazett's table) using ideal weight.

†Intra-auricular pressure.

tip is withdrawn to the axillary region and further attempts made to pass it to its proper position. When the tip is in the right auricle, if blood is to be collected through the catheter, the tubing of the saline reservoir is first disconnected and a large syringe filled with a little saline is adapted to the 3-way stopcock. Two or 3 cc of blood are drawn into this syringe, thus washing the catheter with right heart blood. Then the valve is turned and the blood for analysis is collected in a second syringe containing mineral oil as an air seal. Fifteen to 20 cc of blood can be collected within 25 seconds by using only the slightest amount of suction. When the blood has been collected, the saline reservoir may be connected again and saline allowed to run slowly into the catheter to keep it open. Duplicate samples may be taken later. Finally, the catheter is withdrawn and examined carefully for any evidence of thrombi.

In our experience we have found no evidence of blood clotting on the smooth outside walls of the catheter. Nor have there been any thrombi seen at the holes of the catheter or within the catheter when it is flushed with saline after being withdrawn. We do not believe that the results are affected by any psychic disturbance. There is no pain involved in the operation, once the needle is in place in the arm vein. The pulse rate does not vary significantly before and during the procedure, and cardiac output determinations as measured by the ballistocardiograph before, during and after the procedure are quite constant.

Table I shows the influence of the catheterization associated with an arterial puncture, in 8 successive passages, upon ventilatory volume and rate, gas exchange and respiratory quotient, pulse rate and cardiac output measured with a ballistocardiograph, and in a few instances upon the venous pressure. The ballistocardiograph used differs slightly in design from that described by Starr, *et al.*,[11] and was developed in the Department of Physiology, New York University College of Medicine.

Protocol of Determination of Cardiac Output by Simultaneous Sampling of Right Auricle and Femoral Arterial Blood and Collection of Expired Air (Tissot).*

F.L. Age 61 Weight 53 kg Height 180 cm. Body surface area 1.66 sq.m.
Carcinoma of stomach.
Date—12/31/40—not basal.
Ventilation = 7.77 lit./min., dry gas 0°C, 760 mm Hg.
CO_2 Output = 2.47 %—192 cc/min.
O_2 Intake = 2.89 %—225 cc/min.
R.Q. = .854
CO_2 Content, vols.%: M.V.B.† = 54.7—art. blood = 51.2—A—V difference = 3.5.

11 Starr, I., Rawson, A. J., Schroeder, H. A., and Joseph, N. R., *Am. J. Physiol.*, 1939, **127**, 1.

O_2 Content, vol.%: M.V.B.† = 10.0 — art. blood = 14.0 — A—V difference = 4.0.

$$\text{R.Q. from blood: } \frac{CO_2 \text{ A—V difference}}{O_2 \text{ A—V difference}} = .875.$$

Cardiac Output, lit./min. from

$$CO_2 \text{ A—V difference} = \frac{192}{3.5} = 5.49.$$

$$O_2 \text{ A—V difference} = \frac{225}{4.0} = 5.63.$$

Cardiac Index = 3.35 lit./sq.m. B.S. area.
Heart rate per minute = 70.
Stroke Volume = 79.5 cc.

*Arterial blood sampling starting and ending approximately 15 seconds after mixed venous blood sampling. Total duration of sampling of both bloods 35 seconds. Expired air collected during blood sampling.

†M.V.B. (mixed venous blood) refers to blood drawn directly from the right auricle.

The protocol of one cardiac output determination by simultaneous collection of blood from the right auricle and femoral artery is included herewith. The number of simultaneous determinations of stroke volume measured by this method and compared with estimations from ballistocardiograph tracings is not large enough to warrant a statement concerning the validity of the ballistic method at this time.

48

Pulmonary 'Capillary' Pressure in Man[1]

H. K. HELLEMS,[2] F. W. HAYNES AND L. DEXTER. *From the Medical Clinic, Peter Bent Brigham Hospital, and the Department of Medicine, Harvard Medical School, Boston, Massachusetts*

UNTIL THE DEVELOPMENT of the technique of venous catheterization by Cournand and Ranges (1), no method was readily available for studying pulmonary circulatory dynamics in man. The introduction of this technique has permitted the elucidation of many problems of the lesser circulation in health and disease, until at present the pressures in the right side of the heart and pulmonary artery are common knowledge. Using this technique, a method has been developed by which the capillary pressure of the human lung may be estimated.

In a previous communication (2), the technique of estimating pulmonary 'capillary' pressure in the lungs of animals was reported. In this paper the method as applied to the human lung is described. In subsequent communications the results obtained in patients with heart and pulmonary disease under conditions of rest and exercise will be reported.

METHODS

Thirteen patients were selected for study who had normal cardiovascular systems as far as could be judged from history, physical examination, X-ray, and electrocardiogram. The majority had primary syphilis and were studied at least 48 hours after the institution of penicillin therapy. Ten were males, three were females, and their ages varied from 18 to 40 years. The subjects were studied in a resting state under fasting conditions. Venous catheterization was carried out under fluoroscopic guidance, the catheter being introduced into a distal branch of the pulmonary artery so as to occlude it. The size of the vessel occluded varied between about 2 and 3 mm. depending on the catheter size. Measurements of the pressure existing distal to the occluding catheter were recorded through the hole in the tip of the catheter with a column of saline and with a Hamilton manometer (3). The pressure recorded in this fashion in this occluded vessel will be referred to as the pulmonary 'capillary' pressure for reasons that will be discussed later. The catheter was then withdrawn so as to lie free in the pulmonary artery and pressures were again recorded.

In 7 individuals with arterial oxygen unsaturation due to a right-to-left shunt within the heart or to pulmonary or hepatic disease (see table 2), blood samples were withdrawn under oil from a systemic artery and through a catheter occluding the lumen of a branch of the pulmonary artery. These bloods were analyzed by the method of Van Slyke and Neill (4) for oxygen content, capacity, and saturation.

Received for publication April 1, 1949.

[1] This study was supported by a grant from The Life Insurance Medical Research Fund.

[2] This work was done during the tenure of a Life Insurance Medical Research Fellowship.

In 2 patients with atrial septal defect, venous catheterization was carried out as described elsewhere (5, 6). In each case the catheter was introduced through the defect into the left auricle and out into a pulmonary vein so as to occlude it. After recording the pressure, the catheter was withdrawn to the right auricle and introduced into the right ventricle and pulmonary artery where it was wedged into a distal branch where pressures were again recorded.

The zero point for all pressures was taken 10 cm. anterior to the spine with the subject in the supine position. The antero-posterior diameter of the chest was recorded for the convenience of those using other zero points of reference. Mean pressures were obtained with the saline manometer and by planimetric integration of the Hamilton pressure tracings.

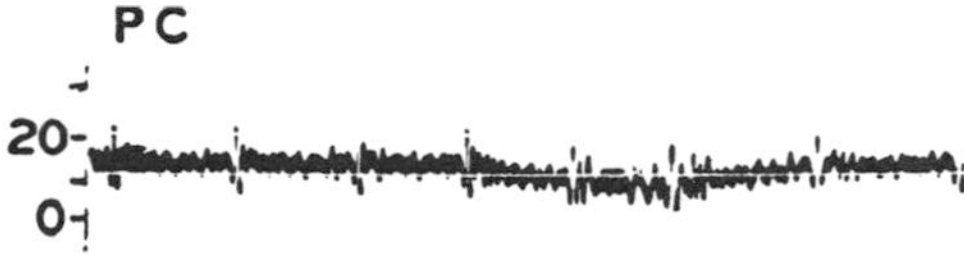

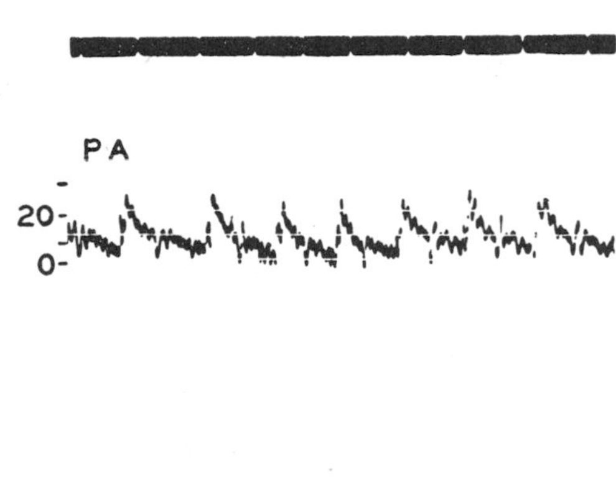

Fig. 1. PRESSURE TRACINGS FROM THE PULMONARY 'CAPILLARIES' (PC) and pulmonary artery (PA) in a normal individual. Note the respiratory variation of pressure and the lack of definite pulsations in the 'capillary' curve. The lower tracing shows the typical pulsatile contour of the pressure in the pulmonary artery. In each tracing, there are numerous artefacts due to motion of the catheter within the heart.

RESULTS

In 13 normal individuals, the contour of the pressure curves obtained through the catheter occluding the pulmonary artery was distinctly different from that obtained when it lay free in the pulmonary artery. As can be seen from figure 1, no definite pulse wave was visible but there was frequently a considerable respiratory variation in the pressure, the pressure being lower on inspiration than in expiration by an average of 8 mm. Hg (table 1). In these 13 patients, the mean pressures at rest averaged 10 mm. Hg with a variation from 7 to 15 (table 1). The pulmonary artery pressures varied between 19 and 30 mm. Hg systolic and 6 and 12 diastolic with an average pressure of 24/10.

TABLE 1. PULMONARY ARTERY AND PULMONARY 'CAPILLARY' PRESSURES, PRESSURE GRADIENT, AND PULMONARY VASCULAR RESISTANCE IN 13 NORMAL INDIVIDUALS

CASE NO.	PATIENT	A-P DIAMETER OF CHEST	PULMONARY ARTERY PRESSURE, MM. HG				PULMONARY 'CAPILLARY' PRESSURE, MM. HG				PRESSURE GRADIENT BETWEEN PULMONARY ARTERY AND PULMONARY 'CAPILLARIES'
			Systolic	Diastolic	Mean		Inspiration	Expiration	Mean		
					Hamilton	Saline			Hamilton	Saline	
		cm.									*mm. Hg*
1	*R. A.*	19.0	23	10	18	17	6	13	10		8
2	*E. B.*	21.0	28	12	21		2	22	15	11	6
3	*A. C.*	15.5	23	10	17	16	8	16	13	11	4
4	*M. C.*		25	12	17		5	10	8		9
5	*J. D.*	21.0	25	12	17	19	8	10	9	12	8
6	*E. F.*	20.0	26	10	15		2	12	7		8
7	*N. F.*	21.0	30	9	18		5	14	11		7
8	*H. H.*	17.5	19	7	11	17	3	10	7	12	4
9	*U. M.*	18.0	23	6	13	16	5	12	9	11	4
10	*J. M.*		25	10	16	15	10	14	13	12	3
11	*M. N.*	15.0	24	10	17	17	8	16	12		3
12	*W. P.*	19.0	22	6	14		6	12	9	10	5
13	*F. R.*		23	10	13		3	10	7		6
Average.............			24	10	16		5	13	10		6

TABLE 2. OXYGEN SATURATION OF PULMONARY 'CAPILLARY' BLOOD IN PATIENTS WITH SYSTEMIC ARTERIAL OXYGEN UNSATURATION

CASE NO.	PATIENT	DIAGNOSIS	SYSTEMIC ARTERY			PULMONARY END ARTERY		
			O_2 content	O_2 capacity	O_2 saturation	O_2 content	O_2 capacity	O_2 saturation
		Arterial oxygen unsaturation resulting from a right-to-left cardiac shunt						
			cc/l.	*cc/l.*	*per cent*	*cc/l.*	*cc/l.*	*per cent*
1	*A. D.*	Tetralogy of Fallot	171	257	66	234	238	98
2	*V. R.*	Tetralogy of Fallot	233	285	82	276	285	97
3	*J. C.*	Tetralogy of Fallot	151	163	93	165	166	99
		Arterial oxygen unsaturation of pulmonary or other origin						
4	*M. G.*	Mitral stenosis						
		Pulmonary congestion	169	188	90	177	180	98
5	*M. D.*	Aortic stenosis, anemia						
		Pulmonary congestion	101	113	89	110	113	97
6	*S. A.*	Hepatic failure	203	224	91	202	204	99
7	*W. M.*	Emphysema	167	207	81	195	200	98

The mean pulmonary artery pressure as determined by planimetric integration of the pressure curves was 16 mm. Hg at rest with variations between 11 and 21. The gradient of pressure between the pulmonary artery and the pulmonary 'capillaries' varied between 3 and 9 mm. Hg with an average of 6.

Blood samples withdrawn through a venous catheter occluding a branch of the pulmonary artery in patients with arterial oxygen unsaturation from various causes were found to be fully saturated with oxygen (table 2).

In 2 patients with atrial septal defect in whom pressures were recorded through the catheter first wedged into the pulmonary vein and then into the pulmonary artery, the pressures recorded on the two sides of the pulmonary capillary bed are shown in table 3, and it will be seen that the values were identical.

TABLE 3. PRESSURES IN PULMONARY ARTERY, IN OCCLUDED PULMONARY ARTERY, AND IN OCCLUDED PULMONARY VEIN OF PATIENTS WITH ATRIAL SEPTAL DEFECT

CASE NO.	PATIENT	PULMONARY ARTERY PRESSURE, MM. HG			PULMONARY END ARTERY MEAN PRESSURE, MM. HG		PULMONARY END VEIN MEAN PRESSURE, MM. HG	
		Systolic	Diastolic	Mean	Hamilton Manometer	Saline Manometer	Hamilton Manometer	Saline Manometer
1	*S. W.*	41	21	30	10	11	11	11
2	*V. E.*	29	9	20	11	7	11	7

DISCUSSION

In a previous communication (2) evidence was presented that in dogs the pressure beyond the point of occlusion of a small branch of the pulmonary artery was about 2 mm. Hg less, and that the pressure measured on the capillary side of a small occluded pulmonary vein was about 2 mm. Hg more than the true pulmonary capillary pressure. This relationship held over a wide range of capillary pressure. The validity of this method of determining the pressure in the pulmonary capillaries is based on the following evidence (fig. 2).

1) The pulmonary arteries ramify and finally end in the capillaries, there being no pre-capillary anastomoses with adjacent pulmonary arteries (7, 8). This is supported by the physiological observation that in normal individuals blood withdrawn through a catheter occluding the lumen of a branch of the pulmonary artery is fully saturated with oxygen (9).

2) There is normally an anastomosis between the bronchial arterial and pulmonary arterial circulations in the capillary bed of the lung (7, 8). No evidence for the existence of any significant pre-capillary anastomoses has been found because, as shown in table 2, in individuals with oxygen unsaturation of the systemic (and therefore bronchial) arterial blood, whether of shunt origin in heart or lung, full arterial oxygen saturation has been found in the blood samples withdrawn through a catheter occluding a branch of the pulmonary artery. If there were any significant pre-capillary anastomoses of the bronchial arteries with the pulmonary arteries, the samples withdrawn through the catheter would have had some degree of oxygen unsaturation.

3) There are no valves in the pulmonary artery, vein, or capillaries anatomically (7, 10) or physiologically (2), so that there is free retrograde flow, cross-flow, and transmission of pressure from the pulmonary capillaries to the catheter wedged into the pulmonary artery.

4) The capillary bed of the lung contains such a rich network of vessels that blood may actually be aspirated back from the capillaries through the catheter occluding the pulmonary artery (9).

In two patients with atrial septal defect, the identity of pressures recorded on the capillary side of an occluded pulmonary artery and vein further support the interpretation that these pressures are close approximations of the true

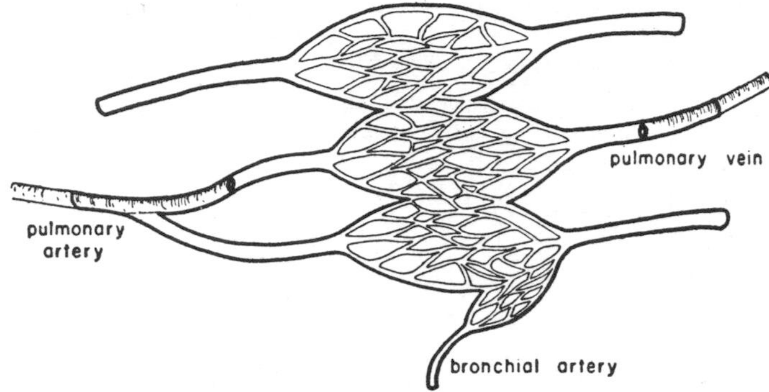

Fig. 2. DIAGRAM OF THE PULMONARY CAPILLARY CIRCULATION as applied to this study showing catheters wedged into the pulmonary artery and pulmonary vein. For a more detailed description and diagram of the pulmonary circulation, see Bruner and Schmidt (8).

pulmonary capillary pressure (see table 3). Any error on the arterial side will be in the direction of a lower reading than the true capillary pressure (2). In dogs, this amounts to only a few millimeters of mercury (2). For this reason, the term 'capillary' pressure is enclosed in quotation marks.

The average pulmonary 'capillary' pressure obtained in the manner described was 9 mm. Hg in 13 normal patients. The gradient of pressure between pulmonary artery and 'capillaries' averaged only 6 mm. Hg at rest.

SUMMARY

A venous catheter has been introduced into the pulmonary artery of man and wedged into a distal ramification so as to obstruct its lumen. Blood samples withdrawn through this catheter in individuals with systemic arterial oxygen unsaturation were fully saturated with oxygen, indicating the lack of any significant pre-capillary admixture of bronchial with pulmonary arterial blood. Pressures recorded through the catheter in the position described have been found to be identical with those recorded through a catheter wedged into a pulmonary vein in two patients with atrial septal defects. It is therefore believed that both pressures are close approximations of the true pulmonary capillary pressure.

The pulmonary 'capillary' pressure was found to average 10 mm. Hg with a variation between 7 and 15 in 13 normal patients. The mean pulmonary artery pressure in these individuals averaged 16 mm. Hg with variations between 11 and 21. The gradient of pressure between pulmonary artery and pulmonary 'capillaries' varied between 3 and 9 mm. Hg with an average of 6.

The authors are indebted to the Godfrey M. Hyams Trust, through whose generous contribution the equipment necessary for the fulfillment of this study was purchased.

We wish to express our appreciation to Miss Barbara Jacobs and Mrs. Harriet Kriete for their technical assistance.

REFERENCES

1. Cournand, A. and H. A. Ranges. *Proc. Soc. Exper. Biol. & Med.* 46: 462, 1941.
2. Hellems, H. K., F. W. Haynes, L. Dexter, and T. D. Kinney. *Am. J. Physiol.* 155: 98, 1948.
3. Hamilton, W. F., G. Brewer, and I. Brotman. *Am. J. Physiol.* 107: 427, 1934.
4. Peters, J. P. and D. D. Van Slyke. *Quantitative Clinical Chemistry.* Baltimore: Williams & Wilkins, 1943, Vol. 2.
5. Dexter, L., F. W. Haynes, C. S. Burwell, E. C. Eppinger, R. E. Seibel, and J. M. Evans. *J. Clin. Investigation* 26: 547, 1947.
6. Dexter, L., F. W. Haynes, C. S. Burwell, E. C. Eppinger, M. C. Sosman, and J. M. Evans. *J. Clin. Investigation* 26: 561, 1947.
7. Miller, W. S. *The Lung.* Springfield: Charles C Thomas 1943.
8. Bruner, H. D. and C. F. Schmidt. *Am. J. Physiol.* 148: 648, 1947.
9. Dexter, L., F. W. Haynes, C. S. Burwell, E. C. Eppinger, R. P. Sagerson, and J. M. Evans. *J. Clin. Investigation* 26: 554, 1947.
10. Karsner, H. T. and A. A. Ghoreyeb. *J. Exper. Med.* 18: 507, 1913.

49

Reprinted from *Acta Physiol. Scand.*, **12**, 301–306, 309–312, 316–320 (1946)

Observations on the Pulmonary Arterial Blood Pressure in the Cat.

By

U. S. v. EULER and G. LILJESTRAND.

Received 9 August 1946.

The well-known regulatory influence exerted on the general blood pressure by impulses deriving from the sinus and aortic reflexogenic zones raises the question as to whether the pulmonary arterial blood pressure is subject to regulatory forces of a similar or different kind. The lungs, being placed in series with the general circulation, would scarcely be dependent on the maintenance of a certain blood pressure level in order to ensure the blood supply to the organ itself, as is the case for a number of organs in the general circulation, notably the central nervous system and the kidneys. On the other hand, there would seem to be reason for some regulation in so far as a high level of pulmonary capillary blood pressure might be harmful on account of the risk of pulmonary oedema.

The existence and rôle of pulmonary vasomotor nerves, which might convey such regulatory influences, has been the subject of numerous investigations, beginning with BRADFORD and DEAN (1889), FRANÇOIS-FRANCK (1895), HENRIQUES (1892), TIGERSTEDT (1903), and others, and more recently by DALY and his co-workers (BERRY and DALY, 1931, DALY and EULER, 1932).

In order to obtain reliable figures for the pulmonary arterial blood pressure, it would seem necessary to keep the animal under as physiological conditions as possible concerning the respiratory functions, and this would involve measurements during spontaneous respiration and a closed thorax. Experiments of this kind are comparatively few. DALY (1937) and later KATZ and STEINITZ (1940) measured the pulmonary arterial blood pressure by the use of the London technique. In several cases, however, the blood pressure in the right ventricle in animals with a closed thorax has been measured.

The earlier experiments concerning the pulmonary circulation have mostly been undertaken with open thorax, though care has been taken in many instances to avoid pneumothorax and to retain spontaneous respiration. Of course, this does not ensure natural conditions with regard to the intrathoracic pressure, since the mediastinal wall is not a rigid structure as is the thorax. However, many of the results add valuable information as to the response of the pulmonary vessels to nervous and chemical stimuli. LICHTHEIM reported, as early as 1876, that at least 3/4 of the total vascular bed of the pulmonary arteries could be excluded without causing any change in the systemic blood pressure. The experiments were performed on curarised dogs, but in one instance also on a non-anaesthetized, spontaneously breathing rabbit with a unilateral pneumothorax. LICHTHEIM also observed a rise in the pulmonary blood pressure of about 50 per cent on compression of the left pulmonary artery, and conlcuded that the right heart was forcing the same volume of blood through the expanded remaining vessels as through the whole lungs before compression. Vasomotor regulatory influences acting on the systemic circulation were disregarded as a possible cause of the maintenance of the blood pressure level, since there was no sign of even a temporary change in the systemic blood pressure on compression of a pulmonary artery. These results were confirmed by TIGERSTEDT (1903) who stated that compression of the hilus of one lung did not cause any change in the systemic blood pressure. The pulmonary arterial pressure was not measured in his experiments, but the maximal pressure in the right ventricle was only slightly raised or changed, and he therefore advanced the opinion that previously excluded parts of the pulmonary vascular bed were switched into the circulation on compression of the vessels to one lung.

One of the important observations by TIGERSTEDT prompted the statement that no definite relation could be found between the systemic and the pulmonary arterial blood pressure. The relation showed variations between 1: 13 and 1: 1.3 in the rabbit. Generally the absolute pressure varied between 11 and 25 mm Hg, though as low a value as 8 mm was found at a systemic pressure of about 100 mm Hg. The maximal pressure observed on occlusion of the aorta was in no case higher than 51 mm Hg.

The effect of stimulation of the pulmonary vasomotor nerves has been studied by a number of investigators, and more recently by DALY and his co-worker on the dog's isolated perfused lungs. They found that vagal stimulation generally caused a moderate vasodilatation, and stimulation of the stellate ganglion vasoconstriction. On the isolated perfused rabbit's lung EULER (1932) showed that vagal stimulation, similar to injection of acetylcholine, caused a rise in pulmonary arterial pressure, and injection of adrenaline likewise produced a slight rise.

Two questions seem to merit special interest with regard to the hemodynamics of the pulmonary circulation. One is the reaction of the lung vessels to a greatly increased flow, as will occur for instance in muscular work, and the second is in what way the lung vessels react to variations in the blood gases. These problems have been subjected to a study on anaesthetized cats breathing spontaneously with closed thorax or in some cases artificially ventilated.

Methods.

In all experiments cats weighing 3—4 kg were used, anaesthetized with 0.05—0.06 g chloralose per kg intravenously through a brachial vein. Arterial systemic blood pressure was recorded from one carotid artery.

In order to record the pulmonary arterial pressure the technique of MELLIN (1904) was used in principle, with slight modifications. The thorax was opened widely on the left side between two ribs at the level of the pulmonary artery, and artificial respiration given. By opening the pericardium the pulmonary artery was exposed, care being taken not to sever the nervous tissue between the pulmonary artery and the aorta. The pulmonary artery was compressed near its origin by means of a pair of forceps. When completely compressed, a rapid fall in the general blood pressure ensued and a short longitudinal slit was then made in the pulmonary arterial wall by means of fine scissors. The special cannula described below (see Fig. 1) was then quickly inserted and the blood stream through the artery released. The cannula consisted of two well-fitting, concentric metal tubes which could

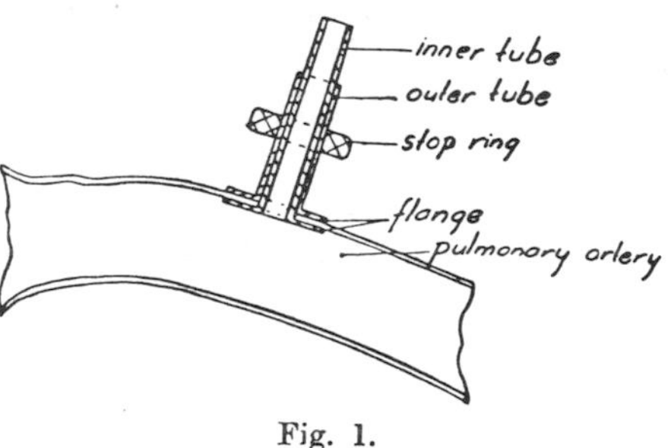

Fig. 1.

be moved one within the other. Both were fitted with slightly curved flanges at their ends, giving a good contact surface. When inserting the cannula, the flange of the inner tube was inserted into the lumen of the vessel. Then the outer tube was slid down so that its flange pressed against the flange of the inner tube, thereby gripping the edges of the incision in the vessel wall. The outer tube was fixed in this position by a stop ring. When the cannula was properly inserted, no bleeding occurred. The cannula was then slightly supported in order to prevent compression or kinking of the vessel, and the thorax closed at an inflated state of the lungs. Spontaneous respiration was soon resumed and normal mechanical conditions in the thorax were restored.

For the recording of the pulmonary arterial blood pressure, the cannula was connected with a vertical 30 cm glass tube of the same bore as the cannula (about 3 mm) which was connected to a piston recorder. The actual pressure in mm blood could thus be read at any time and the tracing calibrated at desired intervals. Clotting was prevented by pure heparin, kindly placed at our disposal by Dr. E. Jorpes.

As a control, in several instances, the pressure was recorded simultaneously from the left auricle. Various gas mixtures were administered either through a Lovén respiratory valve when the animal was breathing spontaneously, or by attachment of gas bags to the Starling pump.

Muscular work was induced by placing the electrodes of an "Innervator" apparatus, giving alternating current at a frequency of about 50 Hz and with rhythmically varying strength, low on the back and on the lower belly.

Denervation of the sinus region was performed by tying off the tissue between the external and the internal carotids.

Results.

1. Pulmonary Arterial Blood Pressure under Normal Experimental Conditions.

Beutner (1852), in Ludwig's laboratory, seems to have made the first observations on the pulmonary blood pressure. In the cat he found values of 7.5—24.7 , on an average 17.6 mm Hg. In our preparations, where the spontaneous respiration after closure was satisfactory, but also in those cases where adequate artificial respiration was instituted and the general systemic blood pressure was at an ordinary level, the pulmonary arterial blood pressure was fairly constant. The following table shows the approximate, typical level of the systemic and pulmonary pressures in the 9 experiments where conditions were considered satisfactory.

The relation between the pulmonary and the systemic arterial pressures thus varied between 1: 13—14 and 1: 5, on an average 1: 7—1: 8 during normal steady conditions. This compares well

Nr	Systemic B. P. mm Hg	Pulmonary B. P.		Breathing
		cm water	mm Hg	
1	115	22	16	Artificial
2	150	30	22	Spontaneous
3	160	16	12	»
4	120	20	15	»
5	90	23	17	Artificial
6	120	22	16	Spontaneous
7	150	25	18	»
8	150	23	17	»
9	135	24	18	»
Average:	132	23	17	

with the observations of Beutner for cats and of Tigerstedt for rabbits where no fixed relation between the pressures was found. The latter author gave the limits for the relative pressures of 1: 13 and 1: 1.3, though it should be remarked that the lower ratios corresponded to either unusually high pulmonary pressure or low systemic pressure or both, indicating abnormal conditions.

In the majority of experiments, the pulmonary pressure levels remained quite steady apart from the oscillations produced by the respiratory movements, and this is clearly seen in most of the tracings. In one experiment (nr 4) large waves appeared, however, with a frequency of about 2 in 3 minutes (Fig. 2). The waves had an amplitude of about 5 cm water but in spite of these considerable variations they were hardly reflected at all in the systemic pressure, as seen in fig. 2. This seems to contradict the explanation given by Aalkjaer (1935), who considered the

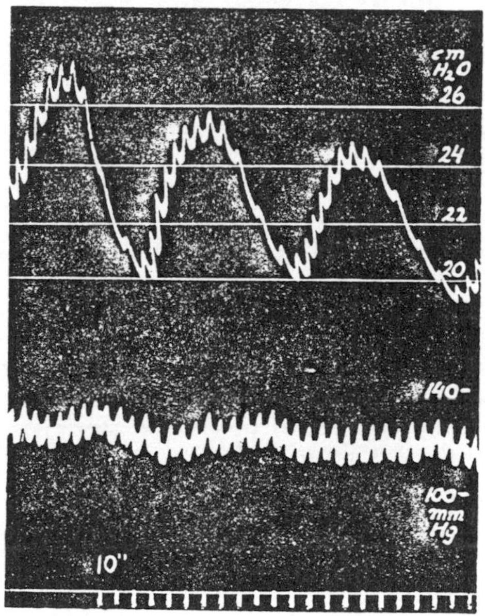

Fig. 2. Cat. 2.9 kg. Chloralose. Upper curve pulmonary arterial pressure with spontaneous waves, lower curve systemic blood pressure. Spontaneous breathing, closed thorax. Time 10 sec.

rhythmical variations in the pulmonary blood pressure to be due to similar variations in the systemic pressure. The waves gradually disappeared when the systemic pressure fell to some 70 mm Hg. It seems reasonable to assume that the effects on both systems are the result of rhythmical activity in the vasomotor centre. Other types of waves occurring independently of the systemic pressure have also been noted (see fig. 3).

Towards the end of an experiment there was mostly a tendency for the pulmonary arterial pressure to rise. Doubtless the reason for this must be found partly in a relative insufficiency of the left heart, resulting in pulmonary congestion, and partly in commencing asphyxial changes in the blood which will increase the pulmonary arterial pressure (see below, p. 309).

[*Editor's Note:* Material has been omitted at this point.]

3. Effects of Inhalation of Gas Mixtures of Varying Oxygen and Carbon Dioxide Content.

The influence of variations in the blood gases on the systemic blood pressure has been subject to numerous observations under varying experimental conditions. The discoveries of HEYMANS and his co-workers (1932) concerning the reflex control of blood pressure through the medium of the chemoreceptors constitute the most important recent contributions to this problem. Recently EULER and LILJESTRAND (1946) have studied the effects of blood gas variations on the systemic blood pressure of the cat and summarized the results.

With regard to the effects of the blood gases on the pulmonary blood pressure, this question may be said to merit special interest on account of the gas exchange in the lungs.

We have tested in repeated experiments the effects of gas mixtures rich and poor in oxygen, as well as rich in carbon dioxide.

a) *Oxygen-lack and pure oxygen.* If the animal is made to breathe a mixture containing 10—11 per cent oxygen in nitrogen, an increase of the pulmonary arterial pressure was invariably

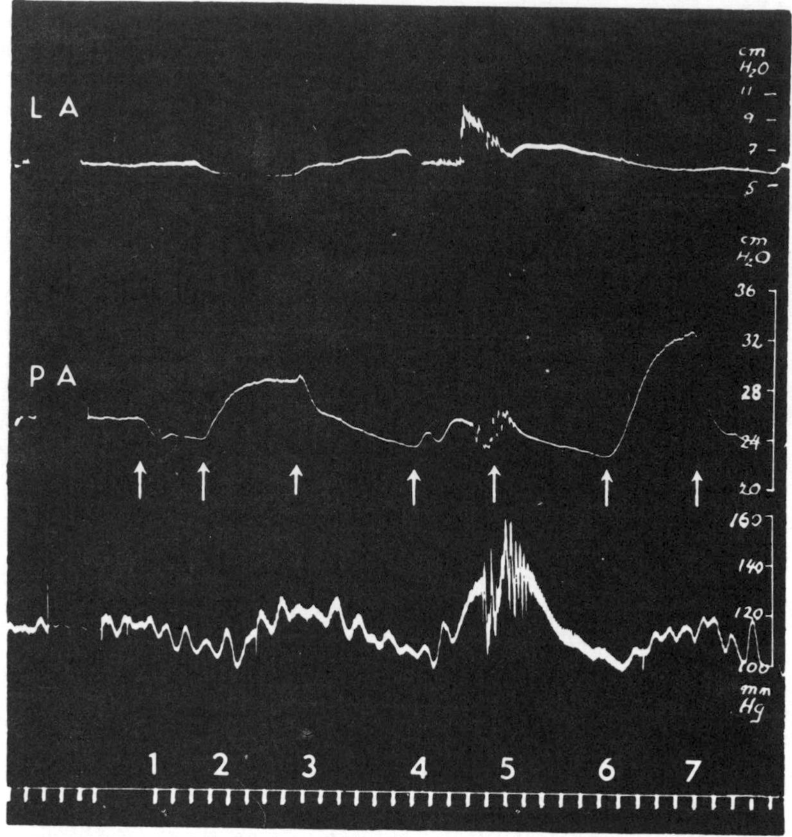

Fig. 6. Cat. 3.9 kg. Chloralose. Uppermost curve pressure in left auricle, middle curve pulmonary arterial pressure, lower curve systemic blood pressure. 1. O_2 (from air). 2. 6.5 p. c. CO_2 in O_2. 3. O_2. 4. 18.7 p. c. CO_2 in O_2. 5. O_2. 6. 10.5 p. c. O_2 in N_2. 7. O_2. Artificial respiration, open thorax. Time 30 sec.

observed. This effect has not been influenced to any perceptible degree by vagotomy or by extirpation of the stellate ganglia, and must be regarded as a direct effect on the lung vessels unless a reflex mechanism of altogether unknown nature comes into play. Also breathing of pure oxygen caused a distinct fall in pulmonary arterial pressure as illustrated in fig. 6. The considerable increase in the minute volume of the heart during moderate muscular work led to a rise in the pulmonary arterial pressure about equal to that observed during rest, when air was inspired instead of oxygen (fig. 4). It must be concluded that this

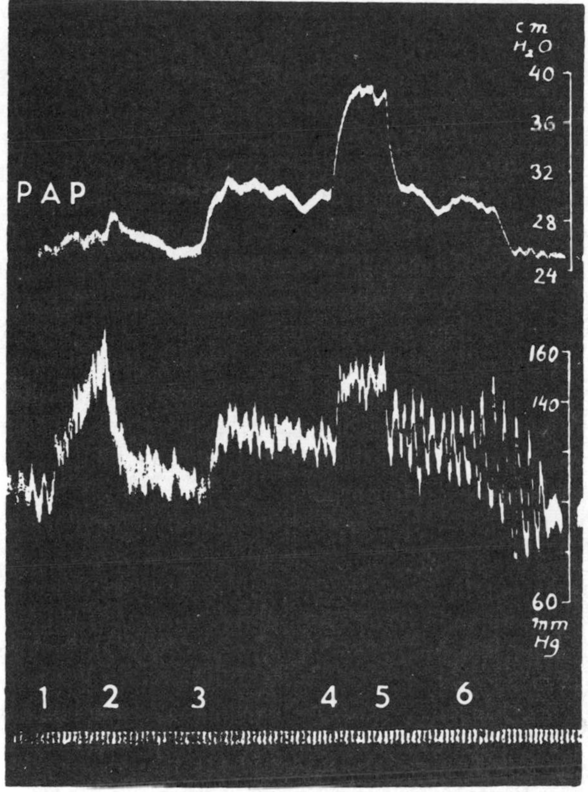

Fig. 7. Cat. 3.5 kg. Chloralose. Upper curve pulmonary arterial pressure, lower curve systemic blood pressure. 1. 20.5 p. c. CO_2 in O_2 from O_2. 2. O_2. 3. Air. 4. 10.5 p. c. O_2 in N_2. 5. Air. 6. O_2. Spontaneous breathing, closed thorax. Time 10 sec.

latter effect is in the main caused by other factors than an increase of the blood flow.

From our observations it can be inferred that even during normal experimental conditions there will be a certain degree of vasoconstriction in the lung arteries caused by the desaturation of the venous blood. Fig. 4 illustrates that this effect is added to that of muscular work, indicating different mechanisms in the two cases.

b. *Carbon dioxide.* When the gas inhaled by the experimental animal was changed from oxygen to a mixture of 6.5 per cent carbon dioxide in oxygen, a moderate increase in pulmonary arterial blood pressure ensued. Higher concentrations of carbon dioxide were also tested with the same result. In some of these experiments, the carbon dioxide gradually increased since the animal was breathing pure oxygen from a spirometer with no means for the absorption of the carbon dioxide. The rise in pulmonary blood pressure was, however, relatively moderate and less than the increase in systemic pressure. Thus in one experiment the latter increased from 134 mm Hg at an alveolar carbon dioxide of 8.67 per cent to 186 mm at 19.80 per cent alveolar carbon dioxide *i. e.* 40 per cent, whereas the pulmonary pressure only increased from 17.2 cm blood to about 20 cm or 16 per cent. The effect of oxygen lack occurred independently of section of the vagodepressors or removal of the stellate ganglia and seems to be a direct action on the vessels. A similar kind of direct action of the blood gas content, though acting conversely, is shown by the placental arteries, which contract vigorously under the action of oxygenated blood (SCHMITT 1922). Also the effect of carbon dioxide noticeably differs from that generally found. The higher percentages were not, however, accompanied by a rise in the left auricular pressure and the lower oncentrations (6.5 p. c. CO_2 in O_2) could even cause a slight lowering of the pressure in the left auricle (Fig. 6). During asphyxia the marked rise in pulmonary blood pressure might occur with only a minute rise in the left auricular pressure (from 3 to 4 cm blood). A comparison of the effects of various blood gases on the systemic as well as the pulmonary blood pressure is found in fig. 7.

In the experiments on the effect of muscular work on the pulmonary circulation, it was noted that the rise in blood pressure was definitely greater when the animal was breathing air than during oxygen inhalation. This is obviously due to an increased degree of desaturation of the venous blood during muscular work in the former case.

[*Editor's Note:* Material has been omitted at this point.]

5. Effects of Nerve Stimulation.

In a few experiments the vagosympathetic nerves in the neck and the stellate ganglia were stimulated for observation of their effect on the pulmonary pressure. Generally, the effects were quite small and inconstant, in agreement with the general conception that the nervous regulation of the lung vessels is of minor importance.

a. *Vagal stimulation.*

This was effected by means of condenser shocks from a thyratron stimulator, using various frequencies and strengths of stimulation. It was found that weak stimulation at a frequency of about 20/sec. on the right vagosympathetic caused a moderate fall in pressure without affecting the systemic blood pressure greatly (Fig. 9). In other experiments, the effect on the systemic blood pressure was a profound but brief fall, followed by a moderate rise in pressure. In this case the pulmonary pressure also fell instantaneously (inhibition of the right heart) and then quickly rose to a level some 10—20 per cent higher than it was before stimulation, and then returned in 1—3 minutes' time to the normal. It is difficult to judge, from the latter type of response, whether the effects are to some degree true vasomotor effects, or caused solely by the alterations in the hemodynamics of the heart and rest of the circulation, or whether the effect is influenced by simultaneous stimulation of sympathetic vasoconstrictor fibres (HENRIQUES 1892, ANDERSSON 1905, TRIBE 1914, LE BLANC and DE LIND V. WYNGAARDEN 1924).

b) *Stimulation of stellate ganglia.*

This was done in two experiments, and in one case a small but definite rise occurred. In the other experiment the effects were too small and inconsistent to permit any definite conclusion as to their effect. The small effects are in agreement with the results of previous investigators on the lung vessels of other animals.

Discussion.

The main object of this investigation has been to study those mechanisms by which the pressure in the pulmonary artery and the blood flow in the lungs are regulated. The fact that all the blood expelled by the right ventricle is driven through the same organ, and for one common purpose, constitutes the paramount difference between the lesser circulation and the systemic blood flow. This also leads to different demands with regard to the pressure regulation within the two systems. The systemic blood pressure in the aorta and its main branches must be kept within rather narrow limits even at very great alterations in the general blood flow, and at the same time the distribution of the circulating blood must be regulated according to the greatly varying needs of the different organs. This is made possible by the cooperation of local factors inducing a dilatation of the arteries of the working organs, and an adaptation of the general tone of the arterial system to the prevailing conditions. As is well known, the tone exercised by the vasomotor centre is in its turn controlled by impulses from the baro- and chemoreceptors of the carotid and aortic regions. The function of the pressure regulation for the pulmonary artery also seems to serve the purpose of ensuring the necessary blood flow through the different parts of the lungs and of preventing too great a rise of the pressure. An increase of the blood flow is accompanied by a rise of the pulmonary arterial blood pressure, as is clearly illustrated by the results obtained after occlusion of the vessels to one lung. But, whereas in this experiment the blood flow is approximately doubled, the relative increase of the pressure is only about 20 per cent. This demonstrates the great distensibility of the pulmonary vascular bed. The observation mentioned above, that the small extra pressure caused by injection of a few ml of Ringer's solution in the pulmonary artery was followed by a definite and somewhat lasting fall of the pulmonary pressure, may also illustrate this distensibility. It will consequently be expected that an adaptation to muscular work will be possible with only a moderate rise of the pulmonary arterial blood pressure. This corresponds well with our results. The degree of oxygen unsaturation of the mixed venous blood (and its carbon dioxide tension) will also be of significance for the level attained. Since this factor already comes into play during ordinary rest, and to a greater extent during muscular work, the increase of pulmonary arterial pressure caused by the augmentation of the blood flow alone should be smaller than the one actually observed in our experiments.

It is also required, however, that the blood becomes distributed to the different parts of the lungs in such a way, that the alveolar air will give off oxygen and take up carbon dioxide fairly evenly throughout the lungs. Mechanical factors, *e. g.* variations in posture, will easily influence this distribution (cp. Rich and Follis 1942). If the blood flow becomes inadequate in relation to the ventilation in some parts of the lungs, the corresponding alveolar air will become richer in oxygen and poorer in carbon dioxide than the rest of the lungs. But this will lead to a dilatation of the blood vessels of that part of the lungs with a redistribution of the blood as a consequence. It is interesting to note that oxygen want and carbon dioxide accumulation have exactly the reverse local effects on the vessels of the systemic and pulmonary circulations respectively; in both cases, however, they seem to be adapted for their special purposes. They cause a dilatation of the vessels of the working organs which need a greater blood supply than during rest, but they call forth a contraction of the lung vessels, thereby increasing the blood flow to better aerated lung areas, which leads to improved conditions for the utilization of the alveolar air. This will also imply that oxygen breathing during muscular work will facilitate the blood flow through the pulmonary vascular bed and allow a greater minute volume at a lower pressure, *i. e.* with less strain on the right heart.

We have concluded from our experiments that the increased pulmonary arterial pressure during oxygen-want is due to a direct action on the pulmonary vessels — in contrast to the corresponding effect on the systemic blood pressure which is produced through the stimulation of the chemoreceptors, whereas the direct action on the vasomotor centre itself is depression. Accumulation of carbon dioxide acts in the same direction as oxygen-want, though less pronouncedly. Probably the site of action is in the vessels themselves, as is the case with the placental vessels.

The only evidence we have obtained of a nervous control of the pulmonary blood pressure consists of the rhythmical variations observed. It is also characteristic that the mechanisms described enable a regulation which seems to be relatively independent of the simultaneous regulation of the systemic pressure. It is quite possible, however, that a certain connection exists between a nervous control of the pulmonary arterial pressure and the corresponding regulation of the systemic blood pressure, as indicated by the results obtained by Schwiegk (1935).

Summary.

The pulmonary arterial blood pressure was recorded in anaesthetized cats by means of a special cannula, according to MELLIN's technique. In most experiments the thorax was closed and the animal was breathing spontaneously.

The pulmonary arterial pressure in 9 experiments averaged 23 cm water, or approximately 17 mm Hg, at an average systemic pressure of 132 mm Hg. The average ratio thus was about 1: 8, with the limits 1: 5 and 1: 14.

Pressure variations of 1—2 cm blood synchronous with the breathing were regularly recorded. In one case, slow large waves of 1—2 minutes duration and about 5 cm amplitude were observed.

Even great variations in the systemic blood pressure, elicited from the pressoregulating reflex mechanisms, were hardly accompanied by variations in the pulmonary arterial pressure.

During muscular work a moderate rise in pulmonary blood pressure generally occurred, greater when air was breathed than when oxygen alone was administered.

Clamping the pulmonary artery to one lung did not cause any change in systemic pressure (confirming LICHTHEIM and TIGERSTEDT) but caused a moderate rise in pulmonary arterial pressure.

Breathing of pure oxygen lowered the pulmonary arterial pressure and oxygen-lack raised it. Carbon dioxide 6.5—20.5 per cent in oxygen raised the pressure sligthly, but constantly. These effects were not influenced by vagotomy.

The effect of injections of adrenaline, nor-adrenaline, acetylcholine and histamine and of stimulation of pulmonary nerves were studied in some cases.

The experiments seem to warrant the conclusion, that the regulation of the pulmonary blood flow is mainly mediated by a local action of the blood and alveolar gases leading to an adequate distribution of the blood through the various parts of the lungs according to the effeciency of aeration.

References.

AALKJAER, V., Skand. Arch. Physiol. 1935. *71*. 301.
ANDERSSON, H. K., J. Physiol. 1905, *33*. 414.
BERRY, J. L. and I. DE B. DALY, Proc. Roy. Soc. B. 1931. *109*. 319.
BEUTNER, A., Z. f. rat. Med. 1852. N. F. *2*. 97.

BRADFORD, J. R., and H. P. DEAN, Proc. Roy. Soc. B., 1889, *45*. 369.
DALY, I. DE B., J. Physiol. 1937. *91*. 14 P.
DALY, I. DE B., and U. S. v. EULER, Proc. Roy. Soc. B., 1932. *110*. 92.
EULER, U. S. v., J. Physiol. 1932. *74*. 271.
EULER, U. S. v., Acta Physiol. Scand. 1946. *12*. 73.
EULER, U. S. v., and G. LILJESTRAND, Acta Physiol. Scand. 1946. *12*. 279.
FRANÇOIS-FRANCK, Ch.-A., Arch. Physiol. 1895. *7*. 816.
HENRIQUES, V., Skand. Arch. Physiol. 1892. *4*. 194.
HEYMANS, C., J. J. BOUCKAERT, U. S. v. EULER and L. DAUTREBANDE, Arch. int. 1932. *43*. 86.
KATZ, L. N., and F. S. STEINITZ, Amer. J. Physiol. 1940. *128*. 433.
KNOLL, PH., Sitz.ber. Acad. Wiss. Wien, 1888, *97*. III. 207.
LE BLANC, E., and C. DE LIND VAN WYNGAARDEN, Pflügers Arch. 1924. *204*. 601.
LICHTHEIM, L., Die Störungen des Lungenkreislaufes, Berlin 1876.
MELLIN, G., Skand. Arch. Physiol. 1904. *15*. 147.
RICH, A. R., and R. H. FOLLIS, Tr. A. Am. Physic. 1942. *57*. 271.
SCHMITT, W., Z. Biol. 1922. *75*. 19.
SCHWIEGK, H., Pflügers Arch. Physiol. 1935. *236*. 206.
TIGERSTEDT, R., Skand. Arch. Physiol. 1903. *14*. 259.
TRIBE, E., J. Physiol. 1914. *48*. 154.

50

Reprinted from *J. Clin. Invest.*, **41**(3), 519–525, 527–529, 530–531 (1962)

REGIONAL PULMONARY FUNCTION STUDIED WITH XENON^{133} *

By W. C. BALL, Jr.,† P. B. STEWART, L. G. S. NEWSHAM and D. V. BATES

(From the Joint Cardiorespiratory Service and Department of Radiology, Royal Victoria Hospital, McGill University, Montreal, Canada)

(Submitted for publication August 15, 1961; accepted November 9, 1961)

Although there are many tests of pulmonary function in common usage, most of these measure only over-all function and are incapable of describing separately the behavior of different parts of the lung. Pulmonary arteriography has proven to be a valuable procedure for estimating the distribution of blood flow through the lungs but does not provide quantitative results. By bronchospirometry it has been possible to measure separately the ventilation and oxygen uptake of the two lungs or even of individual lobes, but considerable skill is required to obtain valid results, and the measurements must be made under conditions which are quite unphysiological. Both arteriography and bronchospirometry, furthermore, are unpleasant for the patient and are not without hazard.

The use of a radioactive tracer gas for assessing regional ventilation was reported in 1955 by Knipping and co-workers (2). They recorded external counting rate over multiple areas of the chest during breathing of air containing xenon^{133} and were able to show the presence of unventilated or markedly underventilated areas in certain patients. In subsequent publications (3–8), these and other workers extended their observations and described a method of displaying the results pictorially but did not attempt to estimate regional ventilation quantitatively.

More recently, Dyson and co-workers (9) have described the use of oxygen^{15} with external counting for determining the relative ventilation and perfusion in different regions of the lung. The initial counting rates after a single breath of radioactive gas were used to compare ventilation in symmetrically located counting fields, and the rates of removal of isotope from the counting fields were used as a measure of relative perfusion. Findings in normal subjects (10, 11) and in patients with mitral stenosis (12) have been published, and the clinical usefulness of this type of information in patients with pulmonary disease has been clearly shown (13).

This paper will describe and illustrate the application of a method for measuring regional ventilation and perfusion using xenon^{133} and external counting. Quantitative results are obtained by the use of a combined single-breath and rebreathing technique together with the intravenous administration of dissolved xenon^{133}.

METHODS

Xenon^{133} was shipped by air every 3 weeks as 300 mc of the highly purified gas sealed in a 10-ml glass ampule.[1] The gas was diluted to 30 ml with carbon dioxide and transferred into a lead-shielded mercury-displacement reservoir for dispensing in small amounts. Xenon is a chemically inert gas about three times as soluble as oxygen and one-seventh as soluble as carbon dioxide at body temperature ($\alpha = 0.0845$ ml xenon per ml H_2O at 760 mm Hg). The isotope $_{54}Xe^{133}$ decays to stable cesium with a half-life of 5.27 days, emitting a negative beta particle of maximum energy 0.347 Mev. This is absorbed by less than 1 mm of tissue and is therefore of no usefulness in external counting. The nucleus formed by beta decay may reach a stable state either by emitting a gamma ray of energy 0.081 Mev or by the process of internal conversion, which is accompanied by the emission of a *K* X-ray of energy approximately 0.030 Mev. The gamma- and X-ray energy is sufficiently low that adequate protection from radiation and shielding of the detecting instruments can be accomplished with 1/16 inch of

* Presented in part at the Forty-fifth Annual Meeting of the Federation of American Societies for Experimental Biology, Atlantic City, N. J., April 14, 1961 (1). The equipment used in this study was largely paid for by a Dominion Provincial Grant. The investigative work has been supported by a Block Term Grant from the Medical Research Council of Canada, and during the past year by generous support from the John A. Hartford Foundation.

† Postdoctoral Research Fellow of the National Heart Institute. Present address: Department of Medicine, The Johns Hopkins Hospital, Baltimore 5, Md.

[1] Produced as a fission product at the Radiochemical Centre, Amersham, England, by neutron bombardment of uranium^{235} (14).

lead, except in the case of the storage and dispensing apparatus, which is shielded with 3/16 inch of lead. The total radiation dosage to the lungs of a normal subject in the complete study to be described does not exceed 40 mrads, although a patient with delayed intrapulmonary mixing may receive a total lung dose of as much as 120 mrads. Both of these amounts are small in comparison with doses received during many ordinary diagnostic roentgenographic procedures.

Apparatus. The subject was seated in a chair with an adjustable seat and head rest. The arms were placed on a horizontal shelf immediately in front of the subject at the level of the manubrium in order to rotate the scapulae outward. Behind the chair were mounted six scintillation counters [2] fitted with 4-inch cylindrical lead collimators and placed for each patient to correspond to fixed positions on a previously taken 6-foot posteroanterior chest film. Measurements on the film and on the subject were made, using the spine of the seventh cervical vertebra as a reference point; the upper zone counters were centered 1.5 inches below the highest projection of the lung, the lower zone counters 0.75 inch above the highest projection of the higher diaphragm leaf, and the middle zone counters halfway between. At each vertical level the counters were placed equidistant from the midline and in the center of the lung projection at that level.

Figure 1 shows the isocount curves in air for the scintillation counters, superimposed in correct position on a drawing of the chest. It will be noted that each counter responds to radiation from a truncated cone of lung, with a sensitivity that decreases quite rapidly with depth.

Pulses from each counter were fed through suitable amplifying and discriminating circuits and were then recorded on separate channels of a multichannel magnetic tape recorder [3] by a nonreturn-to-zero pulse-recording technique. The threshold of each discriminator was adjusted to accept only pulses corresponding to a photon energy of 0.025 Mev or more; hence both gamma rays and X-rays from the xenon^{133} were recorded. Outputs from the tape playback heads were fed to counting-rate meters,[4] which were connected to record on a 4-channel Sanborn direct writer. The tape recording was monitored during the study and could later be played back with any combination of tape speed, counting-rate meter range and time constant, and Sanborn gain and paper speed which by trial and error produced the best display of each portion of the data. For the standard study to be described, a counting-rate meter time constant of 1 second was used in all cases. All counting rates were estimated to the nearest 100 cpm from the Sanborn tracing and were corrected for background and dead-time loss. Dead time of the recording system at a tape speed of 7.5 inches per second was found to be 100 microseconds.

The subject breathed through a rubber mouthpiece

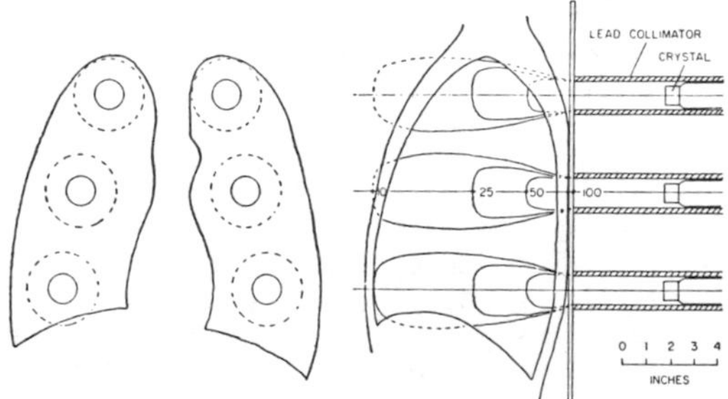

FIG. 1. DIAGRAM ILLUSTRATING POSITION OF THE SCINTILLATION COUNTERS IN POSTEROANTERIOR AND LATERAL PROJECTIONS, WITH ISOCOUNT CURVES SUPERIMPOSED ON THE LATERAL VIEW. Numbers on the isocount curves refer to a counting rate of 100 per cent at the end of the collimator.

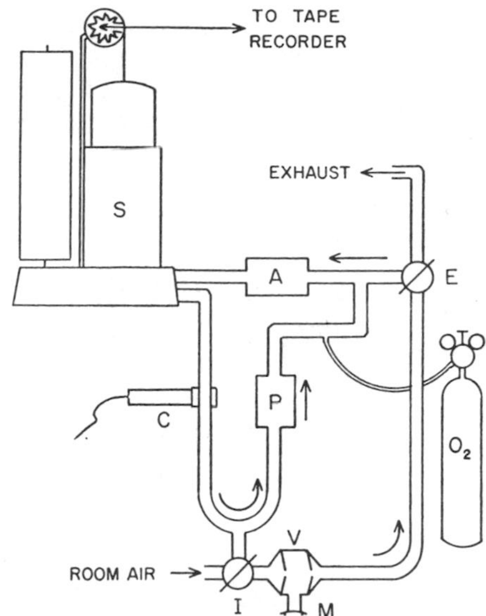

FIG. 2. SCHEMATIC DRAWING OF THE CLOSED SPIROMETER CIRCUIT. M, mouthpiece; V, valve box; I inspired air valve; E, expired air valve; C, scintillation counter for monitoring concentration of xenon in inspired air; P, pump for circulating gas mixture; A, carbon dioxide absorber; S, spirometer. A potentiometer on the spirometer wheel permits a continuous recording of spirometer volume.

[2] Assembled from type 3D2 thallium-activated sodium iodide crystal (Harshaw Chemical Co., Cleveland, Ohio), type K-1716 photomultiplier tube (Du Mont Labs., Clifton, N. J.), and type T-108 linear amplifier (Engineered Electronics, Inc., Santa Ana, Calif.).

[3] Series 3170 30-channel magnetic tape instrumentation system (Minneapolis-Honeywell Regulator Co., Beltsville, Md.).

[4] Tullamore model 2 CRM-2 linear count rate meter (Victoreen Instrument Co., Cleveland, Ohio).

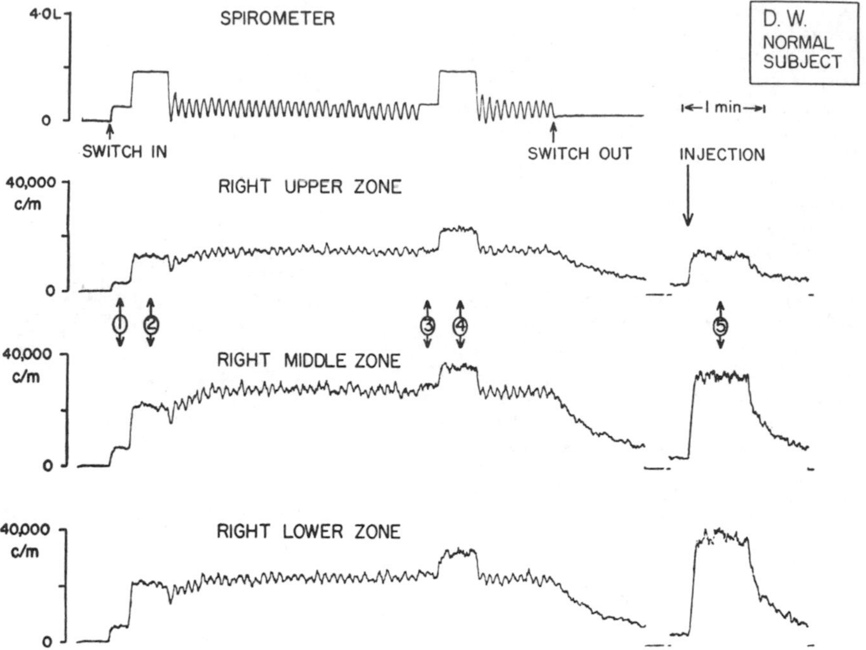

FIG. 3. A PORTION OF THE TRACING FROM A NORMAL SUBJECT, AS PLAYED BACK FROM THE TAPE, SHOWING SPIROMETER TRACING AND COUNTING RATE FROM EACH OF THE THREE CHEST COUNTERS ON THE RIGHT SIDE. Arrows indicate the beginning and end of closed-circuit breathing, and also the intravenous injection of xenon solution. Numbers 1 and 2 refer to the counting rate plateaus which correspond to the small and large initial breaths, numbers 3 and 4 to the plateaus which correspond to the same breath-holding maneuvers after equilibration, and number 5 to the counting rate plateaus during a full inspiration after the intravenous injection. The continuous recording of concentration of xenon in inspired air, together with the counting-rate curves from the left side of the chest are played off separately and are not shown.

and valve box either from room air to an exhaust line for disposal of radioactive waste gas or from a closed spirometer circuit, as shown in Figure 2. The spirometer [5] was fitted with a potentiometer to permit continuous recording of spirometer volume on a channel of tape by means of a standard frequency-modulation technique. The pump circulated the gas mixture on the inspired air side of the circuit at the rate of 36 L per minute to insure rapid mixing. Concentration of xenon in inspired air was monitored continuously by means of a scintillation counter [6] mounted over the inspired air line. Prior to each study sufficient xenon[133] was added to the closed circuit to bring the initial concentration to approximately 0.5 mc per L. During rebreathing, carbon dioxide was removed by a soda-lime absorber and oxygen was added at a rate sufficient to maintain a constant volume.

[5] Stead-Wells 10 L spirometer (Warren E. Collins, Inc., Boston, Mass.).

[6] Similar to those used as chest counters, but containing type 6199 photomultiplier tube (Radio Corp. of America, Harrison, N. J.).

Solutions of xenon[133] for intravenous injection were prepared by agitating a small bubble of a stock xenon-carbon dioxide mixture in a 10-ml syringe fitted with a 3-way stopcock and containing 5 ml of sterile normal saline. Any residual bubble was expelled and the total amount of xenon[133] in the solution determined by counting with the syringe in fixed geometric relationship to a scintillation counter [7] connected to a laboratory scaler.[8] After injection the syringe was again counted, and this count subtracted from the original count. The total amount of xenon[133] injected varied from 0.5 to 1.0 mc.

Procedure. The method of determining regional ventilation and perfusion can be shown with reference to a portion of the tracing from a normal subject (Figure 3). When the subject had been properly placed in the chair and instructed in the breathing maneuvers, the mouthpiece was inserted, a nose clip applied, and the subject allowed to breathe room air from 20 to 30 seconds, during which time background counts were recorded. At the

[7] See footnote 6.

[8] Model 2950 scaler (Picker X-Ray Corp., White Plains, N. Y.).

end of a normal expiration he was quickly switched into the closed spirometer circuit, allowed to inspire a normal tidal volume of air-xenon mixture, and at the end of inspiration was instructed to hold his breath. After several seconds he was instructed to inspire fully and again hold his breath. The counting rates (plateaus 1 and 2, Figure 3) for each lung zone depend upon the amounts of radioactive gas entering the lung within each zone. The subject rebreathed from the closed circuit until examination of the monitored tracings showed that equilibrium had been reached. The breath-holding maneuvers were then repeated, giving two additional counting rates (plateaus 3 and 4, Figure 3) for each zone. Since these external counting rates correspond to known concentrations of xenon within the lung, they can be used in conjunction with the initial breath plateaus to determine the concentration of xenon in each zone after tidal and deep initial breaths (see below). When the pattern of respiration had returned to normal the subject was switched back to breathing room air, and washout curves from each zone were recorded.

After most of the xenon had been washed out of the lungs, a no. 18 needle was introduced into an antecubital vein, and the 5 ml of normal saline containing dissolved xenon[133] was injected rapidly and flushed in with 20 ml of normal saline. As the injection was made the subject was instructed to take a slow, deep breath and hold it without exerting positive pressure. The solubility of xenon is such that nearly all of the injected dose diffuses into the alveoli on the first circulation, giving a counting rate (plateau 5, Figure 3) for each zone which depends upon the amount of labeled blood brought to the lung within that zone. When the subject resumed breathing of room air, washout curves were again recorded.

Calculations

Because of the complexity of the geometry in body-surface counting, the relationship between concentration of xenon within the lung and the observed external counting rate will differ for different subjects and for different counter positions in the same subject. For each counter, however, with a fixed degree of inflation of the lungs and hence geometry of the system, the external counting rate will be directly proportional to the concentration of xenon within the lung. This relationship is determined for each counter in every subject at two levels of inspiration by means of the breath-holding maneuvers after rebreathing, when the concentration of xenon within the lung is equal to the concentration in the spirometer circuit and can be measured directly. From this relationship it is possible to calculate the concentration of xenon within each lung zone at the time either initial breath plateau is inscribed or within each lung zone after the intravenous injection of xenon. For example, the concentration of xenon, F_2, in a given lung zone after initial full inspiration is given by the equation

$$F_2 = U_2 \cdot \frac{F_4}{U_4}$$

where U_2 is the external counting rate over that zone after the initial breath, F_4 the known concentration of xenon in the lungs after rebreathing, and U_4 the external counting rate during full inflation after rebreathing (subscripts refer to numbered plateaus in Figure 3).

In order to permit direct comparison of data from different studies, each regional concentration as calculated above is expressed as a percentage of the simultaneous mean concentration of xenon in the lungs as a whole or, in other words, as a percentage of the concentration that would have been found if the initial breath of xenon had been uniformly distributed throughout the known lung volume. Thus, for the initial breaths, a "distribution index" Y is defined as

$$Y = \frac{F}{F_I(V_I - V_D)/(V_I + \mathrm{FRC})} \cdot 100\%$$

where F is the calculated concentration of xenon within a zone after initial breath, F_I the concentration in inspired air, V_I the volume of gas mixture inspired, V_D the instrumental dead space (100 ml), and FRC the functional residual capacity determined by closed-circuit helium dilution (15). Using the calculated concentration corresponding to plateau 1 (Figure 3), this equation gives for each lung zone a distribution index for quiet breathing; using the concentration which corresponds to plateau 2, a distribution index for deep inspiration is obtained. Similarly, using the concentration corresponding to plateau 5,

$$Y = \frac{F}{X/(V_I + \mathrm{FRC})} \cdot 100\%$$

where X is the total quantity of xenon injected intravenously, and Y is the distribution index for perfusion.

Each of these indices expresses the total amount of xenon *per unit volume* delivered into the counting field as a percentage of the total amount per unit volume delivered to the lungs as a whole, and hence is a measure of the relative ventilation or perfusion *per unit volume* of lung. If distribution were entirely uniform in relation to lung volume and no dead space were present, all indices should be 100. Since these indices are calculated from the ratio of two external counting rates, they are independent of counter sensitivity, volume of lung within each zone, and absorption of radiation by the chest wall.

It would be anticipated that the rate of washout from areas with reduced ventilation as shown by the distribution index would be delayed in comparison with better ventilated areas. Quantitative analysis of these washout curves is made difficult by the fact that the early portion of the curves is influenced by respiratory movement and the later part by return of dissolved xenon from other tissues to the lung and by radiation from xenon within the chest wall. However, since these regional washout curves, when analyzed in conjunction with the distribution indices for quiet breathing, are theoretically capable of providing information concerning the degree of nonuniformity within a zone, they are currently under further study.

Errors

1. Linearity and precision of calibration of the tape-recording system (after correction for dead-time loss), the counting-rate meters, and direct writer were tested by a pulse generator and laboratory scaler and were found to be within 2 per cent for all measurements.

2. Errors due to the random nature of radioactive decay depend upon the counting rate and the duration of counting. For normal subjects these errors are less than 2 per cent for all plateaus except those corresponding to the small initial breath where, because of low counting rates, the error varies from about 2 to 8 per cent. This fact makes the distribution indices for quiet breathing inherently less precise than those for deep inspiration or perfusion. These errors may be larger in patients, due to shorter periods of breath holding, but rarely exceed 5 per cent for other than the small initial breath plateaus.

3. During rebreathing, some xenon dissolves in the blood and is carried to other tissues including the posterior chest wall within the counting fields. The extent to which this tissue xenon would contribute to total equilibrium counting rate was estimated by counting over the hand and calf during equilibration. These counting rates rose in roughly linear fashion during the first 10 minutes of rebreathing, reaching approximately 1 and 2 per cent (hand and calf, respectively) of the simultaneous counting rates over the chest. Since the calf is considerably thicker than the posterior chest wall, and since the effect of more remote structures such as heart and anterior chest wall is diminished considerably by their distance from the counters, it was concluded that counts from these extrapulmonary structures would not exceed 2 per cent of the simultaneous counts from normally ventilated lung after as much as 10 minutes of rebreathing. In studies where shorter periods of rebreathing were required, the error would be correspondingly less.

If a counting field contains a large volume of unventilated lung so that the equilibrium counting rate is low, the per cent error due to xenon dissolved in tissues will be greater. However, the likelihood of significant error from this cause will be immediately obvious by comparing the equilibrium counting rate with that obtained from other areas.

Failure to reach complete equilibrium during rebreathing will result in a falsely low value for the equilibrium counting rate and consequently a falsely high distribution index. In patients with poor intrapulmonary mixing, failure to ventilate lung spaces within a counting field during rebreathing will result in an index which describes ventilation and perfusion per unit volume of ventilatable lung.

4. The error due to Compton scatter of radiation from the opposite lung or from an adjacent zone of the same lung was estimated with the use of a pressed-wood model of the thorax, by counting from all zones with a small xenon source placed in various positions within the thoracic cavity. If distribution is uniform there is no error introduced by scatter, but if one lung is underventilated, scatter from a normally ventilated opposite lung produces counts over the underventilated lung sufficient to raise the distribution index by as much as 2 U. Normally ventilated lung in a zone immediately adjacent will raise the distribution index by as much as 5 U. It should be noted that the effect of scatter is always to minimize the degree of unevenness actually present.

5. For the calculation of distribution indices, inspired air volume must be estimated from the spirometer tracing, and an independently determined functional residual capacity must be used. The accuracy of the recorded spirometer tracing is about $\pm$ 40 ml, which may cause error in estimating V_I for the initial tidal volume, especially if this volume is small. Errors of this sort, however, do not alter the relative but only the absolute values of the calculated indices and would therefore not influence the interpretation of results. Similarly, error in estimating the amount of xenon injected, or failure of the entire dose of injected xenon to diffuse into the alveoli, would affect only the absolute values of the perfusion indices and not their relative magnitude.

When tidal volume is small the amount of inspired xenon delivered to the central portion of anatomical dead space will be relatively larger, and the indices obtained for peripheral counting fields will be proportionately reduced without altering their magnitude relative to each other.

6. In the calculation of xenon concentrations within the lung it was assumed that the volume of inspired gas was identical for plateaus 2, 4, and 5, and for plateaus 1 and 3. Some variation in inspired volume occurred, but allowance for this was made by correcting the equilibrium counting-rate plateaus on the assumption that the ratio of external counting rate to total amount of xenon in the lungs remained constant for different degrees of lung inflation. This assumption was tested in normal subjects over a wide range of V_I, and the maximal error in counting rate thus corrected was 5 per cent for variations in inspired volume of as much as 500 ml.

7. The largest potential source of error in this method is gross body movement during the study, especially in dyspneic patients, who tend to move their shoulders during efforts at deep inspiration, and also in patients who equilibrate slowly and are therefore required to remain immobile for longer periods. Every effort was made to avoid changes in body position during the study by the use of head and arm rests, and by making certain that the subject was comfortably seated at the start.

RESULTS

Normal subjects

Twenty-one normal subjects, 17 male and 4 female, ranging in age from 23 to 44, have been studied by the technique described. Indices for quiet breathing were not obtained in two subjects because of equipment malfunction, and perfusion indices were not obtained in three subjects because of leakage or infiltration of the

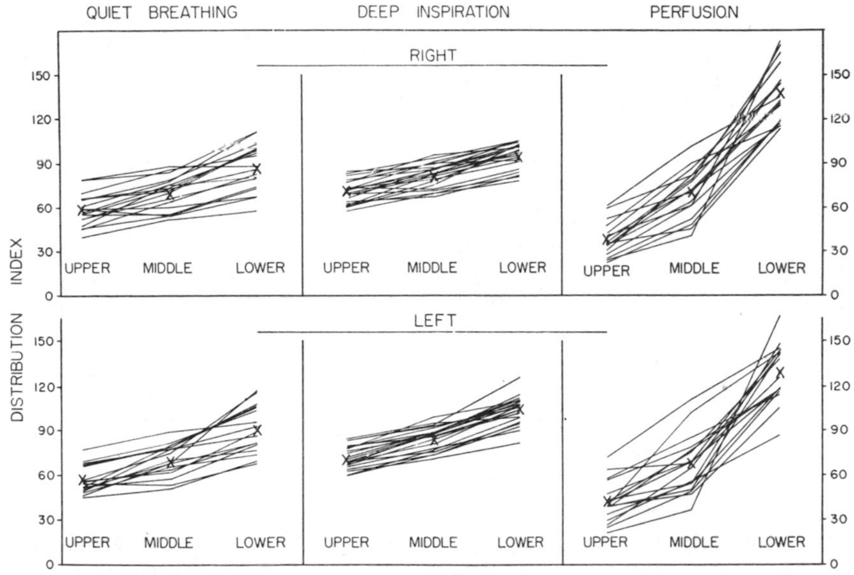

FIG. 4. REGIONAL DISTRIBUTION OF INSPIRED AIR DURING QUIET BREATHING AND DEEP INSPIRATION, AND OF PULMONARY BLOOD FLOW IN 21 SEATED NORMAL SUBJECTS. The distribution indices are computed in such a way that all values would be 100 if distribution were entirely uniform (see text for details). X indicates the mean value for each group of observations.

injectate. In addition, quiet breathing indices have been excluded in one case because the volume inspired (220 ml) was not sufficient to clear instrumental and anatomical dead space, and perfusion indices in another subject were considered invalid because of a shift in body position between the rebreathing and injection parts of the study.

The individual results, expressed in terms of the distribution index, are plotted in Figure 4. Despite the variability among different subjects, there occurred for nearly every subject a progressive increase in the magnitude of the distribution index from upper to middle and from middle to lower zones, indicating that both the ventilation and perfusion per unit lung volume increased progressively from apex to base.

Mean values for these indices with their standard deviations are shown in Table I. It will be noted that the mean indices are all lower for quiet breathing than for deep inspiration; this is due to the fact that a larger fraction of the total amount of xenon inspired lies within the major airways, where it does not contribute to the external counting rates. Variations in the ratio of anatomical dead space to tidal volume are also a major factor in increasing the variability of the indices for quiet breathing among different subjects.

From the mean indices it will be seen that for quiet breathing the ratio of ventilation of the lower zones to ventilation of the upper zones is 1.55, while the corresponding ratio for deep inspiration is 1.41. Although this difference is small it was present in nearly every subject, and by statistical analysis of the paired data was shown to be significant (right lung, $p < 0.001$;

TABLE I

Mean distribution indices and their standard deviations in 21 normal subjects

	Quiet breathing		Deep inspiration		Perfusion	
	R	L	R	L	R	L
Upper	58 ±11	57 ±9	71 ±8	71 ±7	38 ±12	42 ±14
Middle	70 ±11	70 ±10	81 ±8	85* ±8	70 ±17	67 ±20
Lower	87 ±16	91 ±16	95 ±9	104* ±10	137* ±20	129 ±19

* Significantly greater than the corresponding index on the opposite side.

left lung, $p < 0.05$). In addition, the index for deep inspiration for the left lower zone was greater than the corresponding index on the right in all 21 subjects and, although the mean difference is only 9 per cent, this is highly significant ($p << 0.001$). Similarly, the index of 85 for ventilation of the left middle zone on deep inspiration is significantly greater than the index of 81 on the right side ($p < 0.001$), and the index of 137 for perfusion of the *right* lower zone is greater than the index of 129 on the *left* side ($p < 0.01$). The indices for ventilation of the lower zones during quiet breathing do not differ significantly ($0.3 < p < 0.4$). In contrast to the relatively small difference in ventilation of lower versus upper zones, the perfusion indices indicate that the lower zones were 3.3 times as well perfused as were the upper zones.

Technically satisfactory duplicate studies on different days have been performed on four of the above subjects. The mean difference between the paired distribution indices varied from 3 to 8 U (over-all mean 6 U) for different zones, indicating a high degree of repeatability in normal subjects.

[*Editor's Note:* Material has been omitted at this point.]

DISCUSSION

It has been recognized for many years that there is significant nonuniformity of ventilation and perfusion in the lungs of the normal subject in the erect posture. The study of foreign-gas equilibration and washout curves by a variety of techniques, and also the continuous analysis of gas concentrations during a single expiration have provided clear evidence of unevenness in ventilation (17), but until recently there was no direct evidence that this unevenness was regionally distributed.

Regional unevenness of perfusion was suggested by the studies of Martin, Cline and Marshall (18), who found that the concentrations of oxygen and carbon dioxide in expired air from upper and lower lobes differed significantly in the erect subject. By lobar bronchospirometry Mattson and Carlens (19) demonstrated a substantial decrease in oxygen uptake by the upper lobe when the subject assumed the erect posture, and attributed this finding to changes in the distribution of blood flow through the lung under the influence of gravity. Further indirect support for this interpretation was provided by Riley and colleagues (20), whose studies showed a significant increase in physiological dead space in normal subjects on changing from the supine to the erect position.

The recent work by West and Dollery (10) has provided more direct and quantitative data concerning regional ventilation and perfusion in the normal seated subject. By the use of externally placed scintillation counters they were able to measure the rate of removal of oxygen^{15}-labeled carbon dioxide from different regions of the lung after a single breath of the radioactive gas, and have shown this to be a measure of regional perfusion. From the initial counting rates over different regions after a single 900-ml breath of radioactive gas, ventilation was compared in symmetrical areas, and by the use of cadaver measurements and volume calculations an approximate comparison of ventilation per unit volume was made for different levels. Comparison of a lower counting field (at the level of the fifth rib anteriorly) with an upper counting field (at the level of the first rib interspace) in 16 normal subjects showed the ratio of the mean values for ventilation to be approximately 1.4 : 1 and for perfusion approximately 8 : 1.

Corresponding ratios for a comparable vertical separation of counting fields in the present study were 1.55 : 1 for ventilation during quiet breathing, 1.41 : 1 for inspired air on deep inspiration, and 3.3 : 1 for perfusion. The ventilation results are in excellent agreement with those of West and Dollery, and confirm that the lower portions of the lung are better ventilated than the upper portions in the seated subject. Regional differences in the mechanical compliance of the lung and chest wall may be in part responsible for this observation. An alternative explanation, however, is suggested by the work of Swenson, Finley and Guzman (21), who demonstrated a marked and almost immediate decrease in the ventilation of one lung when the pulmonary artery on that side was obstructed, and showed further that this effect could be abolished by allowing the non-perfused lung to breathe 6 per cent carbon dioxide. Regional differences in gas tensions resulting from nonuniform blood flow in the seated subject might thus be responsible for the regional differences in ventilation that were observed in the present study.

The ratio of lower zone to upper zone perfusion measured with radioactive xenon was smaller than that found by West and Dollery (10), but this is in part due to the much narrower counting fields made possible by coincidence counting with oxygen^{15} (9), and to the effect of scattered radiation on counting rates observed over the upper zones in our studies (see Methods). It is also possible that the taking of a full inspiration at the time of injection may have increased perfusion in the upper lung zones. Preliminary observations of the effect of different respiratory maneuvers on the distribution of pulmonary blood flow have produced inconclusive results, but in some apparently normal subjects quite striking changes in distribution have occurred with a deep inspiration or with a Valsalva maneuver. Further study of this problem is clearly necessary.

It is of interest that on deep inspiration the ventilation of the middle and lower portions of the lung was found to be significantly greater on the left side than on the right (Table I). This is presumably due to the difference in resistance to diaphragmatic descent offered by the abdominal contents on the two sides, and correlates well with the fluoroscopic observations of Wade (22), who found that the left diaphragm descends more than the right during deep inspiration. The possibility that a similar but less marked difference is present in the lower zones during quiet breathing is not excluded by our data, and our failure to show a significant difference may be the result of the somewhat greater variability of the quiet breathing indices due to lower counting rates.

The mean distribution index for perfusion was significantly greater for the *right* lower zone than for the *left* lower zone (Table I). Although it is possible that this small difference is the result of a systematic error in equilibrium counting rates over the left lower zone because of dissolved xenon in the heart, this seems unlikely in view of the distance between the heart and the chest counters, as well as the relatively slight solubility of xenon. West and Dollery (10) found clearance rates to be considerably greater at the right base than at the left in normal subjects, but this difference appeared to be due largely to interference with counting rates on the left by the presence of radioactive blood within the heart.

[*Editor's Note:* Material has been omitted at this point.]

SUMMARY AND CONCLUSIONS

1. A radioactive isotope of the inert gas, xenon, has been used in conjunction with externally placed scintillation counters to estimate separately the function of six different regions of the lung. By comparison of external counting rates after a single breath and after rebreathing an air-xenon mixture, it has been possible to compute an index of relative ventilation that is independent of the volume of lung within the counting field. Determinations were made at two levels of inspiration in order to compare the distribution during normal quiet breathing with the distribution after a single full inspiration. By the intravenous injection of dissolved xenon^{133} during breath holding, the relative perfusion of lung in different regions has been determined.

2. In 21 seated normal subjects, it was found that *a*) the lower portion of the lung is somewhat better ventilated than the upper portion, but receives a much greater fraction of the total pulmonary blood flow; *b*) the distribution of inspired air is slightly more uniform on deep inspiration than during quiet breathing; *c*) the middle and lower portions of the lung are better ventilated on the left than on the right during deep inspiration; and *d*) the lower portion of the lung is probably better perfused on the right than on the left.

3. Forty patients with various cardiac or pulmonary disorders have been studied, and four illustrative cases are presented. Two of these illustrate the differences in regional distribution of disordered function that may occur in patients with pulmonary emphysema. The third patient demonstrates the value of the technique in assessing lobar function after transposition surgery,

and the fourth patient illustrates normally distributed ventilatory function despite a disturbed distribution of perfusion in uncomplicated mitral stenosis.

4. The advantages and disadvantages of this method in comparison with the oxygen^{15} technique of West and co-workers (9–13) are discussed.

5. It appears that the xenon technique described is capable of extensive application to both investigative and clinical problems.

ACKNOWLEDGMENTS

We wish to thank the memebrs of the Medical and Surgical Staffs of the Royal Victoria Hospital for referring their cases to us for study. The technical problems involved would not have been circumvented without the assistance of Mr. L. D. Pengelly, Mr. L. S. Bartlett, Miss D. K. Witts, Miss M. MacLeish, and Dr. C. K. Hargrove of the Department of Radiology. We are also grateful to Dr. E. P. Radford for his advice on techniques for recording the experimental data on magnetic tape, and to Dr. H. Venrath for the benefit of his experience with the use of xenon^{133}.

REFERENCES

1. Ball, W. C., Jr., Stewart, P. B., Newsham, L. S., and Bates, D. V. Studies of regional pulmonary ventilation and perfusion using xenon^{133}. Fed. Proc. 1961, **20**, 420.
2. Knipping, H. W., Bolt, W., Venrath, H., Valentin, H., Ludes, H., and Endler, P. Eine neue Methode zur Prüfung der Herz- und Lungenfunktion. Die regionale Funktionsanalyse in der Lungen- und Herzklinik mit Hilfe des radioaktiven Edelgases Xenon 133 (Isotopen-Thorakographie). Dtsch. med. Wschr. 1955, **80**, 1146.
3. Knipping, H. W., Bolt, W., Valentin, H., Venrath, H., and Endler, P. Technik und Möglichkeiten der regionalen Ventilationsanalyse mittels des radioaktiven Edelgases Xenon^{133} (Isotopen-Thorakographie). Z. Tuberk. 1957, **111**, 259.
4. Knipping, H. W., Bolt, W., Valentin, H., Venrath, H., and Endler, P. Regionale Funktionsanalyse in der Kreislauf- und Lungen-Klinik mit Hilfe der Isotopenthorakographie und der selektiven Angiographie der Lungengefässe. Münch. med. Wschr. 1957, **99**, 1, 46.
5. Venrath, H. Die Lungenfunktionsprüfung mit Hilfe von Isotopen *in* Lungen und Kleiner Kreislauf, W. Lochner and E. Witzleb, Eds. Berlin, Springer-Verlag, 1957, p. 144.
6. Bolt, W., and Rink, H. Studien zur regionalen Analyse der Lungenventilation und Lungenzirkulation. Thoraxchirurgie 1958, **29**, 5.
7. Fucks, W., and Knipping, H. W. Bildliche Darstellung der Verteilung und der Bewegung von radioaktiven Substanzen im Raum ("Röntgen ohne Röntgenröhre") unter Berücksichtigung einiger Probleme der Herz- und Lungenklinik. Atomkernenergie 1958, **6**, 209.
8. Trippe, H. Zur Diagnose regionaler Ventilationsstörungen der Lunge mit Hilfe von Xenon^{133}. Cologne, Photostelle der Universität zu Köln, 1959.
9. Dyson, N. A., Hugh-Jones, P., Newbery, G. R., Sinclair, J. D., and West, J. B. Studies of regional lung function using radioactive oxygen. Brit. med. J. 1960, **1**, 231.
10. West, J. B., and Dollery, C. T. Distribution of blood flow and ventilation-perfusion ratio in the lung, measured with radioactive carbon dioxide. J. appl. Physiol. 1960, **15**, 405.
11. Dollery, C. T., Dyson, N. A., and Sinclair, J. D. Regional variations in uptake of radioactive CO in the normal lung. J. appl. Physiol. 1960, **15**, 411.
12. Dollery, C. T., and West, J. B. Regional uptake of radioactive oxygen, carbon monoxide and carbon dioxide in the lungs of patients with mitral stenosis. Circulat. Res. 1960, **8**, 765.
13. West, J. B., Dollery, C. T., and Hugh-Jones, P. The use of radioactive carbon dioxide to measure regional blood flow in the lungs of patients with pulmonary disease. J. clin. Invest. 1961, **40**, 1.
14. Wilson, E. J., Dibbs, H. P., Richards, S., and Eakins, J. D. Preparation of xenon-133 radiography sources from spent fuel. Nucleonics 1958, **16**, no. 4, 110.
15. Bates, D. V., and Christie, R. V. Intrapulmonary mixing of helium in health and in emphysema. Clin. Sci. 1950, **9**, 17.
16. Bates, D. V., Pare, J. A. P., and Meakins, J. F. The clinical usefulness of routine tests of pulmonary function. Canad. med. Ass. J. 1960, **83**, 192.
17. Fowler, W. S. Intrapulmonary distribution of inspired gas. Physiol. Rev. 1952, **32**, 1.
18. Martin, C. J., Cline, F., Jr., and Marshall, H. Lobar alveolar gas concentrations: Effect of body position. J. clin. Invest. 1953, **32**, 617.
19. Mattson, S. B., and Carlens, E. Lobar ventilation and oxygen uptake in man. Influence of body position. J. thorac. Surg. 1955, **30**, 676.
20. Riley, R. L., Permutt, S., Said, S., Godfrey, M., Cheng, T. O., Howell, J. B. L., and Shepard, R. H. Effect of posture on pulmonary dead space in man. J. appl. Physiol. 1959, **14**, 339.
21. Swenson, E. W., Finley, T. N., and Guzman, S. V. Unilateral hypoventilation in man during temporary occlusion of one pulmonary artery. J. clin. Invest. 1961, **40**, 828.
22. Wade, O. L. Movements of the thoracic cage and diaphragm in respiration. J. Physiol. (Lond.) 1954, **124**, 193.
23. Briscoe, W. A., Cree, E. M., Filler, J., Houssay, H. E. J., and Cournand, A. Lung volume, alveolar ventilation and perfusion interrelationships in chronic pulmonary emphysema. J. appl. Physiol. 1960, **15**, 785.

51

ON ABSORPTION IN AIRWAYS

Gabriel-Constant Colin

This excerpt was prepared expressly for this Benchmark volume by Julius H. Comroe, Jr., from Traité de Physiologie Comparée des Animaux, *Vol. 2, 2nd ed., J.-B. Baillière et Fils, Paris, 1873, pp. 108–111*

The mucosa of the respiratory tracts is, of all the mucous membranes, that which possesses the property of absorption to the highest degree.

The first part of this mucosa, which covers the large airways, nasal cavities, sinus, larynx, and trachea, has mainly a sensory and protective role. It is the second part, spread out over the bronchi and the pulmonary alveoli, that, because of its thinness and permeability, possesses an incomparable power of absorption.

The bronchopulmonary mucosa, essentially designed for the absorption of oxygen that arterializes the blood and for the exhalation of carbonic acid and water vapor, is able to take in at the same time everything that might be associated with inspired air: carbon monoxide, hydrogen sulfide, arseniuretted hydrogen (arsine), water vapor and various liquids, vapors, effluvia, volatile viruses, particles volatilized from a multitude of bodies, soluble particles that are found in suspension in the air, and, finally, substances that penetrate accidentally or are deliberately placed in the respiratory paths.

The exceptional activity and excessive rapidity of absorption across the bronchi and pulmonary alveoli are based on four factors: (1) the immense expanse of the mucosa; (2) the thinness of the membrane, whose capillary beds are very superficial; (3) the characteristics of the epithelium, which are reduced to a single layer of cylindrical cells with moving cilia in the small bronchial tubes and to flattened polygonal cells in the pulmonary alveoli; and (4) the working of the thoracic pump, which in a single stroke during inspiration brings gas, vapors, and liquids for absorption over the whole of the bronchial branches and their terminal alveoli.

Pulmonary absorption occurs most rapidly with gases because, besides inspiration, which tends to draw them directly into the terminal parts of the bronchial tree, the tendency for dissemination of their molecules, favored by heat, distributes them in an instant over the whole surface of the mucosa. Oxygen changes the color of the blood of the asphyxiated animal in a few seconds; after two or three inspirations of hydrocyanic gas, a small animal drops dead; in a few inspirations, the chemist exposed to inhalation of arsine can absorb a toxic dose. One knows by numerous accidents how quickly sulfuric acid fumes, ammonium sulfhydrate, and noxious gases in deep shafts and sewers kill persons who breathe them.

All vapors behave pretty much the same as gases. Vapors of ether and of chloroform produce anesthesia in a few minutes; those of essences (perfumes of flowers) demonstrate by the promptness of their effects on the nervous system how rapidly they enter the blood. Alcoholic vapors released from the dregs of grapes or of decanted wine can produce a momentary intoxication; those of carbon disulfide cause digestive troubles and produce a characteristic odor in the feces.

Substances that can be volatilized are absorbed in the airways in much the same manner. Iodine, employed in the form of a tincture in the treatment of wounds and of tumors, enters as much through the inspired air as through the skin in the regions in which it is applied. Panizza has found it in the blood and urine of kids that have breathed its vapors. Phosphorus is often absorbed by workers who deal with it to the point of rendering their breath luminous in the darkness. Mercury, which is volatilized at all temperatures, produces in miners that collect it symptoms that are characteristic of mercurial intoxication. One has seen on an English vessel, loaded with mercury that escaped from its kegs, sailors and animals (sheep, pigs, and cats) who were afflicted with ptyalism, buccal ulcerations, convulsions, and partial paralysis. Our predecessors, who knew some of these facts, proposed as a therapeutic measure in venereal diseases, inhalation of vapors produced by throwing mercury on burning coal, or of cinnabar. All who have employed various fumigations have seen varied symptoms.

Although normally they should not enter the pulmonary system, liquids are also promptly absorbed there. Respiratory movements subject them to a flux and reflux that favor their dispersion and mixing with the products of mucus secretion. Besides, their rapid, partial volatilization in all the air spaces leads to their absorption partly in the form of vapors.

Goodwin has seen that 2 ounces of water injected into the trachea of a dog was promptly absorbed there. Ségalas and Mayer have made similar observations, one in the dog and the other in rabbits. Veterinary students at Lyon, according to Gohier, had to inject 30 liters of water into the trachea of a horse to cause its death, and they poured 40 liters into the trachea of another horse before killing it by suffocation. I have also attempted several experiments of this type, which demonstrate the astonishing activity of absorption in the airways.

After having fixed a tube 1 cm in diameter in the trachea of a horse through an opening in the mid-neck, I poured into this tube warm water (30 to 35 degrees). It went in at the rate of 6 liters/h. The animal developed polypnea and deeper breathing during the 3½ h of the experiment. It was then killed; the trachea and the bronchi were empty; all the injected liquid had disappeared.

In the same manner I poured 25 liters of water into the airways of a second horse over 6 hours, and I removed 6 kg of blood in three bleedings, every 2 hours. The respiratory mucosa absorbed this whole quantity of liquid without the animal appearing to be uncomfortable in any way.

When the introduction of water was more rapid, it produced respiratory difficulties and modifications in the state of the blood, which did not delay death. Thus, in a vigorous, large, upright horse, I have poured cold well water into the trachea by an opening large enough to admit the neck of a bottle. The bottles had a capacity of 750 ml and I poured one after the other without interruption. Until the twenty-fourth bottle, no water escaped either through the wound, nose, or mouth; the horse panted as though it had just come from running; the respiratory rate was 55–60/min. At the fortieth bottle, the animal commenced to stagger, at the forty-second it fell, allowing a large quantity of reddish, foamy liquid to escape through the tracheal opening, mouth, and nose; it died 2 min later. On opening the thorax, it was found that the lung volume was not reduced; it was only emphysematous to an extreme degree. There was a little infiltration but only in the lower parts. The bronchi contained only reddish froth, with no free fluid. The 42 bottles represented 31.5 liters of fluid.

The absorption of water under these conditions slowed up at a rate that could be determined. Thus, in a horse weighing 450 kg, a tube having been adapted to its trachea, I poured into the tube 16 liters of cold water, which were absorbed during the first 22 min; but during the next 63 min, 12 liters were absorbed, a total of 28 liters in 2 h, including an interval of 5 min between the administration of the first and second fractions. Following this procedure, which resulted in considerable polypnea and exaggeration of the respiratory murmur, there developed an anemia demonstrated by extreme pallor of the mucosa.

Other liquids, such as weak alcohol, ether, essence of turpentine, and vinegar, disappeared very quickly from the respiratory passages. I have injected 2 liters of 50 percent alcohol into the trachea of a horse. As soon as forced breathing occurred, it staggered and fell to the ground. After a small quantity of essence of turpentine was injected into the trachea, the odor that characterized the elimination of this substance was promptly detected in the urine.

There is one exception in the fatty oils, which are hardly absorbable except, as one knows, in the intestine. I have seen a cow fall quickly as if asphyxiated when a large quantity of oil was dropped into the airways, and I had thought that this effect was due to the liquid spreading on the mucosa and so forming a barrier to the absorption of oxygen. Since then, some students, having repeated before my eyes the same experiment on a horse, but introducing up to 500 gr of oil into an opening in the trachea, have not produced the result I observed in the cow. Thus, I am now led to attribute the earlier result to spasmodic contraction of the glottis due to oil dropping into this cavity. In horses, the oil produces no difficulty in respiration and the oil is ejected as much through the trachea as through the nose.

Materials in solution and soluble salts are also absorbed with great rapidity in the trachea and bronchi. M. Magendie knew this as a fact a long time ago for strychnine, and other physiologists for several salts in solution.

M. Bouley and I have injected through a very small opening in the trachea of a horse 12 g of alcoholic extract of *nux vomica* dissolved in 200 g of water. In less than 6 min the animal fell to the ground and died 10 min after the injection.

Similarly, into the trachea of a second horse, we have injected 12 g of the poisonous substance in solution. The animal convulsed and fell when the last part of the liquid entered the airways. It died 5½ min after beginning the injection.

Finally, a third horse, whose trachea was open and whose vagus nerves had been cut 48 h previously, received the dose of the same poison. It fell only after 15 min and died 20 min following the injection. The slowness of action of the poison in this last case should be attributed in large part to the congestion of the lung and the accumulation of mucus in the bronchi following the section of the vagus nerves.

Mayer, having injected into the lungs a solution of potassium ferri(σ)-cyanide, found this salt in the blood within 2 to 5 min. The presence of the salt was evident in the left heart before it became detectable in the right heart. Finally, it was present in the urine in 8 min.

Lebkuchner, having filled the airways of a cat with copper ammonium sulfate in solution, recognized this compound in carotid blood at the end of 5 min. Iron sulfate, injected in the same manner, was found after 6 min. Finally, potassium prussiate took only 2 min to appear in the blood of the carotid artery.

I have injected an aqueous solution of 50 g of potassium ferri(σ)cyanide into the trachea of a horse. Blood drawn from the jugular vein contained this salt as early as the fourth minute after the injection.

In like manner, I have injected 200 g of warm water containing 50 g of cyanide into the trachea of a second horse. Three and a half minutes later this salt was found in the jugular blood, and 8 min later it was present in the urine collected from a tube in the right ureter that ran through the upper part of the flank between the psoas muscle and the peritoneum.

52

Reprinted from *Q. J. Exp. Physiol.*, **38,** 255–262 (1953)

5-HYDROXYTRYPTAMINE. PHARMACOLOGICAL ACTION AND DESTRUCTION IN PERFUSED LUNGS. By

J. H. GADDUM, C. O. HEBB, ANN SILVER and A. A. B. SWAN.[1] From the Departments of Physiology and Pharmacology, University of Edinburgh.

(*Received for publication* 23rd *July* 1953.)

THE isolation of the powerful vasoconstrictor substance 5-hydroxytryptamine [Rapport, Green and Page, 1948 *a*, *b* and *c*; Rapport, 1949] was an important advance in the study of the old problem of the pharmacological activity of shed blood [see Gaddum, 1936; Reid and Bick, 1942; Zucker, 1944]. This substance (HT) appears to be mainly responsible for the vasoconstrictor action of beef serum on the perfused rabbit's ear, but is not the only vasoconstrictor substance found in blood; adrenaline, noradrenaline, vasopressin, renin and hypertensin must sometimes be present, and other vasoconstrictors may be there too. According to Bayliss and Ogden [1933], the vasoconstrictor action of defibrinated blood on the perfused kidney of a dog is due to two substances, one of which appears quickly, acts briefly, and is stable in blood, but is removed by perfusion through lungs and kidneys, while the other only appears after $1\frac{1}{2}$ to 2 hours and has a much more prolonged action. The first of these substances may well be HT, but not the second. The smooth muscle-contracting substance (SMC) detected by Zucker [1944] in blood causes vasoconstriction in a perfused cat's tail and excites various other smooth muscles, but has no action on the perfused rabbit's ear, and cannot therefore be HT. The pharmacological effects of serum should not be attributed to HT unless the HT-equivalent is found to be constant when estimated by more than one method.

The work described here was done because experiments by one of us (J. H. G.) had indicated that HT causes pulmonary vasoconstriction in the anæsthetized cat.

METHOD.

The method was similar to that used by Daly [1938] for perfusing monkey's lungs. Cats were anæsthetized with chloralose intraperitoneally (approx. 70 mg./kg.), given 1 ml. of heparin intravenously (5000 units per ml. BDH) and then bled from a cannula in the carotid

[1] Part of this work was done during tenure of a Medical Research Council Studentship for training in research methods.

artery. If heparin is omitted there is a risk that subsequent perfusion of the lungs will fail because of intravascular clotting. Immediately after death the chest was opened and cannulæ tied into the pulmonary artery, left auricle and trachea. Ligatures were tied to close off all extrapulmonary systemic vessels through which blood might escape by way of the bronchial vascular system. At this stage the lungs were removed from the chest and transferred to a respiratory chamber where perfusion and ventilation by negative pressure were begun. In some of the later experiments the lungs were ventilated by positive pressure from a Starling "Ideal" pump. The maximum ventilating pressure was kept constant at 8 to 10 cm. water by the overflow system devised by Konzett and Rössler [1940]. The airtight chamber containing the lungs was used as a plethysmograph and lung ventilation recorded by a Krogh spirometer.

Perfusion with the heparinized blood already collected was maintained at constant volume inflow. In experiments where the effects of HT on the lungs were observed, two flow rates were used, 95 ml. per min. with small and 125 ml. per min. with larger cats. In later experiments on destruction of HT during perfusion the rates ranged from 20 to 200 ml. per min. Blood temperature was kept constant at 33° C. A Dale Schuster pump was adapted for small volumes by using a small rubber teat as pulsator and fitting it with a glass pump chamber. The glass parts of the pump containing rubber flutter valves were fitted with Quickfit joints. With these modifications the total capacity of the pump and connections was 10 to 15 ml. All glass surfaces in contact with blood were coated with a film of silicone (General Electric Drifilm 9987—or 5 per cent solution of BTH "Teddol" in carbon tetrachloride). Pulmonary arterial pressure, venous reservoir volume and tidal air were recorded. The venous reservoir volume is an indirect measure of lung blood volume provided allowances are made for capacity changes in the manometers [Daly, 1938]. Glucose (0·5 ml., 20 per cent solution) and heparin (0·2 ml.) were added at intervals to the venous reservoir.

The substances tested were injected into the rubber tubing leading into the pulmonary artery cannula through a long two-headed needle constructed so that the test dose could be washed in by a following injection of saline. The dead space of the needle was between 0·1 and 0·15 ml., and the total volume of injection was kept constant at 0·4 ml. except on a few occasions when larger doses of the test substances were employed. The same routine was followed for each injection, which lasted 3 to 5 sec. The interval between injections was usually 5 minutes.

Estimates of the concentration of HT in plasma were made by a method developed by Amin, Crawford and Gaddum [1952]. The blood was collected in siliconed centrifuge tubes standing in ice, and quickly centrifuged. A measured volume of plasma was then mixed with

19 volumes of cold acetone. The resulting precipitate was removed in a centrifuge and the acetone extract dried *in vacuo*. The residue was dissolved in de Jalon's solution [Gaddum, Peart and Vogt, 1949] and compared with a standard solution of HT by its action on a rat's uterus suspended in 3 ml. of de Jalon's solution containing atropine (1 mg./l.) at 30° C.

A synthetic preparation of 5-hydroxytryptamine creatinine sulphate was presented by Messrs. Upjohn. Doses are given in terms of the base, by dividing the weight of the salt by 2·3. Dihydroergotamine and lysergic acid diethylamide were presented by Messrs. Sandoz.

Results.

HT, although a powerful vasoconstrictor, does not always cause a rise of blood pressure. In our preliminary experiments with anæsthetized cats the usual effect was a fall of carotid pressure, sometimes followed by a rise when large doses were injected later in the experiment. Both pressor and depressor effects have also been observed by others [Rapport, Green and Page, 1948 *d*; Freyburger *et al.*, 1952; Page, 1952; Reid, 1952]. We thought it possible that the initial depressor effect in our experiments was due to a rise of resistance in the pulmonary circulation. A record of the pressure in a branch of the pulmonary artery showed a rise of pressure within 3 sec. after the injection of HT into the jugular vein, followed 12 sec. later by a fall of carotid pressure. The time relations suggested that the second effect was a consequence of the first. These experiments are not recorded in detail since similar conclusions have already been reached by Reid [1952].

The speed with which the pulmonary pressure rose suggested direct action of the pulmonary vessels, and this was confirmed by experiments on perfused lungs. In all these experiments the intra-arterial injection of HT produced both broncho- and vaso-constriction (fig. 1). The reduction in tidal air caused by doses of 10 to 20 μg. varied from 12 to 80 per cent. The vasomotor response was also variable. The sensitivity of the blood vessels and bronchi were not associated. When the pulmonary arterial pressure was at a constant base-line, the maximum variation between responses to successive injections of the same amount of HT was 22 per cent.

Experiments on anæsthetized dogs [Freyburger *et al.*, 1952] and on cats [Reid, 1952] and isolated guinea-pig ileum [Gaddum, 1953 *a*] showed that the sensitivity of the reactive tissues to successive injections of HT decreased at least temporarily, but in isolated lungs we did not observe an effect of this kind with minimum test intervals of 4 min. This was true of both bronchomotor and vasomotor responses.

An injection of adrenaline given immediately before HT abolished or reduced the bronchoconstrictor response in all our experiments, but had a less constant effect on the vasomotor response. The changes in the bronchoconstrictor response due to adrenaline and their time relations are illustrated by the result in fig. 2. In this experiment 20 μg. of adrenaline was injected; before this HT had reduced tidal air by 20 per cent: 5 min. later it had almost no effect but within 35 min. its activity had returned to the previous level. We have observed this effect on the bronchi with doses of adrenaline ranging from 10 to 50 μg.

Fingl and Gaddum [1953] have observed that some of the effects of HT are antagonized by dihydroergotamine (DHE). In three experiments DHE was therefore added to the blood reservoir after a number of consistent responses to HT had been obtained, and the effect on subsequent injections of HT was then observed. The effect of DHE in a concentration of 1 μg. per ml. blood was first to reverse and then to abolish the vasomotor response to 20 μg. of HT. Larger doses could still produce vasoconstriction though the response was small. The bronchoconstrictor response was completely abolished. Lysergic acid diethylamide (LSD), which is structurally related to the ergot alkaloids, was found by Gaddum [1953 *b*] to antagonize the effects of HT on the rat's uterus. It also antagonized the effects of HT on the lungs in a concentration of 1 μg. per ml. blood. This result is illustrated in fig. 3, which also shows that the lungs still responded to the bronchoconstrictor action of histamine.

Adrenaline itself caused a rise in pulmonary arterial pressure in four experiments, a fall in two experiments, and in one experiment a rise in the early stage of perfusion and later a fall. It always caused bronchodilatation although the changes in tidal air were small. After DHE adrenaline invariably produced vasodilatation and the bronchodilatation normally observed.

The HT-Equivalent of the Plasma.—The method used for estimating HT in the plasma is thought to be fairly specific. Histamine does not cause contraction of the rat's uterus. Ordinary amounts of acetylcholine are inactive in the presence of the concentration of atropine used in the bath. Oxytocin and substance P are insoluble in 95 per cent acetone. Potassium could not be present in sufficient amounts to affect the result. The only substance known to be present in the body in sufficient concentrations which contracts the rat's uterus, is active in the presence of atropine, and soluble in 95 per cent acetone, is HT. The conclusion that the effects were really due to HT was tested by the use of specific antagonists. In one experiment 0·1 μg. of LSD was added to the bath at the end of the experiment. In the presence of this drug the effects of HT and of extract were completely abolished, but the muscle still gave a large response to 1 mU of oxytocin (fig. 4*b*).

There is no real reason to doubt that HT actually was present in the amounts shown in Table I, but since the evidence is not conclusive, the results are presented as HT-equivalents instead of HT-concentrations.

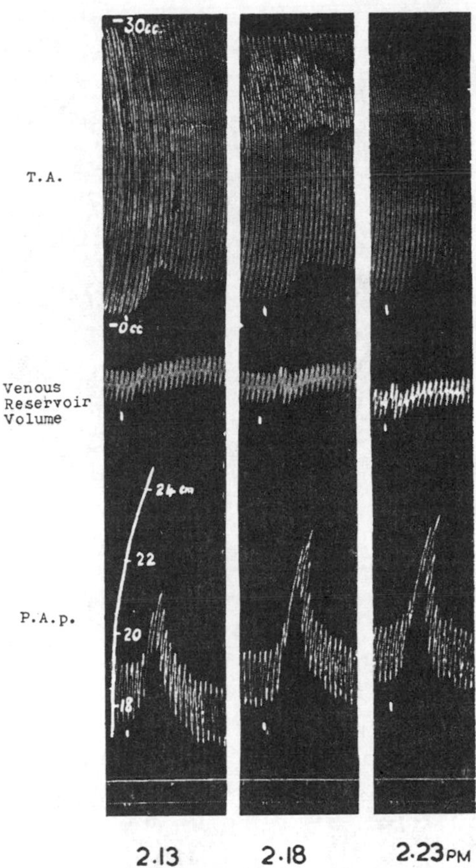

FIG. 1.—Isolated perfused lungs. HT intra-arterial injection 20 μg. 5-hydroxytryptamine. Negative pressure ventilation. TA tidal-air. P.A.P. pulmonary arterial pressure.

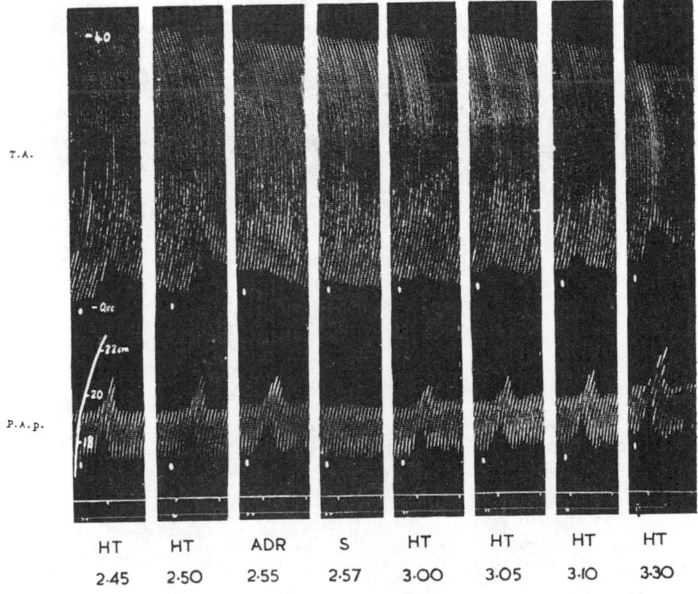

FIG. 2.—Isolated perfused lungs. Effect of adrenaline on the response to 5-hydroxytryptamine.

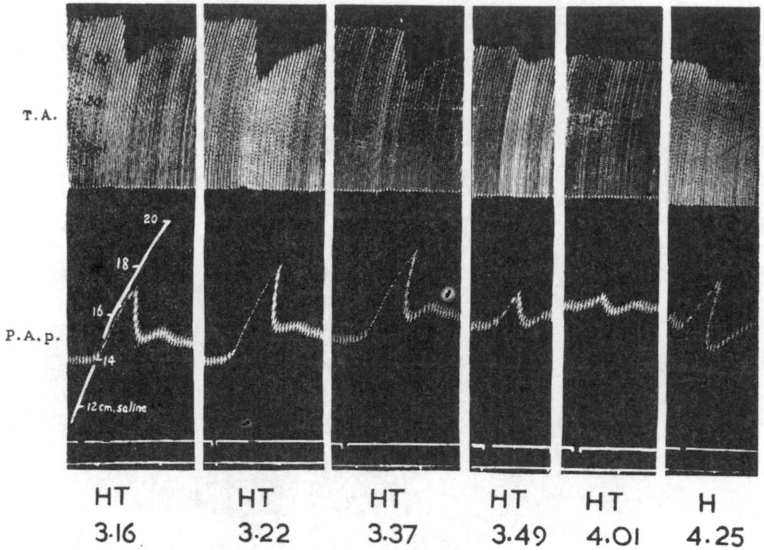

Fig. 3.—Isolated perfused lungs. HT intra-arterial injection 10 μg. 5-hydroxytryptamine. H 20 μg. histamine. At 3.31 p.m. lysergic acid diethylamide added to venous reservoir. Find concentration 1 μg./ml.

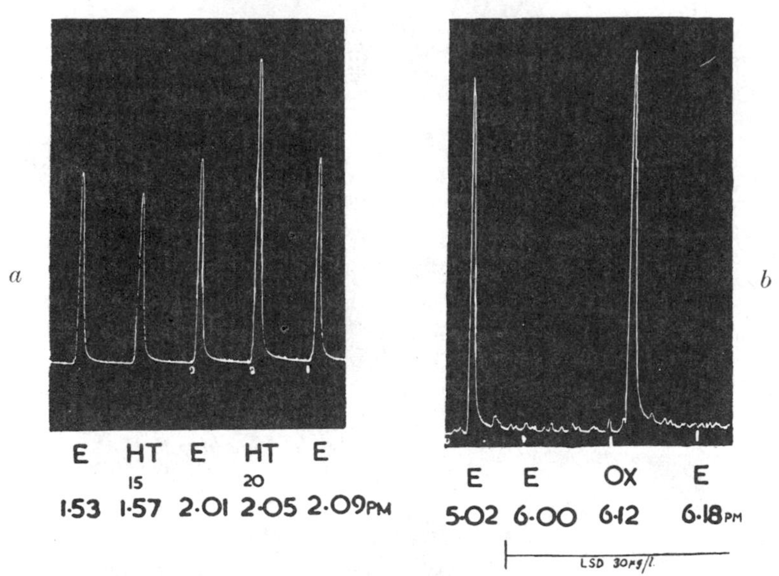

Fig. 4*a*.—Isolated rat uterus. Assay of HT-equivalent of plasma. E = Extract equivalent to 0·015 ml. blood. HT = 5-hydroxytryptamine. Small figures give doses in nanograms (ng.) of the base.

Fig. 4*b*.—E = Extract of different blood sample from that used in fig. 4*a*. Ox. = 1 mU oxytocin. Lysergic acid diethylamide (LSD) 30 μg./l. added at vertical mark.

When blood was run directly from the artery of the anæsthetized cat into a cooled siliconed centrifuge tube and quickly centrifuged the HT-equivalent of the plasma was low (25 μg./l.), but when blood was collected without special precautions the HT-equivalent rose in a few minutes to about 1000 μg./l. These observations are in keeping with the view that HT is normally present in platelets and is easily

TABLE I.

(Time in minutes—HT equivalent (μg./l.).)

Experiment.	1.		2.		3.		4.		5*a*.		5*b*.	
	Time	HT	Time	HT	Time	HT	Time	HT	Time	HT	Time	HT
	0	1100	0	750	0	750	0	333	0	1000	..	..
					8	750	12	167	22	575	..	..
					15	450	24	42	44	230	..	..
					60	100	60	10	..	..	..	..
HT added to increase concentration by amount shown (μg./l.)	1	(1000)	1	(5000)	..		..		..		0	(1000)
	2	1600	2	6000	..		..		..		1	1200
	17	1300	18	2500	..		..		..		21	30
Initial blood vol. (ml.)	..		..		100		145		135		120	
Circulation rate (ml./min.)	..		..		26		66		20		200	
Halving time (min.)	..		..		20		11		22		4	
Per cent removed per circulation (100*k*)	..		..		13		14		21		10	

released [Reid and Bick, 1942; Humphrey and Jaques, 1953]. In experiments 1 and 2 known amounts of HT were added to the reservoir at the beginning of the experiment. This produced an increase in the HT of the plasma which did not differ significantly from the expected increase. Experiment 2 shows that the lungs did remove this added HT. In experiments 3 and 4 no HT was added, but when the lungs were perfused the HT-equivalent of the plasma fell.

In experiment 5 the lungs were first perfused at 20 ml. per min. and the fall of the HT-equivalent of the plasma was followed. HT was then added to the blood and the rate of perfusion was increased to 200 ml. per min. The rate of disappearance of HT was then found to be increased.

In experiments 3–5 the logarithm of the HT-equivalent was plotted against time and the points were found to lie approximately on straight lines. These results therefore indicate that the fall was exponential.

The halving time was estimated graphically and is given in the table. The figures show that the more rapid the circulation the more rapid was the fall of HT-equivalent.

The figures in the last row of the table were calculated as follows:—

x = concentration of HT.
k = proportion of HT removed by the lungs in one circuit.
V = volume of blood in the circulation (ml.).
v = circulation rate (ml. per min.).

The rate of disappearance of HT $= \frac{d(xV)}{dt} = -kvx.$

By integration $\log_e x = -kvt/V$.
If the halving time is t', then

$$k = 0{\cdot}693\ V/vt' \quad (\text{where } 0{\cdot}693 = \log_e 2).$$

The estimates of $100k$ obtained in this way indicate, as might have been expected, that when the circulation was rapid the percentage of HT removed in each circuit was less than when the circulation was slow. The data are, however, insufficient to establish this point with certainty.

Discussion.

Our results with perfused lungs confirm the evidence that HT causes pulmonary vasoconstriction and bronchoconstriction and show that such effects can be caused by a direct action on the lungs. Both were antagonized by ergot alkaloids.

These effects resemble the vasoconstrictor action of defibrinated blood in perfused lungs from rabbits [Tribe, 1914; von Euler, 1932], cats [Newton, 1932] and dogs [Daly, 1938], and the bronchoconstrictor action in perfused lungs from cats [Newton, 1932], guinea-pigs and dogs [Hemingway, 1931 *a*; Daly, 1938]. Both appear to be due to substances liberated in the blood after it has been removed from the body. There is evidence that HT is normally present in platelets [Reid and Bick, 1942] and may be liberated when these break up. These effects of shed blood may therefore all be due to HT, and this theory is supported by the fact that the effects on the dog's pulmonary vessels and the guinea-pig's bronchi were antagonized by ergotoxine [Daly, 1938]. The new facts about HT and ergot alkaloids provide an easy explanation of this antagonism which seemed strange when first found. On the other hand, the experiments described here were all done with cats and scarcely justify the discussion of effects on other animals. If the estimates of the HT-equivalent really do represent concentrations of HT, the amount added to the reservoir in experiment 1 of the table was about equal to that already present. The fact that this caused increased vasoconstriction and bronchoconstriction shows that concentrations similar to those occurring naturally are effective. It is thus reasonable to conclude that this effect of shed blood on cats' lungs is mainly due to HT.

There can be little doubt that many of the other vasoconstrictor effects of shed blood are also due to HT. For example, Heymans, Bouckaert and Moraes [1932] found that the vasoconstrictor effects of defibrinated blood on perfused dogs' heads, frogs' legs and rabbits' ears were antagonized by ergotamine; these effects were probably due to HT. On the other hand, some of the vasoconstrictor effects of shed blood are not completely suppressed by dihydroergotamine [Hebb and Linzell, 1951]. This fact confirms the conclusion discussed above that shed blood may contain other vasoconstrictor substances besides HT.

The estimates shown in the table were made because it is possible that HT has been responsible for some of the difficulties encountered by those who have used defibrinated blood in perfusion experiments. Experiments on dogs' kidneys perfused with blood were much hindered by "vasotonins", until it was shown that they disappeared if a heart-lung preparation was included in the circuit [Verney and Starling, 1922; Eichholtz and Verney, 1924]. The lungs played a part in this detoxication of the blood, and even the kidneys themselves had some such effect [Hemingway, 1931*b*; Bayliss and Ogden, 1933]. There is no reason to believe that the lungs remove vasotonins more rapidly than other tissues, but they do remove them, and if HT is the main vasotonin, it should disappear when the blood is perfused through lungs. Our results confirm that this does happen.

Summary.

1. 5-Hydroxytryptamine (HT) caused vasoconstriction and bronchoconstriction in cats' lungs perfused with blood. These actions were antagonized by dihydroergotamine or lysergic acid diethylamide.

2. The HT-equivalent of the plasma was estimated by extraction with acetone and assay on rat's uterus in comparison with synthetic HT. This was low immediately after bleeding, but rose rapidly to about 1 mg. per litre.

3. The HT-equivalent of the plasma fell exponentially during perfusion with a halving time of 4–20 min.

4. When the rate of circulation was increased the rate of disappearance of HT rose.

REFERENCES.

AMIN, A. H., CRAWFORD, T. B. B., and GADDUM, J. H. (1952). *Communication to the British Pharmacological Society.*
BAYLISS, L. E., and OGDEN, E. (1933). *J. Physiol.* **77,** 34 *P.*
DALY, I. DE B. (1938). *Quart. J. exp. Physiol.* **28,** 357.
EICHHOLTZ, A., and VERNEY, E. B. (1924). *J. Physiol.* **59,** 340.
EULER, U. S. VON (1932). *J. Physiol.* **74,** 271.
FINGL, E., and GADDUM, J. H. (1953). *Fed. Proc.* **12,** 320.
FREYBURGER, W. A., GRAHAM, B. E., RAPPORT, M. M., LEAY, P. H., GOVIER, W. M., SWOAP, O. F., and VANDERBROOK, M. J. (1952). *J. Pharmacol.* **105,** 80.
GADDUM, J. H. (1936). Gefässerweiternde Stoffe der Gewebe. Leipzig: G. Theime.
GADDUM, J. H. (1953 *a*). *J. Physiol.* **119,** 363.
GADDUM, J. H. (1953 *b*). *J. Physiol.* **121,** 15 *P.*
GADDUM, J. H., PEART, W. S., and VOGT, M. (1949). *J. Physiol.* **108,** 467.
HEBB, C. O., and LINZELL, J. L. (1951). *Quart. J. exp. Physiol.* **36,** 159.
HEMINGWAY, A. (1931 *a*). *J. Physiol.* **71,** 201.
HEMINGWAY, A. (1931 *b*). *J. Physiol.* **72,** 344.
HEYMANS, C., BOUCKAERT, J. H., and MORAES, A. (1932). *Arch. intern. pharmacodyn.* **43,** 468.
HUMPHREY, J. H., and JAQUES, R. L. (1953). *J. Physiol.* **119,** 43 *P.*
KONZETT, H., and RÖSSLER, R. (1940). *Arch. exp. Path. Pharmak.* **195,** 71.
NEWTON, W. H. (1932). *J. Physiol.* **75,** 288.
PAGE, I. H. (1952). *J. Pharmacol.* **105,** 58.
RAPPORT, M. M. (1949). *J. biol. Chem.* **180,** 961.
RAPPORT, M. M., GREEN, A. A., and PAGE, I. H. (1948 *a*). *J. biol. Chem.* **174,** 735.
RAPPORT, M. M., GREEN, A. A., and PAGE, I. H. (1948 *b*). *J. biol. Chem.* **176,** 1237.
RAPPORT, M. M., GREEN, A. A., and PAGE, I. H. (1948 *c*). *J. biol. Chem.* **176,** 1243.
RAPPORT, M. M., GREEN, A. A., and PAGE, I. H. (1948 *d*). *Science,* **108,** 329.
REID, G. (1952). *J. Physiol.* **118,** 435.
REID, G., and BICK, M. (1942). *Austral. J. exp. Biol. med. Sci.* **20,** 33.
TRIBE, E. M. (1914). *J. Physiol.* **48,** 154.
VERNEY, E. B., and STARLING, E. H. (1922). *J. Physiol.* **56,** 353.
ZUCKER, M. B. (1944). *Amer. J. Physiol.* **142,** 12.

AUTHOR CITATION INDEX

Aalkjaer, V., 364
Adam, N. K., 241, 254
Adams, H., 111
Adams, W. E., 236
Aeby, 234
Alexander, H. L., 190
Ameuille, P., 341
Amin, A. H., 388
Andersson, H. K., 364
Archer, R. J., 241
Armstrong, B. W., 205, 334
Aschoff, L., 340
Avery, M. E., 281

Baldwin, E., 190
Ball, W. C., Jr., 374
Barcroft, J., 127
Barr, J. S., 334
Bartels, J., 334
Bartlett, R. A., 211
Bates, D. V., 334, 374
Bates, P. L., 183
Bayliss, L. E., 66, 127, 150, 182, 190, 388
Bedell, G. N., 183
Bembower, W. C., 127
Berglund, E., 255
Bernouilli, E., 111
Berry, J. L., 364
Bertalanffy, F. D., 236, 254
Beutner, A., 364
Bick, M., 388
Birch-Hirschfeld, 171
Blaess, 171
Blair, H. A., 183, 333
Bloomfield, R. A., 333
Bohr, C., 172, 311
Bolt, W., 374
Bondurant, S., 279
Bornstein, A., 311
Botelho, S. Y., 183, 333
Bouckaert, J. J., 365, 388
Bradford, J. R., 365
Bratianu, S., 236
Braune, 171, 172
Breed, E. S., 333
Brewer, G., 351
Briggs, J. N., 263
Briscoe, W. A., 334, 374
Broderson, J., 236
Brodie, T. G., 66
Brody, A. W., 183
Bromer, A. W., 334
Brooks, W. B., 111
Brotman, I., 351
Brown, C. C., 182, 205, 211
Brown, E. S., 241, 262, 279
Bruner, H. D., 351
Buchanan, F., 321
Bunta, E., 111
Burgess, B. F., Jr., 183
Burnum, J. F., 334
Burton, A. C., 334
Burwell, C. S., 351
Buytendijk, H. J., 133, 150

Carlens, E., 374
Carroll, D. G., 334
Carvalho, L. de, 341

Chadwick, L. E., 127, 190
Chase, W. H., 279
Cheng, T. O., 374
Cherniack, R. M., 205
Cherry, R. B., 262
Christie, R. V., 111, 133, 150, 190, 374
Claxton, E. B., 334
Clements, J. A., 241, 262, 279
Cline, F., Jr., 374
Cloetta, M., 111, 172, 234
Cohn, J. E., 334
Colebatch, H. J. H., 66
Comroe, J. H., Jr., 150, 183, 333
Conant, J. B., 12
Conte, E., 341
Cook, C. D., 262
Cornish, E. R., Jr., 150
Costa, A., 341
Cournand, A., 127, 190, 333, 351, 374
Courtice, F. C., 238, 254
Craig, J. M., 262
Crawford, T. B. B., 388
Cree, E. M., 374
Cripps, L. D., 111
Cruft Electronics Staff, 150
Curry, C. F., 255
Czapek, F., 234

Daly, I. de B., 364, 365, 388
Darling, R. C., 190
Dautrebande, L., 365
Dayman, H., 133, 205
Dean, H. P., 365
Dean, R. B., 66, 111, 127, 133
DeGrez, 341
Dern, R. J., 183
Dexter, L., 351
Dibbs, H. P., 374
Dixon, W. E., 66
Dollery, C. T., 374
Donders, F. C., 66
Dräser, 234
Drinker, C. K., 238, 254
Dubois, A. B., 150, 183, 324, 333, 334
Dyson, N. A., 374

Eakins, J. D., 374
Ebert, R. V., 133, 150, 182, 205, 211
Ebner, V. von, 127
Eichholtz, A., 388
Einthoven, W., 66
Ellenberger, 234
Endler, P., 374
Eppinger, E. C., 351
Epstein, F. H., 255
Epstein, P. S., 254
Ernstene, A. C., 334
Esch, 340
Euler, U. S. von, 365, 388
Evans, J. M., 351

Farber, S., 279
Farhi, L. E., 205
Feldman, D. J., 255
Felix, 234
Fenn, W. O., 66, 127, 133, 150, 182, 190
Filler, J., 374
Fingl, E., 388
Finley, T. N., 279, 374
Fisher, P. A., 255
Follis, R. H., 365
Forssmann, W., 341
Forster, R. E. II, 333, 334
Fowler, W. S., 127, 150, 333, 374
François-Frank, Ch.-A., 365
Franke, R. E., 334
Fraser, M. J., 255
Fray, W. W., 111
Freundlich, 234
Frey, W., 234
Freyburger, W. A., 388
Frey-Wyssling, A., 236
Fry, D. L., 133, 150, 182, 205, 211
Fucks, W., 374

Gaddum, J. H., 388
Gaensler, E. A., 133, 150, 205
Galen, 295, 296
Gardner, L., 190
Gardner, R., 279
Gerhardt, D., 111
German, W. J., 334
Gershfeld, N. L., 279
Ghoreyeb, A. A., 351
Gibbons, M., 255
Gibbons, R. A., 255
Girling, F., 334
Gitlin, D., 262
Godfrey, M., 374
Govier, W. M., 388
Graf, P. D., 67
Graham, B. E., 388
Graham, G., 150
Gramiak, R., 205
Green, A. A., 388
Grollman, A., 341
Gross, D., 111
Gruenwald, P., 262, 279
Guerriero, C., 236
Guzman, S. V., 374

Haag, 234
Hagemann, O., 311, 320
Haldane, J. S., 111
Hamilton, W. F., 351
Hansen, E., 127
Harkins, W. D., 262
Harris, J. H., 183
Havel, R. J., 279
Hayek, H. von, 236
Haynes, F. W., 351
Hebb, C. O., 388
Hellems, H. K., 351
Hemingway, A., 388
Henriques, V., 365
Herschen, 340
Heuser, C., 341
Heymans, C., 365, 388
Hickam, J. B., 334
Hiffelsheim, 320
Hinault, V., 341
Hitzenberger, K., 111
Hofmann, 298
Hogg, G., 262
Houssay, H. E. J., 374
Howell, J. B. L., 374
Hüfner, G., 234
Hughes, A. H., 279
Hugh-Jones, P., 374
Humphrey, J. H., 388
Hurtado, A., 111
Husten, 234
Hutchinson, T., 66, 111
Hyatt, R. E., 211

Jackson, C. L., 190
Jäger, 234
Jain, S. K., 205
Jaques, R. L., 388
Jaquet, A., 111
Jerrard, W., 334
Jessop, G., 254
Johnson, J. A., 334
Johnson, R. P., 279
Joseph, N. R., 344
Joslin, D., 133

Kaltreider, N. L., 111
Kaplan, J. G., 255
Karsner, H. T., 351
Katz, L. N., 365
Katz, S., 111
Kety, S. S., 150, 333
Kinney, T. D., 351
Klaus, M., 279
Klein, O., 341
Knipping, H. W., 374
Knoll, P., 365
Kobler, 234
Kölliker, A., 172
Konzett, H., 388
Korner, P. I., 238, 254
Kriete, B. C., 205
Krogh, A., 310, 312, 333
Krogh, M., 312, 334
Kronecker, H., 111

LaMer, V. K., 241
Landois-Rosemann, 340
Langmuir, I., 279
Lanphier, E. H., 333
Laqueur, E., 255
Lauson, H. D., 333
Lawton, R. W., 133
Leathes, A., 279
Leathes, J. B., 236
Leay, P. H., 388
Le Blanc, E., 365
Leblond, C. P., 236, 254
Lee, G. de J., 324
Lefcoe, N., 279
Leith, D. 66
Lell, W. A., 190
Lemoine, J. M., 341
Lenard, 234
Levy, M. M., 150
Lewis, D. H., 183
Lichtheim, L., 365
Lilienthal, J. L., Jr., 334
Liljestrand, G., 127, 365
Lilly, J. C., 333
Lima, A., 341
Lindgren, I., 150, 205
Lindhard, J., 127, 333
Lind van Wyngaarden, C. de, 365
Linzell, J. L., 388
Loeb, L. M., 190
Loeschke, H., 234
Loewy, A., 172
Loosli, C. G., 236
Loria, G., 34
Lovatt Evans, C., 255
Low, F. M., 236
Lubin, R. I., 211
Ludes, H., 373

McCall, C. B., 211
McCann, W. S., 111
McDermott, M., 205
McIlroy, M. B., 182, 205, 211, 262
McIntosh, C. A., 133, 150, 190
McIntosh, H. D., 334
McKerrow, C. B., 205, 211

Macklin, C. C., 66, 236, 238, 241, 255, 279
McLaughlin, M., 279
McLeod, J. J. R., 190
McMorris, R. O. 262
Mallos, A. J., 211
Maloney, J. V., 133
Mani, K. V., 205
Margaria, R., 127
Marshall, H., 374
Marshall, R., 183
Martin, C. J., 373
Martin, H. B., 205
Mattson, S. B., 374
Mead, J., 66, 133, 150, 182, 205, 211, 262, 279
Meakins, J. F., 374
Mellin, G., 365
Michaelis, H., 127
Miller, W., S., 351
Mills, J. E., 66
Mitchell, J. S., 255
Moissejeffe, E., 234
Moniz, E., 341
Moraes, A., 388
Morgan, W. T. J., 255
Muller, A., 127
Muller, E. A., 127
Müller, J., 234

Nadel, J. A., 66, 67
Neergaard, K., von, 67, 93, 111, 127, 133, 150, 182, 190, 205, 234, 241, 255, 279
Neilsen, M., 127
Newberry, G. R., 374
Newsham, L. S., 374
Newton, W. H., 388
Nichol, J., 334
Nickerson, M., 255
Nisell, O. I., 183
Noüy, P. L. du, 254

Ogden, E., 388
Olsen, C. R., 66
Ostwald, W., 234
Otis, A. B., 67, 127, 133, 150, 182, 190, 211

Page, I. H., 388
Paine, J. R., 133
Pappenheimer, J., 333
Pare, J. A. P., 374
Pattle, R. E., 241, 255, 262, 279
Peart, W. S., 388
Permutt, S., 374
Perti, B. L., 205
Peters, J. P., 351
Pflüger, E., 182
Phillips, L. L., 262
Plesch, J., 311
Plesset, M. S., 254
Poincare, H., 279
Polack, B., 111
Porter, A. W., 255
Potter, E., 262
Priestley, J., 45, 111
Prinzmetal, M., 190
Proctor, D. F., 67, 127, 133, 205
Proemmel, D. D., 334

Radford, E. P., Jr., 67, 182, 205, 211, 241, 255, 279
Rahn, H., 127, 133, 150, 182, 190, 205
Ranges, H. A., 351
Ranke, 234
Rapport, M. M., 388
Rauwerda, P. E., 127, 150
Ravina, A., 341
Rawson, A. J., 344
Recklinghausen, H. v., 171
Redenz, E., 234
Reid, G., 388
Rich, A. R., 365
Richards, D. W., Jr., 190, 333
Richards, S., 374
Rienzo, S. di, 133
Riley, R. L., 127, 205, 334, 374
Rink, H., 374
Robb, G. P., 341
Robertson, G. W., 66, 127, 150, 182, 190
Rohrer, F., 111, 127, 133, 150, 182, 234
Ronneaux, G., 341
Rosenbluth, M. B., 255
Ross, B. B., 205
Rössler, R., 388
Russell, A., 255

Sagerson, R. P., 351
Said, S., 374
Sarnoff, S. J., 255
Schaefer, V., 279
Scheele, C. W., 27
Schilling C. W. 111
Schmidt, C. E., 351
Schmitt, W., 365
Schneider, E. C., 111
Schrödinger, 234
Schroeder, H. A., 344
Schulman, J. H., 279
Schwiegk, H., 365
Segal, S., 262
Seibel, R. E., 351
Sellick, H., 66
Selverstone, N. J., 182, 205, 211
Senner, W., 111

Severinghaus, J. W., 334
Shanes, A. M., 279
Shepard, R. H., 334, 374
Short, R. H. D., 236, 255
Siakotos, A., 279
Siebeck, R., 312
Silverman, L., 133
Silverman, R., 262
Silverman, W., 262
Sinclair, J. D., 374
Skrodalis, V., 262
Smith, C. A., 262
Sosman, M. C., 351
Stacey, R. W., 262
Stahel, 171, 172
Starling, E. H., 388
Starr, I., 344
Stead, W. W., 133, 150, 182, 205, 211
Steinberg, I., 341
Steinitz, F. S., 365
Sternberg, C., 234
Stewart, P. B., 374
Stigler, R., 111
Stow, R. W., 334
Strasser, H., 127
Sutherland, J. M., 262
Swenson, E. W., 374
Swoap, O. F., 388

Takishima, T., 66
Terry, R. J., 236
Thornton, T. M., Jr., 236
Tierney, D. F., 279
Tigerstedt, R., 365
Tooley, W. H. 279
Treloar, L. R. G., 190
Tribe, E. M., 365, 388
Trippe, H., 374

Valentin, H., 374
Vanderbrook M. J., 388
Van Slyke, D. D., 351
Vassura, G., 34
Venrath, H., 374
Verney, E. B., 388
Visscher, M. B., 66, 111, 127, 133, 334
Vogt, E., 340
Vogt, M., 388
Volkmann, 340
Vries, Reilingh, D. de, 255
Vuilleumier, P., 67, 127, 133, 182

Wade, O. L., 374
Warren, J. V., 334
Wearn, J. T., 334
Wedd, A. M., 333
Wells, H. S., 133, 211
West, H. F., 190
West, J. B., 374
Whittenberger, J. L., 133, 150, 182, 205, 211, 279
Widdicombe, J. G., 67
Wiggers, C. J., 150
Williams, D. T., 262
Wilson, E. J., 374
Wilson, J. L., 279
Wirz, K., 67, 93, 111, 127, 133, 150, 182, 190, 205, 234
Wolfe, W. G., 67
Worden, R. E., 262

Yates, F., 255

Zschiesche, L. J., 334
Zubin, R. I., 133
Zucker, M. B., 388
Zuntz, N., 234, 311, 312, 320

SUBJECT INDEX

Airflow, measurement by pneumotachograph, 173–174
Airway obstruction
  effect of forced expiration, 191–200, 206–211
  in emphysema, 184–190, 194
  mechanical models, 191–200, 206–211
  mechanisms, 191–200
Airways, regulation
  diagnostic studies, 63
  early studies, 63
  neurophysiological studies, 63
Alveolar ducts
  regulation, 63
  smooth muscle, 231
Atelectasis (*see* Respiratory distress syndrome)
Atomic theory, 12

Barometric pressure
  low, effects, 52–53
  measurement, 36
Boyle's law, 10, 38–41
  airway resistance measured by, 175
Bronchi
  anatomy, 63, 162–166
  calculations of flow resistance, 161–172
  measurements in human lung, 161–172
  regulation of diameters, 63
Bronchograms, tantalum, 63

Capillary action, 212–213
Carbon dioxide
  discovery by Helmont, 7, 13
  rediscovery by Black, 7, 14–16
Cardiac catheterization
  first use in man, 335–340
  of right atrium, 341–345
Chance, role of, in scientific discovery, 20–21
Compliance, pulmonary
  definition, 129
  effect of frequency of breathing, 147
  in emphysema, 79–85, 184–190
  measurement, 130
  regional, 134

Dalton's law, 11, 44–48
Dead space, respiratory, calculations for human lung, 166
Decompression, 51
Decompression sickness, 54
Dephlogisticated air, 20
Distribution of pulmonary ventilation, mechanical factors, 134–150

Elastic properties of lungs
  in emphysema, 77–78, 79–85
  in normal man, 73–74, 79–82
  surface tension component, 214–234
Emphysema
  airway resistance, 184–190
  dynamic compression of airways, 184–190
  intrapleural pressure, 77–79, 79–85
  mechanics of airflow, 184–190
Esophageal pressure, index of intrapleural pressure, 86–91, 92–93

Flow-pressure curves, 206–211

Flow-volume curves, 206–211
Fluid-filled lungs, 216–220

Gases, in solution
  Dalton's experiments, 49–50
  Henry's law, 42–44
Gas laws
  Boyle's law, 10, 38–41
  Dalton's law, 11, 44–48
  Henry's law, 11, 42–44
Gas pressure
  Boyle's law, 10, 38–41
  high and low pressures, 12
  law of partial pressures, 44–48
  total atmospheric pressure, 10, 34–37
Gas sylvestre, 13

Henry's law, 11, 42–44
Hooke's law, 68–72
Hyaline membrane disease (*see* Respiratory distress syndrome)
Hypoxia
  high altitude, 12, 51–54
  Mayow's experiments, 17

Laplace's law, 64
Laws
  Boyle's, 10, 38–41
    airway resistance measured by, 175
  Dalton's 11, 44–48
  Henry's, 11, 42–43, 49–50
  Hooke's, 68–72
  Laplace's, 64
  Poiseuille's, 151–160
Lung
  fluid-filled, 65, 214–234
  functions
    alveolar-fluid absorption, 375–378
    gas exchange, 1, 306, 309
    metabolic, 375–388
  model, 134–150

Mechanics of ventilation
  air viscance and turbulence, 113
  airway resistance, 151, 161–172, 175–183
  early studies, 59
  effects on distribution of ventilation, 134–150
  elastic forces, 112
  maximal inspiratory and expiratory pressures, 96–100
  non-uniform compliance, 134–150
  non-uniform resistance, 134–150
  pressure-volume diagram of thorax and lungs, 94–111
  relaxation pressure, 102–103
  tissue resistance, 113

Nitro-aerial particles, 17–18
Non-respiratory lung functions, 280, 375–378, 379–388

Oxygen
  discovery
    Lavoisier, 9–10, 31–33
    Mayow, 8, 17–19
    Priestley, 8, 22–24
    Scheele, 9, 26–30
  uses
    in medicine, 25
    oxygen torch for melting metals, 24

Phlogiston theory, 8
Pneumocytes, source of surfactant, 65, 235–236
Pneumotachograph, 173–174
Poiseuille's law, 151–160
Pressure, intrapleural
  measured by esophageal balloon, 86–91
  measured by esophageal catheter, 92–93
  normal, 73–74, 75–76, 79–85
  in patients with emphysema, 77–78, 79–85
Pressures
  maximal expiratory, 96–100
  maximal inspiratory, 96–100
  relaxation, 102–103
Pressure-volume relationship
  diagram of lungs and thorax, 94–111
  Hooke's law, 68–72
  relaxation pressure, 95, 102
Pulmonary blood flow
  continuous measurement, 324–334
  regional, 366–374
  total, 284, 310–323
Pulmonary capillaries
  anatomic demonstration, 301–305
  "capillary" pressure in man, 346–351
  function, 306–308, 309
  postulated existence, 298
Pulmonary circulation
  early discovery, 282–283, 287–289, 290–292, 293–300
  effect of hypoxia on resistance vessels, 352–365
  Harvey's experiments, 293–300
  measurement of blood flow
    body plethymograph, 324–334
    continuous measurement, 324–334
    nitrous oxide uptake, 310–323, 324–334
  regulation of blood flow, 352–365
Pulmonary ventilation
  distribution of, mechanical factors, 134–150
  mechanism, early views, 58

Resistance, air flow
calculations *in vitro* (Poiseuille), 151–160
calculations on human lung, 161–172
distribution of resistance, 164
effect of tube diameter, 155–160
effect of tube length, 151–155
measurement by body plethysmograph, 175–183
regional, 134
Resistance, pulmonary, measurement, 129
Resistance, tissue, 113
Respiratory distress syndrome in newborn
deficiency of surfactant, 66, 256–262
relation to pulmonary surface tension, 65, 232, 256–262, 278–279

Scientific revolutions
in chemistry, 7
in physics, 7
Surface tension
in air- versus fluid-filled lungs, 65, 214–234
analysis (Young), 64
calculations, 65
Laplace's law, 64, 212–213
applied to alveolar curvature, 224–228
Bowditch translation and annotation, 64
measured on surface balance, 239–241, 256–262, 263–279
pulmonary edema foam, 65, 237–238, 242–255
surface tension–area diagrams, 268–271
Surfactant, pulmonary
composition, 263–279
function, 237–238, 242–255
in lung extracts, 239–241
measurement using surface balance, 263–279
in pneumocytes, 65, 235–236
properties, 65–66, 237–238, 242–255, 263–279
in respiratory distress of newborn, 66

Tantalum bronchograms, 63
Time constants, 134–150

Work of breathing
early measurements, 75–76
efficiency of breathing, 122–124
maximal work, 124–126
in normal man, 108–110, 117–122

Xenon, radioactive, 366–374

About the Editor

JULIUS H. COMROE, JR., after twenty-one years on the faculty of the University of Pennsylvania, moved to San Francisco in 1957 to become Director of the University of California's Cardiovascular Research Institute (until 1973) and Professor of Physiology. He is co-author of *The Lung,* The Year Book Publishers, Incorporated (1955 and 1962; translated into seven languages) and of *Physiology of Respiration,* Year Book Medical Publishers, Incorporated (1965 and 1974; translated into four languages); he was Editor-in-Chief of *Circulation Research* from 1966 to 1970. He is a member of the National Academy of Sciences, a past president of the American Physiological Society, and is the recipient of two honorary degrees (Karolinska Institute and University of Chicago) and a Fellowship in the Royal College of Physicians, London.